Acclaim for Jacob Levenson's

THE SECRET EPIDEMIC

"It's an ambitious aim for any journalist to tell the larger political story alongside the personalized human one. But to manage it gracefully, moving among so many players and their respective positions, is a particular accomplishment. . . . Arresting."   —*The New York Times Book Review*

"Thoroughly researched and well-written . . . convincing and nuanced. . . . Important reading for people interested in gaining insight into AIDS in the twenty-first century."   —*Chicago Tribune*

"Levenson broadens the view of the U.S. epidemic. . . . A fascinating history. . . . Reads like a thriller, intricately weaving tales of individual characters."   —*The Baltimore Sun*

"Levenson doesn't use numbers to tell the story of AIDS in black America. Instead, he writes of lives touched by AIDS."   —*Chicago Sun-Times*

"An unflinching account that combines first-rate reporting and comprehensive research. . . . A must-read."   —*Tucson Citizen*

"Through the stories of these characters—told delicately and yet powerfully, with a mastery of language, imagery and pacing surpassing that of many novels let alone works of nonfiction—we engage much more profoundly with the issues that shape this epidemic than we ever could with a simple policy book."   —*Salon*

"Offers rich detail on how stigma can still compel people to die silently rather than seek adequate treatment."   —*Out*

"Levenson skillfully weaves personal stories into a narrative filled with information about the day-to-day challenges of health and social workers, as well as families. Passionate and provocative."

—*Black Issues Book Review*

"Like Randy Shilts in his groundbreaking *And the Band Played On,* Levenson writes in an informal, narrative style that concentrates on stories of individuals. . . . An important read, and a book that should be read by everyone in this country who is concerned about the AIDS epidemic.
—*Gay Life*

"The importance of this book at this critical juncture cannot be underestimated. . . . *The Secret Epidemic* promises to open up the range of the public's vision and also public discourse on this public and private health crisis facing the African American community and, indeed, the country as a whole."
—Henry Louis Gates, Jr.

"Reading more like a novel than an academic study, Levenson's book sheds light on how dramatically the AIDS crisis is devastating the black community and how that community still struggles with how to best confront the issue."
—*Metro Times* (Detroit)

"A must-read. . . . A compelling, impassioned, and deeply humane work of writing and . . . an urgent, necessary alarm for anyone who thinks the AIDS epidemic in America has been tamed. Think of this book as the sequel to Randy Shilts's *And the Band Played On*—the arrival of a major author with a hugely important story to tell."
—Samuel G. Freedman

"Levenson forces us to face our own indifference to suffering. He explores the roots of that indifference and reminds us that ignoring distasteful facts merely exacerbates the consequences."
—*Colorado Springs Independent*

"Thoroughly researched, articulate presentations of facts in terms that are both human and broadly epidemiologic. . . . There is a cool ferocity to Levenson's prose. The narrative is simple and straightforward. He doesn't get in the way of his storytellers."
—*The Plain Dealer*

"Levenson paints vivid portraits of the people whose lives have been turned inside out by this modern-day scourge and of those fighting to save them. . . . An engaging read."
—*The Crisis* (NAACP)

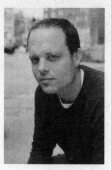

Jacob Levenson

THE SECRET EPIDEMIC

Jacob Levenson has written about AIDS for *Vibe, The Oxford American,* and *Mother Jones,* and he received a grant from the Open Society Institute to work on this book. Levenson studied at the University of California, Berkeley, and he received a master's degree in journalism from Columbia University. He lives in Brooklyn.

THE SECRET EPIDEMIC

THE
SECRET
EPIDEMIC

The Story of AIDS and Black America

Jacob Levenson

ANCHOR BOOKS
A DIVISION OF RANDOM HOUSE, INC.
NEW YORK

FIRST ANCHOR BOOKS EDITION, FEBRUARY 2005

Chapter one previously appeared in slightly different form in *The Oxford American*.

The Library of Congress has cataloged the Pantheon edition as follows:
Levenson, Jacob.
The secret epidemic : the story of AIDS and Black America / Jacob Levenson.
p.   cm.
Includes index.
1. AIDS (Disease)—United States. 2. African Americans—Diseases. I. Title.
RA643.83.L48 2004
362.1'969792'008996073—dc22
2003058038

Anchor ISBN: 0-385-72234-6

Author photograph © Elena Seibert
Book design by Robert C. Olsson

www.anchorbooks.com

Printed in the United States of America
10 9 8 7 6 5 4 3 2 1

This book is for Kazandra,
with love, for her insight,
courage, patience, and honesty.
And to my parents, George and Vicki,
for their guidance and inspiration.

Contents

THE SECRET EPIDEMIC

_____

Tornado Road

1996

SARA JACKSON EASED HER husband Jack's dirt-brown Buick down Tornado Road, which stretched out before her like a red clay river, rippling with thick waves of tire tracks and dipped with shallow pools from the footprints of her cousins, aunts, and uncles, who had lived in this countryside for about as long as anyone could remember. Tall pine trees leaned in over the car, flickering Alabama sunshine through her dusty windshield. The forest soon gave way to a clearing. On the left was a rusted barbed-wire fence strung across an expanse of grass.

Sara rolled the Buick's steering wheel to the right and pulled up in front of her parents' trailer. It was the summer of 1996. She was only sixteen and was entering the eleventh grade, but she and Jack had just married and already moved into their own house a hundred yards farther down the road. They called it the green house. Maybe once it had suggested such a bucolic sentiment, but the southern heat and rain had stripped the paint and warped the wallboards and window frames, so that from the outside it had the dreamy look of a reflection off the waters of a still pond.

Sara couldn't quite articulate why she liked it better here than in the city. Her parents had recently moved her and her younger sister Rebecca back to Choctaw County after they had spent most of their childhood in Mobile. There was less crack, violence, and gang activity in the country. But the presence or absence of those social ills didn't quite capture the innate qualities that distinguished the two places. The country seemed to retain a stability that calmed her. She shared enough blood with the black

3

families who lived in the constellations of trailers and small homes sprinkled across the county that she could comfortably call a good portion of them kin. Her grandmother, who lived in a cottage across from the green house, had bought the land they lived on, with the help of a white family in whose home she'd worked. There was plenty of fishing for trout in the weave of creeks that rushed through the surrounding forest. And there were whole stretches of yard for growing vegetables.

Sara was pleasantly surprised that Jack had followed her to Choctaw. He'd been raised in Mobile and was five years her senior. They'd met through a cousin of hers. He was her second real boyfriend, and she didn't exactly love him, but she was attracted to his etched muscles, loosely curled hair, and light skin. Their relationship was a point of tension between Sara and her mother, Angela, who worried about Jack's temper, the way he hovered over her, wouldn't let her talk to other boys, wanted to keep her in the home, and was pressuring her to have children. On some level Sara knew Angela was right. Sometimes Jack's breathless, pressing affection felt more like obsession than real love. In a way, though, that was what drew her to him.

Sara didn't believe that anyone could love her—maybe, she thought, because her father, Robert, had left them to spend fourteen years in a Texas prison. She had secretly blamed herself for his absence. It was completely illogical—the kind of all-powerful conclusion a two-year-old might dream up to reconcile the confusion of a divorce—but she had felt that way for as long as she could remember. It made her feel that her heart was sealed off, that she was naturally cold and impenetrable, that no one could really become attached to her.

She didn't have to worry about Jack abandoning her, though, not as long as he needed to touch, taste, control, and virtually inhabit every moment of her life. That didn't mean she was submissive to him. They were nearly the same size, and she was capable of fighting him off when she wanted to spend some time with her mama, or daddy, or sister. Rebecca had always been Sara's baby or, as she affectionately called her, Sustuh!! She was more sensitive and trusting than Sara, the one person who Sara felt understood her.

Sara grabbed a bag of groceries off the seat of the car, stepped into the summer heat, walked up the steps of the trailer, and pushed through the screen door. The living room felt darker than it was, because of the stained faux wood-paneling pasted to the walls. To the right was Rebecca's room. She wasn't home. Sara's mother was moving around in the back. She didn't like to hang out for long with Angela—if she did, they'd inevitably light into each other about Jack, or school, or pretty much anything.

Angela had fallen for Sara's daddy, Robert, when she was only seven and he was twelve. She was thirteen when she gave birth to Sara. It was young, even up here in the country, to have a baby. But Angela had figured they'd get married when she was eighteen and settle in with all their other kinfolk. Robert got her pregnant a second time, with Rebecca, when she was fifteen. Soon afterward he was sent to prison for nearly fifteen years. Angela waited for him to be released, and she and Robert were finally wed on Tornado Road last summer. Robert looked tall and lanky in a brown pinstriped suit, a white pressed shirt, and a maroon tie embroidered with the silhouettes of dancing couples. And Angela had seemed distinctively southern in a simple white cotton dress decorated with lace. Robert was working as a logger now, and for the first time probably ever they resembled a normal family.

Any mail for me? Sara called out.

There's something from the health department, Angela yelled from the back.

She found a large envelope on the kitchen table. She was excited—it probably had information about that badge and T-shirt she was supposed to get for the blood donation she'd given at school. She'd volunteered to donate partly because she liked the idea of doing something for the sick, but also for the lure of a citation. For the last three years she'd taken ROTC classes, earning medals for bravery and drill team, and she was preoccupied with the thought of joining the army and fighting for the United States overseas.

She tore open the envelope and stared at the words. Thank you, it read, for your donation. But we are unable to use your blood, because it is contaminated with HIV.

Sara didn't know much about the disease, except that it was deadly. Dazed, she angled past the kitchen table, walked down the narrow hallway, and found her mother in the back of the trailer.

Angela was still young, but she carried herself with the world-weariness of a middle-aged woman whose youth had slowly been leached out of her. Sara numbly handed her the letter and then saw her mother's eyes rush with tears. Sara wrapped herself around Angela. They were nearly the same size: full-figured, round at the cheeks, and square-shouldered. *I must be dreaming,* she thought. *This must be a nightmare.* It'll be all right, Mama, she said. God does things for a reason. Angela continued to weep.

Three days later an identical letter arrived from the county health department. This time it was addressed to Rebecca.

Smoke

2000

W HAT IF THEY'RE DYING? *What the hell am I gonna do about their babies?* The questions raced through David deShazo's mind. He was chain-smoking Marlboros as he drove north out of Mobile, up State Highway 17 into the Alabama countryside. A black garbage bag stuffed with blankets, baby clothes, and toys took up most of the dusty backseat of his Pontiac. The car was cold and reeked of stale smoke; his heater was busted, and he didn't have the two hundred bucks it would cost to get it fixed.

It was eight-thirty Friday morning, November 10, 2000, and he was headed up to Choctaw County to find two black sisters who were infected with HIV. The girls lived with their mother and two baby sons down a dirt road somewhere outside Gilbertown, near the Mississippi border. The caseworker in Selma, who was supposed to be in charge of their case, had told David that morning that they hadn't been heard from in seven months. Now winter was coming, and as best he knew, they didn't have heat, a telephone, or a car to get to the doctor. He just hoped that neither of them had developed full-blown AIDS. He took a draw off his cigarette, squinted through his bug-smeared windshield at the two-lane highway, and tried to fight down a flickering current of anxiety.

His twenty-one years of social work had produced enough dark memories for David to be able to reassure himself that he was prepared for anything he might encounter. The memories had a way of floating through his head and calming him. Sometimes he could all but see that pretty brown-haired girl he was supposed to help at the mental hospital in

Mobile. She had been molested and had sliced herself up with a razor blade until her face was a maze of long thin incisions. Other times he'd remember the elderly he tended to when he worked in home health and hospice, their eyes hollow and searching, as they died alone in old metal trailers scattered like lonely tin coffins across the Alabama countryside. The memories would come, and he'd be released from the anxiety. But sometimes, if he wasn't careful, he'd find himself haunted by the vague suspicion that he'd failed these people. The notion would float around the edges of his consciousness, eroding his confidence, before he'd reject it as irrational. Then he'd wonder whether the suffering these people endured was inevitable or whether somewhere along the line this country had failed them. For a moment he might be gripped by a confused anger over what had become of the Alabama of his childhood. More often, though, he'd imagine what could happen if AIDS continued to spread through the South.

He hadn't really known what to expect when Mobile AIDS Support Services (MASS) hired him to drive deep into the poorest black rural counties of southern Alabama to search out people infected with HIV, convince those he deemed candidates for infection to get tested, and warn others that AIDS was threatening to spread through rural Alabama. In the eighteen months since taking the job, he'd driven more than sixty thousand miles through forgotten Civil War–era towns, talking about the virus to just about anyone who'd listen. He'd caught hate stares at general stores and gas stations, and a county commissioner over in Wilcox had reprimanded him for discussing AIDS without permission at a church meeting. Recently in Coy there had been rumors of a retired army sergeant banishing his infected daughter to an abandoned trailer, then burning her possessions after she died. A few weeks ago the sheriff in Choctaw County offhandedly mentioned that if an infected prisoner ever tried to bite him, he'd empty his pistol into the man and take his chances with a local jury; and he'd heard a smattering of comments from whites that the "niggers" and "faggots" were just getting what they deserved. None of those things really surprised him, though. The silence that surrounded him in these towns unsettled him more. The vast majority of people regarded him with wariness, and often when he talked to them, it seemed as though he were shouting across some unbridgeable chasm.

This country wasn't the New South of peroxided blondes, baseball-cap-wearing teenagers, shiny-headed dads, and bowl-cut little boys, smartly dressed in candy-colored polo shirts, Bermuda shorts, and khaki pants. Nor was it the South of Ted Turner, the Atlanta Braves, Emeril Lagasse, and urban sprawl. That South was comfortable, packaged with the business traveler in mind in cookie-cutter whites, reds, and blues to look like Anywhere, America. This Alabama felt older to him: a place that endured mainly in black and white memories of Martin Luther King Jr. marching on Montgomery; Sheriff Jim Clark greeting civil rights marchers with tear gas, bullwhips, and nightsticks; or maybe George Wallace fervently proselytizing, "Segregation now! Segregation tomorrow! Segregation forever!" Those were the images rehashed on PBS, anyway. But even that wasn't the Alabama David recalled from his childhood in the 1950s and 1960s.

He'd grown up in Jackson, about fifty miles southeast of Choctaw County, and his softly lit memories had a more idealized, small-town American hue to them. Sure, his father, a country doctor, had had "colored" and "white" waiting rooms. David also had a hazy recollection of sitting next to his mother in the deShazo family's pink station wagon when the news crackled over the radio that Lyndon Johnson had signed the Civil Rights Act. She leaned back and wondered aloud why northerners always had to shove ideas down their throats. But that was just the way things were then. He was more likely to recall Carrie, the slender black woman who did most of the work raising the deShazo boys, and how much he loved her; the long rides out into the country with his father to tend to poor colored farmers; and how sometimes his dad would get paid, and other times they'd drive back with a sack of potatoes on the seat of the car and permission to hunt on the patient's land.

Alabama still possessed the same expansive, aching beauty of his youth. The countryside, with its withered cotton fields and mazes of creeks and rivers, felt timeless. An endless procession of churches—some wooden, airy, and antiquated, others no more than creaky one-room buildings—lined the roads, with signs that read out names like New Providence Baptist, Jesus Is Lord Old Zion Missionary, and Little Zion Baptist. They lent the region an air of being protected from the amoral advance of modernity. But it wasn't unchanged. Since taking this job,

David had noticed something unsettled about these country communities. He had trouble capturing it in words, but it seemed inextricably bound to his work. The South was the new frontier of AIDS in America. More people were infected with the virus in the region than in any other part of the country. And now it was threatening to spread slowly and quietly through rural black Alabama.

David, perhaps more immediately than most public health officials, understood what could happen if the AIDS epidemic ripped through the poor black South. MASS employed five caseworkers who were responsible for roughly eight hundred clients in the city and its surrounding five rural counties. Eighty percent of their patients were black, and most didn't have private insurance, Medicaid, or direct access to the new drug cocktails. The caseworkers spent the bulk of their time just trying to get them more medicine. For the sixth straight year they'd exhausted their casework money early and had to cover payroll by patching together a series of small grants and private donations. They needed to hire more staff but could afford to pay people like him a salary of only $23,000, plus thirty cents for every mile he drove on mornings like this, to look for these two girls.

David crossed into Choctaw County, home to sixteen thousand people. Roughly half of them were black, and a quarter of the population lived in poverty. There were no hospitals or infectious disease doctors around here. The road was stained with burnt-orange dirt—clay that made the soil difficult to farm, leaving paper mills as pretty much the only industry in the area. A couple of logging trucks stacked with fresh-cut trees sped by in the opposite direction.

In a sense, David had replaced his father as the modern country doctor. Paying house calls with a clipboard instead of a black bag, he had the job of telling people that they were going to die, getting them on waiting lists for medications, rushing them to the hospital, and making sure they had heat and electricity. At fifty his face was finely lined, and his hair and mustache were a smoky gray. His teeth had yellowed, and he hid his brown eyes behind a pair of rose-colored prescription glasses. The simple way he carried himself in his uniform of faded blue jeans and wrinkled flannel shirts put people at ease. Still, the relationship he had with his clients was more complicated than the one his father had shared with his patients. All morning he'd been running cynical scenarios in his head about what to do with the babies if there was no food in the fridge, or if he suspected the sisters were prostituting themselves to pay the bills.

Gilbertown wasn't much more than a stoplight, a cemetery, a dollar store, and a Foodmart. Large houses soon gave way to scattered wooden shacks and trailers with rusted American cars parked out front. David slowed the car and made a right down a narrow, unmarked dirt road. He'd seen these girls once before, the previous fall, as a favor to the caseworker in Selma who was supposed to be in charge of their case. When he'd spoken to her on the phone that morning, she'd explained to him that she had stopped checking in on them because they told her they didn't need help. Legally, she was in the right. David, though, had a bit of a savior complex. He liked thinking that he had the skills to manipulate, beg, and cheat the welfare system to get the sisters the medications, doctors, and help that might save their lives. It was a shaky rush, one he rarely felt in other social work jobs.

He parked the car at an angle in front of the weather-beaten wooden porch of their white metal trailer, stepped into the crisp bright morning, climbed three rickety steps, and knocked on the door. A husky woman's voice bellowed for him to come on in.

Sara didn't recognize David at first when he pulled back the door, hastily strode to the center of the trailer, and set down his garbage bag. A rush of cold fall air swirled through the stifling living room, which was so hot that it was difficult to breathe. She casually continued to change her eighteen-month-old son, Benny Jr. Her hair was in long cornrows that gathered at her neck and ran down the back of her dirty Michael Jordan T-shirt. Rebecca's twenty-two-month-old son, William, was giggling and waddling back and forth in blue pajamas on the slanted linoleum floor in front of her. Clothes, empty soda cans, and an overturned tricycle cluttered the living room. There was a harsh cough from the attached kitchen. David glanced over. Rebecca was slumped over the back of a metal chair facing an open oven, trying to keep warm. She'd pulled a tattered yellow blanket up over her head, and it was difficult to make out her face. David introduced himself and asked how they were doing.

Sara glanced up from her baby, said hi, flashed a loosely confident smile, and tried to size him up. She'd had bad experiences with social workers. After she and Rebecca were diagnosed, a woman from the Choctaw County Health Department had shown up on Tornado Road asking all their cousins and uncles if they'd been sexually involved with Sara or Rebecca.

David said he'd brought some supplies, then abruptly started firing questions at Sara. What's your income? Have the babies been tested? Sara felt a flash of annoyance but answered anyway. Rebecca received a disability check, she told him, but she got nothing but food stamps. Neither of their babies had been tested in a while. What about insurance? David asked.

"I got to get some because that medicine is real high," she said.

"How long has Rebecca been like that?" David asked, nodding toward the kitchen.

"Something's messing with her eyes," she answered. "She been running a fever for three days."

"What kind of medicine is Rebecca taking?"

"AZT? I don't know," Sara said. "I could show you."

"You getting any medicine, Sara?"

"I get medicine while I'm pregnant, but I save it. I ain't going to get no more when I have the baby."

"You pregnant again, Sara?" he asked incredulously.

"Seven months," she said, shaking her head, smiling, wondering how he didn't notice.

David asked if they were still seeing the doctors in Waynesboro, Mississippi. Sara said yes but that they didn't have a car, and she'd missed her last two appointments because she didn't have any way to get there.

Rebecca coughed again—a coarse hack, heavy with phlegm—stood up, walked slowly past Sara, and pushed through the screen door. Sara went into the kitchen, opened a cabinet, and handed David a plastic basket packed with prescription bottles, many still in sealed boxes. Rebecca took some of them, Sara told David, but there were so many that the regimen often became confusing.

Sara told David that she'd been turned down for Medicaid before she got pregnant. Back then she'd been taking her sister's medications. Rebecca pushed through the screen door and collapsed on the couch with her yellow blanket. David asked Sara if her boyfriend had been tested. He'd tested negative a year ago, she answered, but he hadn't been retested since she got pregnant again. As far as she knew, Rebecca's boyfriend hadn't been tested, either. Then Sara told him that her boyfriend took some of her medications just to be careful.

"Does Rebecca use birth control?"

"Not anymore," Sara answered.

"Do you think she'd use condoms if I left you some?"

"Probably, 'cause one time we got a box full, and I hardly got any for myself," Sara said.

David started into a series of questions about the children but was interrupted by a visitor at the front door. Sara glanced over. It was her aunt Jesse, who was visiting from Mississippi and had dropped by to help with the laundry. Sara introduced her. Jesse nodded and made her way to the back of the trailer.

"I don't want my aunt to know 'cause she talks too much," Sara whispered.

The trailer was in chaos. Dishes were piled in the sink. A couple of flies buzzed around a cold plate of grits and sausage. The couch Sara was sitting on was filmy and damp. There were dark holes in the linoleum floor through which one could see the ground. As David continued to ask questions about the children, Sara rolled an empty medicine box back and forth beneath one of her bare feet.

"Every time she coughs like that, does she throw up?" David asked Sara carefully, looking toward Rebecca.

"Yeah, she does," Sara said.

He turned to Rebecca and spoke to her directly for the first time. "How long has that been happening, Rebecca?"

Silence.

"Rebecca, did you tell the doctor about your stomach?" David asked loudly, as if he were talking to someone who didn't speak English.

"I feel real nauseated," Rebecca whispered. Her delicate mouth was slack, and she was staring off into space with half-closed eyes. David directed a couple more questions at Sara, then knelt in front of Rebecca. He was close enough that he could reach out and lift her thin body in his arms, but somehow he seemed miles away.

"This sickness Rebecca has is really scaring me," he said, looking at Sara, and then, turning back to Rebecca, he asked, "Did the doctor give you any X-rays?"

Silence.

"Rebecca? Rebecca? Did the doctors take any X-rays of your chest?"

Silence.

"Did he say anything about pneumonia?"

Rebecca whispered something.

"Huh?" David said, leaning closer.

"In my ribs."

"You got pneumonia in your ribs?"

Rebecca nodded. A pneumonia infection could kill her within days. David asked Sara if they had any medicine for pneumonia. Before Sara could answer, though, Aunt Jesse interjected from the kitchen that their grandfather, who lived down the road, was supposed to get it from the pharmacy. It wouldn't make any difference, though, she continued, because Rebecca wouldn't take it anyway.

"Please, Rebecca," David said, "we need to get you healthy for William."

Silence.

"What can I do about your medicine problem?" he pleaded.

"You can't," Rebecca answered softly.

Their father might be able to make her take it, Jesse interrupted from the kitchen. Rebecca was his baby, and he could make her do anything. But he was in prison again. Then Jesse's voice broke. She stood up, covered her face, and walked toward the back of the kitchen. She made it to the doorway of the bedroom and collapsed against the wall in tears. David followed and awkwardly draped his arm around her shoulder.

Sara could only make out tidbits of their conversation. "Rebecca needs someone to explain to her that the medicine's good for her," Jesse said loudly. She'd stopped crying, but the words still came out unevenly. "She ain't got that kind of understanding 'cause she grew up too fast."

Sara was frightened that David would tell Jesse that she was infected. Her friends and family knew that something was wrong, but not everyone was sure it was HIV. If it got out that Sara was infected, word would spread quickly through the county. Maybe everyone already knew; it seemed as if people went out of their way not to touch her. Some neighbors didn't bring their children by anymore. And when she shopped at the market, she'd noticed that other customers moved out of line.

She nervously ran her hand across a tangle of thick dark scars on her leg. It was strange to think back now on how Jack had reacted to the news of her infection. He didn't get hysterical, retreat into fear, or even shy away from her. He just grew more possessive. He pressured her to drop out of high school, and at the end of 1996 they moved back to Mobile. Then he got crazed and violent. Maybe he was frightened of her—frightened that she'd infected him. Maybe he felt guilty for infecting her. Or maybe he had just always been unstable. They would scream at each other about everything and about nothing at all. Then sometimes they would physically go at each other until the fight was gone out of both of them. She left him after only a few weeks. She wanted to go back up to Choctaw but was worried that he'd follow her, so she went to Aunt Jesse's in Pascagoula.

It didn't take Jack long to track her there. One January day Sara walked out of Jesse's house and found him standing in the sun in front of his car. He started making overtures about reconciling. "Nope," Sara said. "This fighting has got old, buried, and stinky." She turned around and started back toward the door. Her stomach felt tight and queasy. She glanced nervously over her shoulder as she neared the front steps. Jack had lifted up his black mesh shirt to reveal the curve of his narrow waist and the black handle of a pistol tucked into his tan pants. He pulled it out. She glimpsed the gray barrel before it spit a burst of orange flame.

The base of her back lit up red and hot as if she'd been stung by a scorpion. She lurched forward onto her aunt's front steps. Jack fired again, and she felt a dull, tearing sensation as the bullet ripped through the top of her left forearm and tore out through the bottom of her wrist. Another explosion, and the back of her left calf shuddered dully. Jack pulled the trigger again, and a fourth bullet lodged numbly in her left thigh. He aimed the gun at the back of her head and fired. The bullet flew past Sara's left ear and ricocheted off the cement foundation of the house. She heard the harsh metal-on-metal swoosh of the car door, the rev of his engine, and then silence.

Blood gathered warm and wet, then sticky underneath her white T-shirt and brown shorts. She drew her hands up underneath her face. Through the silver-dollar-sized hole in her wrist, past the mass of skin, fat, and muscles that were loosely oozing out, she saw her hard white bone. *Lord, if you ready to take me,* she prayed, *go on and take me. Just don't let me suffer.* Jesse shuffled out of the house. She begged Sara not to fall asleep. Somehow Sara managed a laugh, then said, "Don't worry—if I do, I'll wake up."

Sara recovered from the shooting, and as she watched AIDS devour Rebecca, she hated that her little sister lacked the same power to face down death. Rebecca had always possessed an innocent quality. Perhaps that was why she had succumbed so quickly to AIDS. She had been hit by her first fevers when she was pregnant with William. Then her boyfriend had left her. At first Sara was gripped by worry as she watched the weight drop off her sister's frame. She used to scream and plead with her to take her pills. But her words seemed just to pass through Rebecca. Looking at her these days—her face drawn, her eyes loose and feverish—made Sara imagine her own death, and that magnified her anxiety. She increasingly withdrew from Rebecca and turned her energy toward her new fiancé, Benjamin Sr.

They had fallen in love when Sara moved back to Choctaw County after she was shot. His mother lived at the end of Tornado Road. He was physically more imposing than Jack, with the stony biceps, pectorals, and shoulders of a professional athlete. But he would never hurt her. He was the one person up here whom she'd told about her diagnosis, and it didn't faze him. Just to be safe, though, they shared what medicine she got: he'd take an AZT pill one day, and then she'd take one the next.

They'd lived in the green house, then upgraded to a trailer across the road. It would never look quite right: the floor slanted to the left, the ceiling was caving in at points, and the row of kitchen cabinets that hung over an old green stove was beginning to bow. The place didn't have any heat or a phone. She'd recently received a letter from the electric company warning her that if she didn't pay her bill, they'd turn off the power. She'd been living there by herself while Benjamin served a short prison term. He was supposed to be out in a week, and she'd been trying to get the place clean for him.

Sara wasn't frightened for her future. She'd be okay so long as she had her family. Her cousin, who owned the trailer, cut them a break on rent. Her grandmother helped out with food, and Benjamin's mother often took care of Benny Jr. whenever Sara could get work. She'd tell them that David was a social worker who'd come to help her get Medicaid. In a sense that was true. Medicaid was what she'd need more than anything else if she was going to live long enough to raise Benny Jr. and her unborn baby.

David walked back into the living room with Jesse. He was worried that he wasn't going to be able to keep these girls alive without help. It was clear to him that Jesse was aware of the girls' infections, and he wanted to enlist additional family and neighbors who could drive Rebecca two hours to Mobile to see a specialist and who would lend a hand with food when Sara had the baby. "I know the doctors in Waynesboro have been good to you," he said, "but it may be time for you guys to see a specialist. How do you feel about that?"

"I'll do anything that'll keep me healthy like I am, 'cause I don't want to leave my children like this," Sara said. But when David asked her if she would consider telling her grandparents or the host of cousins and in-laws who lived in the area that she was infected, she was quiet.

"Do you think folks would turn their backs on you?" he asked.

"They would," Sara said, and her eyes fell.

David figured she was probably right. He'd heard the stories from the caseworkers at MASS about clients getting cold-shouldered out of their churches, fired from their jobs, and abandoned by their families. In some towns it was hard to find a funeral home that would take the bodies of AIDS victims. The social worker who used to handle the agency's rural cases often had to deliver medications to clients at "secret" locations like the parking lot of the Piggly Wiggly.

David was beginning to feel overwhelmed. He needed a break, so he offered to go down to the pharmacy in Gilbertown and pick up Rebecca's medication.

In the car David was shaken. "Keep up the defenses, deShazo," he said to himself, pulling out a cigarette. "Keep 'em up. This is strictly business. Stay in your head." His jaw was set, and his head was thrust slightly forward, a beaten bulldog pose that made him look at once determined and defeated.

When he had landed this job, he had been out of work for a year and a half and was trying to sober up and get over the collapse of his marriage to his second wife, Fran. His last steady work before that had been as a traveling health care worker checking on the homebound elderly who suffered from conditions like cancer, diabetes, and COPD, a circulatory condition that he liked to call Cranky Old Person's Disease. His job was to get them their pills and make sure they made it to their doctors' appointments. It had struck him as pointless. Their families didn't appear to care about them, and it seemed as though they were being eaten to death by loneliness more than old age. Sometimes he liked to think that they deserved to die in isolation. Maybe they had molested or beaten their children. But more often he was afraid that they hadn't done anything to deserve to die alone. Maybe, he thought, their children simply stayed away because, like him, they couldn't stand the stench of poverty and death.

Most nights during that period he stopped by the liquor store and grabbed a six-pack and a fifth of gin on the way home from work. He'd put Jackson Browne or Bonnie Raitt on the stereo—Fran was still with him then, and she didn't care for the harder-edged sound of Dylan or Hendrix—sit on the back deck, and drink. He'd finish the beer within an hour, start on the liquor, and wait for the alcohol to make him feel that he understood his job, his first wife, his relationship with his two children, this landscape, its people, and his place in it. It was a fleeting, dreamlike rush, and it made him feel warm, comforted, and childlike. Most nights he chased after it with shot after shot of gin, until he puked or passed out.

In a sense David had been trying to reclaim his footing ever since he left Jackson, in the summer of 1968, to attend the University of Alabama in Tuscaloosa. During his first semester he joined the ROTC and a fraternity. He imagined that he'd come home after graduation, marry his high school girlfriend, and settle down in some equivalent of the house with the white picket fence. Tuscaloosa, though, was acutely divided over the

Vietnam War and civil rights. The drugs, interracial couples, and protests unsettled David. Most people back home had supported the war and were trying to resist desegregation or, as David called it, "the change." He felt stretched too thin. American society seemed to be cracking. His hometown began to strike him as phony and unreal. It was as if the people there were purposely barricading themselves off from the rest of the country. He quit the fraternity and the ROTC, grew out his buzz cut, became something of a southern hippie, and decided he'd never live in another tight-minded small town.

Thirty years later, when he applied for this AIDS job, he found himself craving the security offered by the country. He'd burned out of three social work jobs, Fran had left him, and his doctor had told him that if he drank again, his pancreas would fail and he'd die. He'd never done AIDS work, but in his interview with MASS he argued that he understood the way people spoke, ate, lived, and prayed in rural Alabama. That, more than any AIDS experience, would be the key to talking sex and drugs in this country. He was hired with seven other social workers to barnstorm thirty-two of the state's poorest rural counties in an effort to identify those at risk and get medical care to the infected.

It didn't take an epidemiologist to see that rural Alabama was a potential tinderbox for an AIDS epidemic. It had some of the worst rates of gonorrhea, syphilis, and chlamydia in the country; those diseases, the Centers for Disease Control (CDC) said, helped facilitate HIV transmission. There was a high incidence of teen pregnancy, which suggested that young women were having a good deal of unprotected sex. And there was a wealth of anecdotal evidence of rampant crack abuse, which had long been tied to HIV infections. Complicating matters, there'd been virtually no AIDS education in these counties. David had been assigned the five counties north of Mobile and was given the simple instruction to blanket them.

He knew he couldn't walk into this country, throw condoms on the table, tell the locals that AIDS was in their town, and show them how to fornicate safely. He would have been pegged as an outsider hawking drugs, homosexuality, and disease, and he would've been welcomed about as warmly as those Yankees who came down south in the 1960s to "disempower folks from their local ways." It wasn't that rural Alabamians were mean, closed-minded, or even simply conservative. It was more that they believed that they had crafted a way of life that kept them insulated from the social and moral crises that were slowly destroying the rest of country. And they were prepared to take a stand against anyone or anything that suggested otherwise.

David understood that. He'd seen it back in 1968, when his mother drove him and his identical twin brother to the courthouse to register for the draft. She wasn't really for the Vietnam War. But that spring the deShazo family had watched blacks burn their own neighborhoods after Martin Luther King was killed, body counts pile up in Vietnam, and news of Robert Kennedy's assassination, all in vivid color on their new RCA television set. Their American way of life felt threatened. Some people in Clarke County fought back by sending their kids to all-white private schools or refusing to do business with blacks. His mother made her statement by showing everyone in the county that she believed in America enough to let her boys get drafted to Vietnam.

So David didn't even mention AIDS during his first five months on the job. He spent two- or three-day stretches on the road just getting to know people. At first he stuck to places that were familiar to him. It seemed like every day he would pass a town, forest, or bridge that stirred some memory of racing cars with his brothers through the Salt Flats on Rockville Road, hunting deer and rabbits, and running to Mississippi with his high school buddies to drink at the bars on the Gulf Shore. He hung out at general stores and gas stations, volunteering to help out with home health, welfare, and Medicare applications. He felt sure of himself in this country. Things still made sense here. Rural Alabama was largely segregated, conservative, and poor, but everyone talked about being kin to everyone else. If he could convince them that AIDS wasn't a sign of moral or spiritual failure, he figured they'd feed, shelter, clothe, and nurse the infected.

After a few weeks of hanging out at county health departments and budget motels, though, he felt that he hadn't really penetrated his territory. So he ordered engineering maps of his counties, which detailed the endless stretches of unmarked road that ambled through the forest. At first it seemed that there wasn't much out there except timber fields and old farmland. But after a while he started to get a feel for where people lived. Some places had names, but they were too hidden to be rightfully called towns. When he found Vredenberg, he thought it was just a deer hunting camp in the woods. But a pockmarked road led to a water tower and a clearing, maybe a half-mile in diameter, lined with rows of old trailers and small wooden houses with peeling paint. Black teenagers with cornrows and bandanas eyed him warily as he drove through the gravel streets. The Vietnam vet who owned the town's one-room grocery told David that he kept a nine-millimeter behind the counter, to protect himself from the crack dealers. Other communities were even more invisible. Coy was just a collection of a hundred or so families scattered around Arthrene Brooks's general store. Arthrene and her husband, Cleo, had moved home to Alabama to get away from the gangs in South Central Los Angeles. But in Coy they found dealers who offered their son free rock cocaine. Girls were prostituting themselves in her parking lot for drugs. One of Arthrene's customers had overdosed. And she'd heard talk about people in town dying of AIDS.

David met many people who'd come back to the country after living in places like Los Angeles, Detroit, and Cincinnati. He understood why they'd returned. When he graduated from social work school in 1979, he was committed to working with the urban poor. His first job had been in child welfare in Mobile. Like that of other midsize cities like Detroit, Oakland, Cleveland, New Orleans, and Newark, Mobile's economy in the late 1970s had been hit hard by white flight. The face of downtown looked as if it had been frozen in 1964. David spent his share of time in various black neighborhoods in and around Mobile. He was trained in clinical social work, and looking back, he probably had some fuzzy notion that he could help families pull together in the hard times. But there was something wrong with those neighborhoods. It wasn't just the chronic urban problems of alcoholism, drug abuse, and unemployment. It felt as if that intangible bond that makes human beings feel connected to one another had disintegrated. How could he make sense of a mother who wouldn't feed her children? Or people who couldn't scratch up friends and neighbors to watch their kids while they searched for work? When friends asked him what he did with children, he'd reply, "You hatch 'em, we snatch 'em." It was around then that he began drinking heavily.

Now, he thought, he had been naïve to think it would be any better here. This landscape and its people had been largely forgotten after the

last civil rights workers left thirty years ago. The air was leaden with resignation, even defeat. Some people eked out a living in the logging industry
or paper mills. But many "retired" at thirty-five and just waited for their
welfare checks. It was if there was nothing for them to struggle for anymore, and the only thing they had left to hold on to was their faith that
they were safe here in this hidden world.

David heard rumors of AIDS everywhere he went. But the girl who
was sick was always in the next town over, the one with all the drugs and
prostitution. He couldn't persuade anybody to climb into his dusty blue
Pontiac and head down to the local health department to have blood
drawn. People were wary of the government, but they seemed to be even
more scared of one another. No one wanted to be recognized with him
and risk word getting out that they had AIDS. Maybe they'd test, they
would tell him, if it was just him and them under the pecan tree up on the
hill.

He carried a list of statistics everywhere he went now. There were
dozens to draw from: 54 percent of all new HIV cases were African American; the CDC had estimated that as many as one in fifty black men were
infected with HIV; the disease had become the number-one killer of both
black men and women between the ages of twenty-two and forty-five;
black women were the fastest-growing group of AIDS victims; and infection rates were higher among young gay black men than for any other
group in the country. But the numbers sounded abstract and far away.
Like these people themselves, the epidemic felt elusive, quiet, and hidden, as if it had no place or source. He was like a man who had wandered
deep into a cloud of swirling smoke, in search of a fire that didn't exist,
and it wasn't clear if he would ever make his way out. He drew wary looks
from both races, as though neither was really sure what to make of him.
Whites, who he'd observed had come to view overt racism as impolite,
stopped him with suspicious questions like, Who are you? What are you
doing? Tell me again why you're here. And he'd found himself constantly
reassuring blacks that he hadn't come to buy their land, search out drug
dealers, or even "accuse" them of having AIDS. At times he felt that he
was operating at a distance from both worlds and lacked a language to
break through to either—an experience that seemed to expose the fundamental gulf that had opened up between the races in post–civil rights

America. Forgotten towns settled after the Civil War, crack cocaine in the woods, "niggers" and "faggots" and general stores, Holiness churches, sweet gum trees, and rural ghettos—it was all so frightening, beautiful, and American—and riper for an AIDS epidemic than he'd ever imagined.

Fluorescent lights shone brightly off the Gilbertown Pharmacy's cold white tile floor, giving it a sterile feel that made it seem far away from the Jacksons' trailer. David picked out a plastic pillbox that he hoped would make it easier for the girls to stick to their medication regimen and took it to the counter, where a heavy-boned white woman with feathered brown hair told him that she'd heard Rebecca was in bad shape and that everyone at their church prayed she was saved. Then she mentioned that they had a couple of other women and a man who ordered HIV medication, too. David tried to digest this new information without working himself up into one of his anxious fits. To begin with, he couldn't believe the Jackson girls were sleeping with their boyfriends, or that there was so much confusion out here that Sara thought feeding her boyfriend AZT, a drug that helps prevent pregnant women from passing the virus to their unborn babies, was going to do a thing to keep him safe. They could be starting a mini-epidemic.

AIDS could move pretty quickly through a county like Choctaw. The virus wasn't like the flu, which people caught the first time they were exposed. HIV spread most easily through stable social groups, like the ones found in small towns where people inevitably shared sexual partners. These sexual networks, as the doctors at the CDC called them, could be traced out on paper like genealogical trees. David had recently heard about a case in a Mississippi town where two teenage girls were diagnosed with HIV during a routine screening for STDs. Investigators from their county department of public health interviewed them and traced out a web of forty-four people. They tested several and identified a total of seven infections. They'd all contracted the virus heterosexually.

When David got back to the trailer, Sara had righted the tricycle and put some of the clothes on the floor away. Rebecca was sitting up and talking on the phone. She flashed a smile and for an instant looked like any other teenager. David arranged the pillbox and sat back down in front of her. She was holding William tightly in her arms on the couch and was rocking him back and forth.

"Do you ever feel like there's no reason to live, Rebecca?" he asked.

"Sometimes," she said, and stared at the ground.

"Is there anybody you can go to when you feel like that?"

"There ain't nobody but myself," she said. Her eyes were glassy, but she stopped herself short of crying.

David got ready to leave. The bright afternoon light had faded to a soft yellow. He scheduled an appointment to come back next week and asked the girls to arrange it with Angela so she'd be there, too.

Then he pulled onto State Highway 17, stuck Jimi Hendrix in the tape deck, and began thinking about the chaos of it all. Why hadn't their doctor given Rebecca medication for her depression? How would he deal with their doctors in Waynesboro (which was across the border in Mississippi), the politics of infringing on another agency's territory, a girl who was on the verge of death, a new baby on the way, a couple of boyfriends who might be infected, an illness that was a secret, and a town that was at risk?

If Sara wasn't approved for Medicaid after she had the baby, David would apply for free medications from one of the major pharmaceutical companies. He also wanted to get the sisters on a program that would help pay for electricity and heat. But it'd be tough to ask for it without mentioning AIDS. Maybe he could use his United Way business card to cut a deal with the local utility company. He wanted to find a nurse in the area with some HIV experience, who would check up on Rebecca. That would involve getting Rebecca approved for Alabama's home health care program, which would require a medical history from her doctor and the cooperation of the Choctaw County Health Department. She might be dead by then. It was dark when David reached Chatom, merged onto Interstate 65, and accelerated south back toward the Gulf of Mexico, Mobile, and home.

Heading in the opposite direction, Interstate 65 cuts northeast through the forests of Alabama for three hundred miles to Montgomery, home of the Confederate White House and the Alabama state legislature. From there it curves northwest to Huntsville, where—that same evening—state representative Laura Hall was preparing for the first meeting of Governor Don Siegelman's blue-ribbon commission on AIDS. The commission faced a profound set of problems: the federal AIDS programs didn't provide enough coverage for the infected; the state legislature had put little money toward the epidemic; and many of Alabama's AIDS patients were dying without regular medical care. It had taken Laura and Randy Russell, the director of AIDS Alabama, the state's largest AIDS organization, eighteen months to persuade the governor's staff to approve the commission. Now Siegelman wanted the commission to produce a report by spring with solutions to the state's growing AIDS epidemic.

Siegelman was taking a risk by lending his name to the project. He had been elected as one of Bill Clinton's New Democrats in 1998 and was the state's first Democratic governor since George Wallace. Alabama's economy was beginning to founder, the state's schools were already teetering on the edge of insolvency, and the committee was likely to make recommendations that would cost significant money.

Complicating the problem, most Alabamians, including the state's lawmakers, didn't know much about AIDS. Over the course of the first stage of the epidemic, between 1981 and roughly 1995, Alabama's infected tended to die quickly and were either too poor, too ashamed, or too isolated to make much political noise about their condition. Then in the mid-1990s a slew of new medications, popularly hailed as a panacea for the epidemic, hit the market and started to prolong the lives of AIDS patients. Consequently, between 1990 and 2000 the number of infected people living in Alabama—a state of four million—tripled to nearly nine thousand. They had virtually no resources to care for themselves. The average AIDS patient in the state made roughly $7,000 a year. Only a scant few had private insurance.

Medicaid and the federal AIDS Drug Assistance Program (ADAP) were the two programs that provided AIDS patients with access to doctors and life-saving drugs, but they were difficult to access. Alabama, like a number of southern states, set stringent qualifying standards for its social welfare programs. The federal government had set up ADAP on the assumption that states would keep it afloat by matching federal funding. Alabama hadn't put any money toward ADAP until 2000, when Laura

Hall persuaded the legislature to kick in half a million dollars. That wasn't enough money, and ADAP in Alabama had been capped. The waiting list had peaked out earlier in the year at 430. Those patients were dependent on local agencies like MASS to find them medications. Most often that meant the social workers had to fill out monthly applications to compassionate care programs set up by pharmaceutical companies. In 2000, for instance, MASS had "begged" for $1.8 million worth of medications from the pharmaceutical industry to cover its clients. And there was talk that some agencies had to secretly give out drugs they'd illegally stockpiled from the medicine cabinets of the dead.

The problem wasn't limited to Alabama. The expense of the new medications, coupled with the epidemic's continued shift into poor communities of color, had frightening implications for the future of AIDS in America. Ten states had capped enrollment for their ADAPs in 2000. The CDC estimated that a third of Americans infected with HIV were unaware of their infection. Just to wipe Alabama's ADAP waiting list clean, Laura's AIDS commission would have to convince the legislature to give the program $6 million in state money. Even that would be only a temporary solution for the people who had already sought support. What concerned Laura more was that she knew there were black families like her own in Alabama with infected men, women, and children who were too frightened even to ask for help.

On Tuesday morning, November 14, 2000, four days after his first visit to the Jacksons, David picked his way along Highway 17 toward Choctaw County. The Pontiac didn't like pushing fifty, and some of the local cops up here weren't too friendly to outsiders. He'd been thinking about the girls all weekend and trying to keep his fear and sorrow in check. But sitting alone in his apartment on Saturday, he had broken down. When the tears subsided, he found himself angry. He was trying to brace himself with that anger this morning. *This girl ain't gonna die. She ain't gonna die,* he thought to himself. *If I have to break every goddamned rule in social work, these girls are going to have a chance.* The sentiment kept playing through his head in an endless loop, almost like a mantra. But the truth was that he didn't even know if Rebecca had made it through the weekend.

Sometimes he wondered if he did this work out of conviction or out of some twisted need to play hero. After all, who'd put himself through this for $23,000 a year? He felt as if he were waist-deep in the rotting edges of society, in the dark spots where the foundation had been eaten away. He grabbed a polished red apple from under his seat and, with one hand on the wheel, carved it with a cheap serrated knife. He was in Washington County, about twenty-five miles south of Gilbertown.

When he pulled up to the Jacksons' trailer, it looked deserted. The door was padlocked, and empty Budweiser cans were piled on the ground to the right of his car. A chair on the porch was turned on its side. Turning, he saw a dust-brown, four-door, late 1970s Chevrolet coming up the road. Sara was in the backseat with her baby, Benny. David walked over to her window. "Where's Rebecca?" he asked. Sara got out of the car and told him: Rebecca had collapsed on Saturday, just stopped breathing. She was in the hospital in Waynesboro. She ducked back into the backseat of the Chevy and said she'd be back later in the afternoon.

David got back behind the wheel of his Pontiac and pulled off in the direction of Waynesboro. The road was narrow, and sunlight played wildly off the trees and through the windshield. He came to an unmarked intersection and guessed Mississippi to be to the right. Was the infectious disease doctor in Waynesboro giving Rebecca proper care? he frantically wondered. He hadn't even bothered to prescribe antidepressants for her. David realized he needed to calm down. He started rationalizing: Rebecca's hospital stay would be a good thing; maybe it would even make it easier for him to get her home health care. But that thought relaxed him only for a minute. She had been so depressed when he'd seen her, almost nonresponsive. Maybe, he thought, he could hold up her son as a reason for her to take the medications and hang on a bit longer. How bad had things gotten in this country, he thought, that he had to use her baby as bait to keep her from completely succumbing to hopelessness?

Waynesboro was a flat single-story town of five thousand. After making a couple of wrong turns, he found the hospital. The lobby was almost empty except for a few middle-aged nurses wandering back and forth in green hospital gowns. In the elevator heading up to Rebecca's room, David looked tired and stared nervously up at the blinking floor numbers.

He found Rebecca's door unlocked. She was lying in a fetal position facing the single window. It was a few minutes past noon, yet her small room was dark, lit only by a sliver of sunlight shining through a crack in the blue polyester curtains. The walls were hospital white and green, and the Lifetime channel broadcast in oversaturated red and blue on the television set bolted to the wall. Rebecca had her arms pulled up close to her face; her wrists were covered in black bruises. An IV was hooked up to her right arm, and she was clinging to her blanket like a small child. The hospital frightened her—it was a place where people came to die. Most of the times she had been admitted here she had checked herself out against doctor's orders.

David walked around to the side of her bed and leaned up against the radiator next to the window. "How you feelin', Rebecca?" he asked. She half-mumbled, half-whispered an inaudible reply. "What?" David asked, his voice ringing hard and a bit frantic off the bare walls. He wanted to comfort her, but first he had to reassure himself that she wasn't about to die.

"I'm gonna have surgery tomorrow," she said, her voice raspy.

"What for?" David asked.

"My gallbladder," she said, then was seized by a fit of heavy coughing.

"How old are you, Rebecca?" David asked.

"Nineteen," she answered. She'd just celebrated her birthday.

"You know, Rebecca, there's a lady in Mobile who does nothin' but check on children whose parents are infected."

"He ain't infected," Rebecca said almost angrily.

"I know," he said, "but it may be wise for William to see her anyway 'cause she's a specialist."

"My mama's with him," she said quietly.

"Yeah, I know your mama's there doin' a real good job. Maybe we'll just get your information and deal with your care first. I need you to sign these papers," he said, and handed her a records release form. She signed them, and he knew that there was nothing he could do or say to make the situation better. So he left.

On the drive back to Mobile he passed a hand-painted sign for Pine Grove Cemetery on the corner of a dirt road leading into the forest. He took a deep drag on yet another cigarette. The trees by the edge of the highway had turned late-fall burnt orange and sunflower yellow. He wanted to know where this disease came from, why there was so little out here for this dying girl, and what had happened to America in the thirty years since the promise of the civil rights movement. She was gonna die, he thought, and there wasn't one thing he could do about it.

CHAPTER TWO

_____

Allied

1986–1987

D R. MINDY THOMPSON FULLILOVE hadn't wanted to come to California. She'd agreed to move for her husband Bob's job at UC Berkeley, which is to say she had come for their relationship. Now it was March 1986, and they'd lived in the East Bay for nearly three years. She missed her youngest daughter, Molly, who was back home in New Jersey with Mindy's ex-husband. And she missed working as a psychiatrist helping families at the Morrisania Neighborhood Family Care Center in the Bronx.

Black, teeming, and political, the New York ghetto pulsed with a desperate and tangible energy. The place, the mothers, their children—it had all gotten under her skin. Something electric and vital was happening there, a death struggle, or maybe a life struggle that she hadn't quite been able to wrap her mind around. That energy, whatever it was, was missing from her first San Francisco job: working as a psychiatrist at a mental health clinic in the Tenderloin District, a windswept strip of streets dotted with heroin addicts and prostitutes, just west of San Francisco's glittering downtown. Mindy's father, Ernest "Big Train" Thompson, an East Coast black labor organizer in the 1940s and 1950s, had once told her that one could always find strength and hope in the heart of the ghetto. If that was true, then the Tenderloin wasn't a ghetto, at least not in the Harlem, Watts, and South Side of Chicago sense of the word. It was more like a drainage gutter for the castoffs who couldn't make it in a city that—with its chardonnay drinkers, _haute_ California cuisine, and sparkling views of the Pacific Ocean—was doing its best to make good on Ronald Reagan's promise for a new morning in America. Mindy had recently left the Tenderloin clinic for a similarly drab day hospital in the Mission District, a largely Hispanic community where, as a black woman, she felt like even more of an outsider.

It was nearly eight on a Saturday morning, and sunlight was pouring in through the bedroom window of their Victorian-style house on Chilton Street in Berkeley. She and Bob had just completed their income tax returns and discovered that they owed the government a fairly hefty sum of cash. They both hoped that the grant applications she'd recently submitted to fund a support program for minority medical students at UC San Francisco, where she was a graduate student adviser, would relieve some of the financial pressure on them. More than that, she hoped the grant would put her on the path to It. She had been searching for It most of her life. There wasn't really a better word for it than that. It felt primal. It fed her ambition. It cut through her periodic bouts of depression and gave her the courage to overcome her shyness. It was something she had to say, or maybe It wasn't. Maybe It was a question she had to pose. She didn't know. Probably the best way to describe It was a sense of purpose that had always felt just beyond her reach.

Perhaps It grew out of a lifelong experience of not quite belonging—a life of viewing the world from a point just off center. When Mindy was a girl, Martin Luther King had marched through the South, Malcolm X had raised the flag of black militancy, and Daniel Patrick Moynihan, the Democratic senator from New York, had released his study on the crisis of the black family. Mindy's racial consciousness, though, was forged in the more visceral crucible of her family. She grew up the daughter of a mixed marriage in a black neighborhood in Orange, New Jersey, during the 1950s and 1960s. Each year, with intermingled anger and longing, she watched her mother creep off alone to Ohio to visit Mindy's white grandparents, whom she had never met. By the time Mindy was six, she had seen her father's career as a leader of the burgeoning black labor movement broken by McCarthyism. And when she was seven, her parents had forced her to desegregate the Orange school system. Her early adulthood had been shaped by similar political and racial principles. As an undergraduate at Bryn Mawr, she petitioned the university's administration to hire her father's friend, Herbert Aptheker, the Marxist intellectual, as a visiting professor. At Columbia University College of Physicians and Surgeons, Mindy and a handful of medical students had investigated the treatment of black mental patients at the teaching hospital in North Harlem. And she and her first husband had adopted two black children out of foster care before Mindy gave birth to Molly.

These splinters of racial experience had helped mold her into a quiet, intense young doctor who was determined to accomplish something—which, to her frustration, she still couldn't quite put into words. She was too logical, too practical—too much of a scientist—to employ a notion like *destiny* to describe her search. She was more likely to think of herself as ambitious. At thirty-five she had published articles in two of the country's most prestigious medical journals: an article on black medical students in the *New England Journal of Medicine,* and a piece on race and identity in the *Journal of the American Medical Association.* And she'd done some research on the condition of the black family.

She'd spoken on family structure at a few conferences. Her presentations hadn't gone particularly well—she wasn't political like her father or gregarious like Bob, so the spotlight was a painful place for her. Still, she had presence. She was tall, with long curly hair, a coffee complexion, and rounded cheekbones. Her eyes were tired, dark brown, and gave little room for pretense—which made her gaze seem both disarming and suspicious, so that she often caused people to feel at once understood and uncomfortable. In those sterile lecture halls, though, she'd come across as cold, her words not necessarily irrelevant but somehow missing the mark. She hoped to take this Saturday off, give herself a rest from worrying about her career, and visit with a friend who was in town from New York.

The phone rang, and Bob answered. It was Sala Udin, calling for Mindy. He was a black drug treatment specialist, whom she knew slightly through her position as president of the Northern California Black Physicians Association. Her main impression of him was that he was a politician. She had grown up around politicians and was a bit wary of them.

It was strange that he'd phoned on a Saturday. Not surprisingly, Sala had a sell job for her. The National Institute of Mental Health (NIMH), he told her, was rushing to set up a research center with a mandate to investigate strategies to stop the new AIDS epidemic. The NIMH was one of the four original components of the National Institutes of Health (NIH), and center grants were among the largest blocks of funding they gave to academic investigators. A group of psychologists, doctors, and epidemiologists at UC San Francisco, San Francisco General Hospital, and the San Francisco Department of Public Health were getting ready to submit a center grant proposal. The problem, Sala felt, was that they were all white. He and a group of black and Latino activists were fighting for them to include minority researchers on their team, and they were looking for qualified scientists. He wondered if Mindy was interested.

She hesitated. She'd casually followed the development of the epidemic in the paper. AIDS was that disease that was killing gay men by wiping out their immune systems. San Francisco had been especially hard hit. It sounded horrible and devastating. But outside her general concern for the health of the people in her community, she didn't see what it had to do with her. She wasn't, after all, a public health researcher. She was a psychiatrist, a black, straight, female psychiatrist engaged in examining the crises facing black Americans. Thanks, she told Sala, but she wasn't interested.

Sala persisted. He'd put together a lunch, he told her, with a few other minority researchers to discuss how to get the team at UCSF to include them. It was in a couple of days. She should be there.

Mindy gave in. She'd go. But that would be all. AIDS certainly wasn't It.

Relieved, Sala set down the phone. He, along with a group of activists and community-based public health professionals, had been negotiating for weeks with the two lead investigators from UCSF, Dr. Stephen Hulley and Dr. Tom Coates, to get control over a portion of this grant. So far they'd essentially stonewalled him. Sure, they said, they wanted to involve minorities in their research, but so far they had promised to do so only in an advisory capacity. That was simply unacceptable to Sala. He had seen hundreds of black men and women lost to heroin addiction. Sometimes it seemed half the friends he'd grown up with in Pittsburgh's Hill District had either died or been anesthetized by the drug. Now junkies were getting AIDS through needles. And it wasn't stopping with them. Heroin users were giving it to their lovers and, according to reports, giving birth to babies infected with this disease.

These white scientists, in his opinion, were naïve if they thought they could walk into the ghetto, perform a couple of studies, figure out a way to get addicts to stop using, and thereby prevent AIDS from spreading through the black community. Sala had spent the better part of two decades working in heroin recovery centers. He had watched the drug devastate his sister and younger brother. It had taken all his experience to get his nephew to kick the habit. An unimaginable number of black men and women were probably walking the streets unknowingly infected with HIV. If something wasn't done soon, there were going to be thousands of funerals across black America.

Sala was the director of a center that trained heroin treatment specialists in downtown San Francisco. Treatment and prevention were in a state of disrepair. The nationwide network of inner-city treatment centers financed during the Nixon Administration had been largely defunded—many of those that had managed to survive were struggling to stay solvent. Ronald Reagan's drug-prevention strategy centered largely on his wife Nancy's Just Say No television campaign, which seemed to be targeted mainly at white kids in the suburbs. Sala was part of a group of specialists who had been certified by the National Institute on Drug Abuse (NIDA) to develop and teach culturally sensitive heroin treatment and prevention methods. Their ideas were slowly gaining acceptance in public health circles. Now the AIDS epidemic had upped the ante.

Sala was clear that the best hope of stopping the epidemic before it devastated minority America rested in funding black and Latino researchers to figure out how and why intravenous drug users were putting themselves at risk of AIDS. This wasn't a question of equal opportunity. The investigators were going to have to persuade minority addicts to come clean about their intimate sexual and drug-using habits. Time in this equation equaled lives, and it would simply take too long for white researchers to gain enough access to get that kind of data. Even if they did, Sala doubted that they'd have the expertise to know, for instance, that needle sharing was an integral part of the junkie subculture.

The proposal was due in less than two months. Sala was scheduled to meet with Hulley and Coates in a week. They had told him that they'd consider bringing qualified minority investigators on board, but all the black and Latino doctors, public health researchers, and psychologists whom Sala had reached so far either had full dockets or weren't interested in AIDS. Mindy had been a last resort. She was a junior researcher, but she was Columbia-trained and already was affiliated with UCSF. If they rejected her, he had one more weapon to threaten them with. The NIMH specifically stated that the proposal had to have community approval. Sala had been funded by the National Institute on Drug Abuse; he and his partners were connected to the San Francisco Department of Public Health. He knew how to sabotage their project. It wasn't a move he relished; he was aware that gay white men were dying in alarming numbers in San Francisco, and he doubted that the UCSF doctors were acting with racist intent. But there was limited money to deal with this epidemic, and as best he could tell, little was being done to shield blacks from it.

Confrontation—or at least the threat of it—had, of course, always been an essential element of the civil rights movement. Two decades after the Civil Rights Act, though, it was debatable whether the kind of aggressive rhetoric that inevitably implied the charge of racism was still an effective crowbar to pry open space for blacks in American institutions. To use it required a certain moral authority. And the American public's sense that blacks stood on firm moral ground had been eroding since the 1970s, when in the wake of Jim Crow the face of the inner-city black emerged distorted, as an angry, drug-addled, welfare-dependent single parent. At the same time, however, charging racial insensitivity may have been the only serious card Sala had to play. Blacks and whites had yet to develop a new language or conceptual framework to address the crises that continued to plague black America. Black leaders were scattered and, to varying degrees, intellectually disconnected from one another. It was hard to tell whether they had failed to articulate a post–civil rights vision for race in America, or the nationalist rhetoric of the 1970s had been misguided, or they had simply been defeated. Now, with AIDS, black America was being attacked by a sexually transmitted, drug-use-related disease that called for confronting, and even laying public claim to, its most shameful demons. And there was reason to believe that much of the damage the virus was now wreaking could have been avoided.

SALA HAD PROBABLY BEEN first inspired to go down to Mississippi to register voters by Malcolm X. He'd run away from Pittsburgh as a teenager in the late 1950s, to live with his aunt on Staten Island. Often he trekked up to Harlem on weekends with his friends to catch a street-corner sermon from the civil rights leader. Malcolm often delivered his arguments from the bed of an old pickup truck flanked by a clique of armed young guards standing on point in bow ties and two-button suits. Malcolm's strategy of juxtaposing reason with the implication of violent action stuck with Sala. So when he heard a speech by a Student Nonviolent Coordinating Committee (SNCC) recruiter at a church in Pittsburgh in 1964, he flashed on Malcolm laying waste to blacks who complacently railed against racism from the comfort of the North, while the real war was being fought against attack dogs and fire hoses down South.

The battleground in the South proved less literal than Malcolm agitated for, or than Sala imagined. Certainly some moments had the chaotic tenor of war, like the night the Klan broke into SNCC headquarters, brandishing shotguns and sticks. But Sala was more deeply shaped by the restrained tone of the day-to-day struggle: the courage it took for the farmer he lived with to walk up the steps of the county courthouse to register to vote, knowing that whites could take his land or even kill him; the self-control Sala learned to muster, to be able to ignore the policemen who relentlessly harassed him for minor traffic infractions; and the dignity the farmer's children displayed when they integrated their school.

Sala stayed in Mississippi for just over four years, and when he returned to Pittsburgh's Hill District in 1969, he believed that blacks were poised to become economically and culturally independent. He became involved with the Afro-American Institute, a black nationalist group of intellectuals, artists, and community organizers interested in developing black curricula in the public schools, promoting black arts, and electing black candidates to public office.

Pittsburgh, though, had changed. Growing up, Sala and his friends had belonged to gangs, but crime had been so infrequent that his mother had rarely bothered to lock her apartment. Now he heard gunshots at night. Rioters had burned dozens of buildings in the city, and more stood abandoned, like dark carcasses towering over the empty streets. Black families were reeling from the losses they had suffered in Vietnam. And the Nixon administration was preparing to dismantle Lyndon Johnson's War on Poverty programs. Sala was particularly worried about heroin. The black nationalist movement was based on the essentially optimistic premise that once blacks were unmuzzled by systemic racism, they would build thriving communities across America. Sala only had to look at his sister to see that heroin could cloud that vision. The drug had infiltrated many families. Every block and housing project seemed besieged by dealers. Little had been developed nationally in terms of heroin treatment or prevention. He even heard whispers at the Afro-American Institute that the proliferation of heroin was part of a government conspiracy to kill blacks.

Heroin certainly hadn't been treated as a public health crisis. Surprisingly, that began to change when the Nixon White House made the connection between heroin abuse and crime rates. In August 1969 Dr. Robert DuPont, a young Washington, D.C., psychiatrist, equipped a group of college students with urine cups and took them down to a city jail. Forty-four percent of the inmates they sampled tested positive for heroin. Nixon had campaigned hard on crime and had been embarrassed that the murder and burglary rates in the District had tripled and quadrupled during his first year in office. DuPont proposed that he could bring those numbers down by treating the city's addicts with methadone, a little-known synthetic drug that satisfied heroin cravings. Nixon took the gamble and gave him funds to open a clinic in Washington. Within a year burglaries in the city fell 41 percent. Then in 1971 Congressmen Robert Steele and Morgan Murphy visited Vietnam, returning with a report that 10 to 15 percent of the enlisted men were strung out on the drug.

The numbers were probably exaggerated, but war veterans couldn't be easily dismissed as criminals or degenerates, and the report gave the administration an opening to reframe heroin in public health terms. In June 1971 Nixon told Congress, "Drug traffic is public enemy number one domestically in the United States today and we must wage a total offensive." That summer he established the Special Action Office for Drug Abuse and Prevention (SAODAP) to coordinate all federal drug treatment and prevention activities; then in 1973 he established the National Institute on Drug Abuse to oversee treatment and prevention research. The administration undertook an ambitious project to construct a nationwide network of treatment facilities. For the first time funding for treatment and prevention eclipsed funding for law enforcement. The number of cities with federally funded treatment services jumped from 54 to 214, and soon there were three thousand rehab clinics operating across the country.

Sala hadn't been quite ready to subscribe to vast conspiracy theories, but after watching Hill District drug deals go down in broad daylight, he had come to suspect that the dealers were paying off Pittsburgh's cops. In 1970 he and a small team of activists commandeered a shooting gallery in a condemned building and turned it into a rehab center called House of the Crossroads. Here they housed recovering addicts, organized them into armed teams, and instructed them to patrol the neighborhood and attack dealers. The idea seemed militant, proactive, and empowering. But the dealers beat them back so severely that Sala worried they would kill some of his people. So he applied for federal subsidies and used the money to both treat and employ addicts in an effort to reintegrate them into the community.

Nationally, treatment and prevention worked, and between 1973 and 1975 heroin use fell precipitously. Politically, though, the strategy was founded on shaky ground. Nixon was in a delicate position: he was compelled to condemn drug use as criminal, but at the same time he was attempting to eliminate it with the instruments of public health. Moreover, the partnership between the Republican White House that was administering the nation's new drug war and the black leaders who represented the addicts in treatment was tenuous. Nowhere was this more evident than in the debate over methadone. By the early 1970s DuPont had successfully established methadone maintenance as the most common treatment for heroin addiction. The drug had a number of advantages: it was easy to dispense, relatively cheap, and clearly effective in satiating the hunger for heroin; from a public health perspective, it protected addicts from blood-borne diseases like hepatitis. But it was also an addictive narcotic. Some junkies said their methadone high was just as powerful as the one they got from heroin. Blacks and left-leaning whites attacked the program as everything from a cynical strategy to deflect the cost of expensive inpatient care to a thinly veiled scheme to opiate black Americans. By the time Gerald Ford took office in the wake of Watergate, methadone treatment had lost some of its political luster.

Progressive drug politics weren't entirely dead, however. Recreational narcotics like cocaine and marijuana were gaining some mainstream acceptance. After Jimmy Carter took office, he persuaded NIDA, the Drug Enforcement Administration, and the NIMH to back legislation that would legalize marijuana. But parent and conservative groups struck hard against the initiative and defeated it. The parent groups then turned their attention to bongs and pipes, lobbying to pass federal laws that would make it illegal to purchase or possess drug paraphernalia. When Ronald Reagan ran for office, he recognized that the drug issue had the capacity to galvanize his conservative base. Indeed he and Nancy Reagan's abstinence-only message helped cement a national shift away from progressive drug policy in favor of a more punitive model.

In 1983 Sala resigned his position at House of the Crossroads. The government hadn't fulfilled its early promise to reduce heroin addiction through treatment. And the black leaders who had trumpeted nationalism as a sort of redemptive panacea for the black community had trapped themselves in a confused position, at once isolationist and locked in a struggle against white America over who was to blame for the litany of crises that were dragging down black inner cities across the country. Sala felt burned out. Even his own Off the Pusher campaign now struck him as ultimately painful to the very people he was trying to help. According to the Office of National Drug control policy there were 1.8 million lifetime heroin users in the United States. Hunted by law enforcement, often unable to buy needles, thousands of them huddled together in the shells of the empty, burned-out buildings that still littered America's cities, passing what needles they had from arm to outstretched arm.

SALA NOTICED that he was the only straight black man sitting at the broad table in the brightly lit meeting room. A couple of days had passed since his conversation with Mindy Fullilove. She and Ed Morales, a

Latino psychologist who was the lead academic on the minority team, sat next to him, along with a group of black and Latino activists from the city's gay and drug treatment community. Opposite them were the white scientists from UCSF. The two that really mattered were the psychologist Tom Coates, who had put the project together, and Steve Hulley, a doctor and epidemiologist whom Coates had asked to be the team's principal investigator.

Sala recognized that this was his last opportunity to negotiate, and he had prepared what he considered to be a reasonable proposal. As it stood, the UCSF team had a series of component divisions that included epidemiology, behavior, substance abuse, and policy. Each was headed up by a white investigator. Sala and his allies wanted them to add a minority component that would be based at a drug treatment clinic in Bayview-Hunters Point, the city's largest black neighborhood. The rub, though, was that he wanted the minority component to have control over an equal share of the grant money, which would be difficult to negotiate. One reason was that the researchers he had brought to this meeting were quite junior. Mindy Fullilove had a Columbia pedigree but she had little public health experience. Ed Morales directed the Bayview-Hunters Point methadone program and was an instructor at San Francisco Community College, which had a weak research reputation. The men from UCSF, on the other hand, were respected public health scientists. Hulley, who on top of his duties as principal investigator had been tagged to head up the epidemiology component, was Harvard trained, a professor at UCSF, and had headed major NIH-funded investigations on smoking prevention. Coates, who would lead the behavior component, had stops at Johns Hopkins, Stanford, and now UCSF listed on his résumé; his specialty was cardiology and cancer prevention; and he had been one of the first investigators in the country to win NIMH AIDS research money. Their lieutenants, like Dr. Jim Sorenson, who had been tapped to investigate IV drug users and who headed up the heroin treatment center at San Francisco General Hospital, were equally respected. But Sala faced another, perhaps more formidable, obstacle as well: he wanted them to give NIMH money to community-based researchers. The entire notion was anathema to Hulley and Coates's university-based, scientist-centered vision of public health research.

As the meeting progressed, Sala kept talking, framing and reframing. Coates and Hulley were unfailingly polite, but they simply weren't willing to cede control of the money. The two sides were speaking around each other, and inevitably that sharpened the racial tension that was a subtext of the negotiation. Coates and Hulley had the luxury of bringing in top white scientists to investigate the epidemic as it tore through the Castro and perhaps threatened the population at large. The reality of race in the mid-1980s was that Sala simply did not have a set of black scientists whom he could call on to match them credential for credential. His frustration built, welling up from a deep part of him. This wasn't about racism or even money anymore. These men seemed to him unwilling—or were perhaps unable—either to empathize with the depth of his concern or to appreciate the nuances of his position. He had seen entire families and neighborhoods destroyed. Black men were rumored to be wasting to the point that they looked like skeletons. But, to Sala, these men from UCSF were averting their eyes while hypocritically moving to help their own people.

TOM COATES had received the call from Dr. Marcus Conant in August 1985. "You've got it, Tom," he'd said. Tom told his secretary to cancel the rest of the afternoon, went home to his apartment, sat on his couch, and stared out the picture windows of his living room at the setting sun as it spread over the San Francisco skyline. He could make out the marquee of the Castro Theatre glistening red in the late afternoon light, beyond that the edges of the Embarcadero, and then the silhouette of the Bay Bridge stretching over the darkness of San Francisco Bay. The view was one of the reasons he'd borrowed the money from his parents to buy this apartment. Usually he found it calming and meditative, but that afternoon he felt as if he were looking out onto a dying city. He had to tell his boyfriend he was infected; he didn't know if he could hide it from his parents; he was undesirable, even unlovable; and he felt that he had brought it upon himself—they had all brought it upon themselves. Now he was going to die, most likely alone, and he didn't know what he could do to prevent it.

He was forty and handsome, with a shock of gray-flecked dark hair, a square jaw, and glasses that made him look a little like Clark Kent. San Francisco had seemed like paradise to him. He'd landed his dream job at UCSF studying the applications of psychology in disease prevention. He wasn't exactly out—certainly not at work—but the city's electric collection of gay bars, clubs, and political life offered more than enough safe havens where he could let down his guard and be an openly gay man. For a time it had even seemed that gay men would own the city. Then they had started to die.

Tom had been one of the first to take the new HIV antibody test. It was a difficult decision. There was no cure, no vaccine, no treatment for AIDS, and it was beginning to scare average Americans. Margaret Heckler, head of the Department of Health and Human Services (HHS), the superagency that oversaw both the NIH and the CDC, had announced in 1983 that AIDS was the nation's top health threat. Now that the CDC had developed a diagnostic test for the disease, it was likely to launch a textbook epidemic response. That meant identifying those diagnosed, naming them on a master list, and notifying all their sexual partners.

Tom didn't think the CDC's approach would ever work with AIDS. The CDC was good at surveillance—expert at it. When four cases of swine flu were identified at the Fort Dix army base in February 1976, the CDC immediately placed the entire base under surveillance. Shortly afterward, the cases were written up for the agency's *Morbidity and Mortality Weekly Report (MMWR)*, and the Thursday before publication, reporters were briefed on the outbreak. The CDC's director, Dr. David Sencer, called for mass inoculations, and by the end of the year fifty million Americans had been vaccinated. But AIDS was different. It was a retrovirus that didn't manifest symptoms until its final stages. It didn't even kill you. It just eviscerated your immune system to such a degree that it made even the common cold lethal.

Until just a few months earlier, the only way to identify people who might be carrying the virus was through their sexual or drug habits, especially men who had anal sex with other men and junkies who shot heroin with dirty needles—people whom most of America despised, feared, or at the very least didn't know. It wasn't hard for Tom to imagine a nightmare scenario where gay men like him were effectively ripped out of the closet and branded as pariahs. Their jobs, family relationships, health care, and homes would be jeopardized. Even quarantine was a remote possibility. Worse, the epidemic might very well continue to spread. Simple prevention messages weren't curbing the behavior of gay men. In early 1983 Tom and two San Francisco psychologists, Bill Horstman and Leon McKusick, surveyed six hundred gay men about their sexual behavior. They found that the men knew about AIDS, even about what kinds of sex would get them infected, but only 15 percent had stopped receiving anal intercourse, 20 percent said they had cut down on rimming, and a mere 5 percent had stopped engaging in oral sex.

Tom had been reluctant to center his professional life on AIDS. Studying the disease was like outing himself, and he wasn't sure what that would mean for his career. In the weeks after he was diagnosed, though, he realized he had to devote himself to trying to curb the epidemic.

DR. ELLEN STOVER had her first conversation with Tom Coates about AIDS on a June afternoon in 1983 at the National Institute of Mental Health in Bethesda, Maryland. She knew him slightly from a smoking-prevention project that she'd funded back in the 1970s, but the two San Francisco psychologists he'd brought with him, Steve Morin and Jeff Mandel, were strangers to her. She pulled up a chair across from them at the black Formica meeting table in her tenth-floor office and asked them what was on their minds. The three men wanted to know what the NIMH planned do about the new epidemic. She recalled the television news footage she'd seen of masked, gloved paramedics in sterile white suits gingerly carrying the corpses of gay men out of their New York apartments. Those images could inspire the kind of public panic that swiftly warped into paranoid hatred for gay men or anyone else who Americans imagined were infected. Still, she wasn't exactly sure why they'd come to her. The NIMH wasn't in the infectious disease business.

The San Francisco psychologists had actually been shrewd to approach the NIMH. Ordinarily the doctors and epidemiologists at the

CDC were the first to investigate the outbreak of a disease, identify its cause, and coordinate with local health authorities to contain it. The bio-medical researchers at the much larger National Institutes of Health (NIH) were then saddled with the often more expensive and incremental task of developing treatments and vaccines. AIDS, though, hadn't behaved like most viruses. It disguised itself in a shroud of other diseases. The CDC had been fairly certain since at least 1982 that it had an infectious agent on its hands, but the scientists at the National Cancer Institute still hadn't been able to isolate the virus that caused it. The only sure way they knew to shield people from infection was to change their sexual and drug-using habits. It was the NIMH that held the federal purse strings for behavior research.

Stover was something of an NIMH lifer, with a matter-of-fact personality that helped her get things done in the agency's multimillion-dollar bureaucracy. She didn't know that Tom and his colleagues were gay, but the urgency in their tone struck a chord with her, and after the meeting she briefed her director, Shervert Frazier, on what she'd learned. He said he'd give her some seed money to organize a small research and policy agenda conference, with whatever public health and sexual behavior researchers she could scratch up.

Stover knew that wouldn't be easy. The NIMH had suffered cutbacks in the early 1980s, and sexual behavior research had been completely defunded, which meant that she was going to have to jump-start the field. The NIMH didn't even have an active database of sex researchers. She flipped through her Rolodex and started making phone calls. She didn't get much response. Well-known investigators didn't trust that the federal government would really make another serious investment in research about sexual behavior, and younger scientists thought AIDS was a career dead end. Stover suspected that some of them were hiding behind those excuses because they didn't want to touch such a shameful disease. Eventually she managed to pull together a group of investigators that included Coates, Morin, and the chancellor of UCSF's medical school, Phil Lee, who had been the assistant secretary of health in the Johnson administration and was one of the architects of Medicare.

The problems they faced were profound and systemic. The CDC, which had been marshaled to contain the epidemic, was not staffed, funded, or organized to develop and implement a national plan to stop the spread of AIDS. Disease prevention had always been the neglected arm of the American public health system, and that had never been more true than in the late 1970s and early 1980s when, flush from its success with polio, the scientific community felt that infectious diseases had been largely contained. In 1980, the year before AIDS surfaced, death rates from infectious disease had fallen to their lowest recorded rate in the twentieth century. The CDC had undergone a major reorganization that shifted its resources toward chronic illness.

CDC doctors who were marshaled to investigate the new AIDS epidemic had had to make a substantial effort to garner money and manpower to prove that AIDS was a serious threat to the public health. Now, in 1983, they were being slowed by white-hot public scrutiny. There was concern within the medical community that the Reagan administration would hesitate to pour money into what was apparently a homosexual epidemic; the blood banks were worried that the agency would jeopardize the nation's blood supply by declaring that AIDS could be spread through transfusions; and gay activists were concerned that the CDC's prevention efforts might threaten their civil rights. Even if the CDC managed to navigate those minefields, it didn't have on board behavioral scientists who were formally trained to recognize and investigate the political, cultural, and psychological forces driving the epidemic. Moreover, the agency lacked a strong presence outside Atlanta and was heavily dependent on state and local health departments to carry out prevention work—a strategy that could prove scattershot with a disease like AIDS, which required frank talk about sexuality and drug use.

Clearly, the small class of investigators Stover convened in Washington couldn't address all these problems. They were, however, positioned in academia, politics, government, and the gay community to maneuver more freely around the epidemic than the CDC. First on their agenda was to promote prevention, the only sure way to slow the spread of the disease. They all agreed that the federal government was neither accustomed to nor particularly adept at poking about in Americans' sex lives. So they decided that the NIMH's efforts should be carried out in concert with gay leaders. Gay scientists like Tom could help smooth that relationship. Stover would be their voice in Washington.

After the meeting she patched together a small AIDS research budget at the NIMH. More important, she nurtured relationships with her contacts at the NIH and the CDC. Through her connections she learned that no vaccine or cure was in the pipeline at the NIH. So in 1984, when Bob Gallo at the National Cancer Institute isolated the virus that causes AIDS, boldly predicting that he would develop a vaccine within two years, she pressed the NIMH to invest more money in prevention research.

Two years of effort paid off, and in 1985 Shervert Frazier called her into his office. For some time he and Stover had been concerned that the inherently slow pace of scientific investigation was costing lives. Two years often passed between the time they funded an AIDS study and the date the findings were actually published. And they were both further frustrated that no system was in place to rapidly distribute the most current research either to the people who were directly dealing with the infected or to the many scientists who were working across disciplines to stop the virus. "I want you to link up the entire country," Frazier told her evenly.

As they fleshed out his idea over the following weeks, Stover grew excited. They planned to have the NIMH fund a network of multidisciplinary, university-based AIDS research centers in cities across the United States. These centers in the epidemic hotbeds of San Francisco, Los Angeles, and New York would house virologists, epidemiologists, psychologists, and doctors who would gather and quickly share the freshest information about how, where, and why the disease was spreading. As far as Stover knew, nothing quite like it had ever been undertaken to combat an infectious disease.

TOM COATES didn't tell Steve Hulley that he was infected as they drove down to Stanford for a cardiology conference in early 1986. He didn't tell him that he had been worried about AIDS since an evening back in 1982, when he glanced up from the man he was flirting with at a bar in Pittsburgh, peered at the television, and heard the newscaster report that a strange new syndrome was killing gay men. Or that he'd put down his drink, walked back to his hotel room, and crawled into bed frightened and alone. He didn't tell Steve that he was terrified that he'd die before his parents; that he'd decided not to tell his two brothers and his sister that he was infected; or that his boyfriend was still healthy. And he didn't tell him that he was gay. That information was immaterial.

Ellen Stover had done her part. Now Tom had to write a winning proposal for the review board at the NIMH to get one of her grants to fund an AIDS research center in San Francisco. He needed to persuade Steve to agree to be the prospective center's principal investigator. He knew he was in a delicate position. It was absolutely essential that he and other gay scientists like himself head up the center, though not just for the obvious reason that they had intimate knowledge of the mechanics of gay sex. The sort of investigations that he hoped to undertake were going to drag gay men's sex lives into the public spotlight. Terms like *rimming, fisting, poppers,* and *anal sex* would be thrown around in congressional hearings. None of it was going to be palatable to middle America—unless, of course, he was the one testifying on Capitol Hill, posing the research questions, and parsing the language. But it would never work for him to do it as a gay man, an AIDS victim, or a politico. He had to present himself as an objective scientist, a young whiz kid with a reputation as a rising star in preventive medicine.

Tom had worked with Steve back at Stanford and figured that the tall Iowan had never knowingly spoken to a gay man in his life. But Steve did have major NIH contracts, and Tom felt confident that he could navigate his way to another. So rather than telling him that he expected to die sometime in the next couple of years, he laid out the epidemiology of AIDS and the potential for the center to make a dent in the epidemic.

Steve Hulley waffled for a few days. A patient, measured, and detail-oriented man, he had an instinctively deductive mind that was ordered by the clean lines of scientific logic and seemingly unburdened by much sensitivity toward the messy, often contradictory interior lives of the people around him. It was a quality that probably helped him maintain his decidedly uncynical disposition and also on occasion got him into trouble with people for comments that came across as callous.

He was hesitant to jump into Tom's project. He was already an established figure in cardiovascular health and was building a reputation as a great mentor in American science. Furthermore, he didn't have much experience with gay men. That wasn't because of any personal bias—they'd just never previously been front and center in any epidemiological matter. Still, he'd begun to worry about the severity of the epidemic, and he felt a responsibility to do something about it. He also romanticized the preeminent epidemiologists as da Vincis, men who made marks in diverse fields. In an age of chronic disease, he had considered branching out into physical injury. AIDS felt more vital. With an up-and-coming scientist like Tom as his first lieutenant, the epidemic might offer him the opportunity to cross the threshold into greatness.

They had only a couple of months to develop the proposal for the AIDS research center. Tom had all kinds of policy, psychology, and cultural ambitions for it, but Steve was clear that each element that they pushed had to have a public-health facet. Steve had worried that they had no gay scientists in the fold and called Tom to ask if he had one in mind. "Uh, Steve, I think I qualify," Tom answered. The proposal took shape quickly, and it was impressive in both its institutional and its intellectual breadth. Medical doctors, statisticians, epidemiologists, sociologists, and psychologists signed on from UCSF, UC Berkeley, and the San Francisco Department of Public Health.

Ellen Stover's grant was explicit in its requirement that the research center have full community support. Knowing of Tom's connections in the Castro, Steve wasn't too concerned about holding a couple of public meetings. That was when they ran into Sala Udin and his cohort of activists, who wanted everything from veto power over research initiatives to control over part of the grant money.

Steve recognized the value of community involvement, but the stakes were too high here to bend to political pressure. Science was his religion: in his mind, these would-be politicians had no scientific credibility, membership in a minority wasn't a qualification for federal research money, and the NIMH didn't fund activists. Still, he was afraid to call Sala's bluff. He might very well have sharp enough fangs to defeat the project. In that light, he was a threat to the public health. Steve met with Tom several times to try to come up with a solution. With only a few weeks to go before the submission deadline, they offered Sala a final compromise:

if he found high-quality minority scientists, they'd welcome them onto the team as full partners.

At the final meeting, when Sala unveiled Mindy Fullilove and Ed Morales, Steve wasn't impressed. Mindy would have been okay as junior faculty—she was clearly talented, and she was Columbia-trained—but she lacked adequate research experience. And he was less confident in Ed Morales, the psychologist who would head this prospective minority division. Steve reiterated their position that they'd be happy to bring them on in an advisory capacity. Sala refused.

Steve couldn't understand it. He was interested in public health. To him, many of these people were self-aggrandizing power-mongers. How could Sala or any of his partners claim to represent their constituencies in good faith, then stand here and obstruct vital health research? This was too difficult, too painful. He felt he couldn't do this much longer.

Midway through the meeting, everyone started to talk at once. Voices grew louder. Sala wriggled free of his chair and slammed down his brown leather briefcase. "If we're not included in this proposal, then it is going down," he said evenly. "We're going to sink it."

Steve stood up. Something in him had snapped. Perhaps it was his overriding sense of reason, or perhaps he recognized that his ultimate loyalty was to the health of the public. Hold on, he said. I think we can work something out.

———

FOR MOST OF HER adult life Mindy Fullilove had channeled her energy along traditional political and racial lines. AIDS felt different, almost from the moment Steve Hulley agreed to let her and Ed Morales join the team as the prospective research center's "third world component." Most of the team had been brushed in some horrifying way by the epidemic. People routinely arrived at meetings straight from funerals. Some were even dying from the disease themselves. They worked hastily to write in the minority component of the grant proposal. A young black psychologist, John Peterson, joined the team. Michigan-trained, he was the minority education director for a nonprofit AIDS agency in Oakland and had been an assistant professor at Claremont McKenna College. Over the summer of 1986 Mindy took Steve Hulley's epidemiology course at UCSF and threw herself into both the scientific and the popular AIDS literature.

The epidemic by then was seizing headlines across the country, and the message to the public was clear: AIDS was a gay white disease. Rock Hudson's death in the fall of 1985 was still in the papers; journalists were telling harrowing stories about how AIDS was devastating gay neighborhoods; and doctors and public health officials, in an effort to quell mounting public hysteria, were being quoted in newspapers as saying that most Americans hadn't been exposed to the virus.

But in black and Latino communities, where AIDS was also spreading through dirty needles, the situation was more grave. Thirty-nine percent of all AIDS cases were members of an ethnic minority. Twenty-four percent were black. Seventy-four percent of all women with AIDS were black or Latino. Fifty-seven percent of all pediatric AIDS cases were black. Incidence of AIDS in gay and bisexual black men was 50 percent higher than in homosexual white men. And black U.S. Army recruits were four times as likely as whites to be infected with HIV. The numbers weren't hard to find; they appeared in CDC reports. The Public Health Service had access to them; so did the Department of Health and Human Services. But little had been done to specifically warn minorities about the threat that the epidemic posed to them.

This omission could not be blamed on the fact that the government was ignoring AIDS in general. In 1984 the Public Health Service had put together the Executive Task Force on AIDS to coordinate all of the AIDS activities of America's most powerful public health agencies: the NIH, the CDC, the Food and Drug Administration, the Health Resources and Services Administration, and the Alcohol, Drug Abuse, and Mental Health Agency (which housed the NIMH and NIDA). The Public Health Service projected that the CDC would spend a combined $282.2 million on HIV prevention in 1987 and 1988. Only 6 percent of that was specifically targeted at minorities.

The UCSF team was awarded the NIMH's AIDS research center grant in September 1986. Steve and Tom set up shop at UCSF; Mindy, John, and Ed established their base of operations in a large, brightly lit room on the second floor of the Bayview-Hunters Point Foundation. The clinic was hardly a research facility, but it did offer a laboratory of streets lined with liquor stores, churches, and modest houses that were home to San Francisco's black community. All the participants had been a little uneasy with the title "third world component," so they changed their name to MIRA (which means "look" in Spanish), an acronym for Multicultural Inquiry and Research on AIDS. As far as they knew, they were the first scientists in the country dedicated to studying the minority AIDS epidemic.

Steve Hulley took an immediate interest in Mindy. She was raw and untrained but had an enormous intellectual energy that he took for confidence. Over the winter and spring of 1987 she and Ed held focus groups with black and Latino leaders, developed partnerships with drug treatment centers, and published an article reviewing the extant research on AIDS among minorities. She was racing against the epidemic. San Francisco's three minority neighborhoods—the Mission District, Bayview-Hunters Point, and the Western Addition—surrounded the Castro District. The disease seemed likely to seep out of the gay ghetto and infect black and Latino heroin addicts, but the MIRA team wasn't working with enough hard data to be able to accurately predict how it was going to happen. Although the CDC regularly published the latest AIDS surveillance, AIDS activists had successfully lobbied to keep new HIV infections confidential. The CDC estimated that HIV took five to seven years to incubate into AIDS. That meant that the surveillance data the MIRA team was looking at in 1987 was actually a window onto the epidemic in 1981. Furthermore, quantitative data on sexual behavior and drug use in San Francisco's black and Latino neighborhoods hardly existed, which made it difficult to develop an effective AIDS-prevention strategy. As far as Mindy knew, no AIDS researchers had gathered information from any minority neighborhood in the country. One reason had to do with how AIDS had been first identified and investigated in the early 1980s.

The first cases of what would come to be known as AIDS were reported among gay men suffering from pneumonia in Los Angeles in the spring of 1981. Then came reports that many of the patients had also been diagnosed with Kaposi's sarcoma, a rare cancer usually found in elderly men. Shortly afterward Dr. Jim Curran, the chief of the CDC's Venereal Disease Control Division, was tapped to head up a Kaposi's Sarcoma and Opportunistic Infection Task Force. Despite being short-staffed and underfunded, the task force managed to bring together experts from diverse fields like virology, cancer, and parasitic diseases, in addition to a small team of epidemiological intelligence officers, who were the agency's foot soldiers for disease investigation. Soon after the first gay white cases were written up in the CDC's *Morbidity and Mortality Weekly Report* (*MMWR*), the task force received word that a similar syndrome was showing up in IV drug users in New York and New Jersey. Dr. Mary Guinan was dispatched to New York to investigate the heterosexual cases and Curran flew out there himself to see suspected patients. He had done quite a bit of work on hepatitis B with gay men in the 1970s, and he almost immediately suspected that they had a similar sexually transmitted and blood-borne disease on their hands.

For several reasons, however, many in the scientific community remained unconvinced that AIDS was an infectious disease. First and foremost, no infectious agent had been identified. Many of the IV drug users had been diagnosed postmortem, making it difficult to determine if they had contracted the disease through homosexual contact. It also didn't make sense that AIDS was showing up all over the country among gay white men, and only in New York and New Jersey among IV drug users. If these two groups were really suffering from the same disease, it should have been materializing in IV drug users in the same cities where it was manifesting in gay men. Perhaps, some surmised, this syndrome—which some had taken to calling Gay Related Immune Deficiency, or GRID—was caused by poppers, a drug commonly used by gay men to help facilitate anal sex. Others hypothesized that it was transmitted through semen.

In 1982 the Kaposi's Sarcoma Task Force undertook a cluster study, investigating the spread of the virus by mapping out whom the infected people had come into contact with. They decided to focus on gay men, a group that was far easier to reach and control for than IV drug users. The results clearly indicated that AIDS was indeed caused by an infectious agent. Then in June 1982 the first cases in hemophiliacs, who had caught the virus through blood transfusions, were reported, powerfully suggesting that the virus was also blood-borne. The implications for IV drug users and their sexual partners, though, were largely overshadowed by the threat the new disease posed to the nation's blood banks.

Now it was 1987, and research on the minority epidemic was sparse. Steve urged Mindy to put together a large-scale survey of HIV rates, substance abuse, sexual behavior, and attitudes toward AIDS in San Francisco's minority neighborhoods. Using San Francisco as a model, they hoped the results would yield a national prevention strategy for minority America.

John Peterson had reason to doubt that the study Steve was promoting would reveal much useful data. He had seen the numbers, read the literature, and listened to the public health debates about IV drug users and gay white men. But they weren't the only two groups fueling the epidemic. Black men were silently dying in unknown numbers. John had seen their anguished faces and listened to their tortured questions. They didn't live in nouveau riche gay ghettos like the Castro, or even in San Francisco's aging and slowly depopulating minority neighborhoods. They inhabited black cities like Oakland and Richmond, sometimes with their wives, girlfriends, and children. They belonged to black churches, were working class, and were the children of the great migration from the South. And they secretly slept with other men. These people had no intention of discussing their "risk behaviors" with either black or white researchers. That would be social suicide, a brand of death that for many was more frightening than actual death.

John had known he was gay since he was six years old and had accepted that fact about himself ever since he'd gotten his hands on the works of Sigmund Freud in high school. But his homosexuality had always been secondary to his larger sense of himself as a black man. John's father had been one of the first black men of his generation to own a house in Orlando, Florida. John could read almost as soon as he was able to walk and was one of those kids who'd sooner be found in the segregated library than on the basketball court or football field.

John had never been able to find a comfortable place for himself in gay America. The circle of gay academics he had run with at UCLA and Claremont were intellectually compatible but mostly white. He was not drawn to the Castro; the gay ghetto's monolithic whiteness, its bathhouses, and its promiscuity were off-putting to him. He fancied himself the kind of charming, respectable, conscientious young man that any black mother would want her daughter to marry, and in the fall of 1983 he had moved to the East Bay hoping to find a long-term relationship with a black man in a black community. No tenure-track position was waiting for him at Berkeley or Stanford, so he parlayed his academic experience into a job as an AIDS educator at the Berkeley Gay and Lesbian Community Center, one of the first clinics to offer AIDS services in Alameda County.

Little action had as yet been taken against AIDS in Alameda County. John and the six other full-time staff members he worked with at the community center were largely responsible for providing AIDS services for Oakland, Berkeley, and Richmond, some of the most densely black cities in America. But few blacks visited the center. It wasn't surprising, given that the center had the word *gay* in its name. So he'd held an AIDS awareness meeting at a black Oakland bar that doubled as a cruising joint for black gay men a few nights out of the week. Maybe twenty-five people had attended, but word about it filtered through the city. Black men who had sex with men began to trickle into the clinic. John tried to field their frightened questions. Some said they weren't gay. Others thought they were safe because they also slept with women. They were worried that someone might find out they had sex with men. They wanted to know whom they could talk to. All John could do was reassure them that they were safe speaking to him and that in his eyes, at least, their sexuality was acceptable. But he couldn't tell them that it was safe to seek help from their families. They faced potentially serious consequences for disclosure. Many had little money and were dependent on the social safety nets woven by black churches and extended families to help with food, clothes, electric bills, and health care. Loss of these benefits would be just the tangible cost; these men also stood to lose their families, their churches, their children, and their identities.

The amazing thing, to John, was that hardly anyone seemed to know these men existed. When he settled in at MIRA, he reviewed the scientific and public health literature on gay black men. One study had been conducted by Alfred C. Kinsey's research team, who had done early work on human sexuality in the 1950s. Their bit on gay black men, though, was virtually useless. In fact, barely anything substantive had been written about black sexuality in general.

It was strange, especially considering that black sexuality was such a flashpoint for race relations. Both blacks and whites had used images of the black sexual beast—from Bigger Thomas to the racist archetype of the black rapist—as currency in the race wars. "Medical studies" at the turn of the century recommended that castration was a better punishment for blacks than lynching. Prohibiting miscegenation and protecting white women had been the central goals of fanatical racism. Even the Tuskegee experiment had been centered on syphilis, a sexually transmitted disease. Now a disease that was spread sexually had been killing blacks in significantly disproportionate numbers for seven years, and nobody at the federal level had funded any serious investigations into black sexuality.

Mindy's understanding of the dynamics of race in America had been shaped by her experience of segregation. When she was a kid in East Orange, New Jersey, her parents had been known as progressives, which in the 1950s parlance meant socialists or—depending on what circles you ran in—Reds. It had been her father's idea for seven-year-old Mindy to desegregate the Heywood elementary school in a nearby white neighborhood. Mindy, playful as a girl, was terrified to leave her black block on Olcott Street with its familiar clapboard houses. In the weeks leading up to the first day of school, she threw impotent screaming fits that were followed by a searing pain that hit her eyes and stomach, making bright light almost unbearable.

At the Heywood Avenue Elementary School nobody called her "coon" or "nigger," and she wasn't beaten or tormented. As best Mindy could tell, she didn't exist in the minds of any of the kids—and that terrified her. She wrestled with that fear for five school years, as she trudged into the alien world of white Orange. During that time she loved to celebrate the Jewish holiday of Purim at her friend Sally Crystal's house. At Purim Jews tell the story of Esther, who risked execution by begging her husband, King Ahasuerus, to prevent Haman from massacring the Jews. Mindy knew what it must have felt like for Esther to face death, aware that the survival of her people rested on her shoulders. Mindy loved to dance the part of Esther. As she twirled around Sally's living room, her fear dissipated, and she imagined the Jewish queen's power as though it were her own. In the fall of 1987 those remembrances were distant childhood memories, but the pain of dislocation and the isolation she had endured at Heywood Avenue Elementary School, combined with that distinctly childhood sense of overresponsibility, lingered with her.

Mindy had often understood her search for It as ambition and a grandiose need to be somehow "great." Perhaps for that reason her pursuit had always been somewhat awkward. AIDS had finally given her clarity. Thousands stood to die: in an immediate sense their survival depended on her team's ability to mobilize the public health system. More broadly, the conspicuous blackness of the epidemic was going to force her to examine the significance of race in America in the era after the overtly institutional structures of racism had weakened and the problems plaguing blacks were increasingly understood to be rooted in poverty. The success of that task rested on her capacity to make sense of and translate the black experience in the post–civil rights landscape. This experience was foreign to her in the sense that it belonged to the next generation, one that could no longer be easily categorized and understood within the boundaries of segregation, yet was still deeply informed by its legacy. Part of the problem she faced was that her team was focusing on the epicenter of the epidemic in San Francisco, when the center of the Bay Area's black community was Oakland, which lay fifteen minutes away.

CHAPTER THREE

The Heir

1942–1990

DESIREE RUSHING SAT IN her living room in Oakland, California, held the single white sheet of paper in her long thin black fingers, and felt no fear. Printed in black and white, there in the middle of the page, were the words *false positive*. She didn't know what the phrase meant. It was 1988, and she'd been late enough times over the years to her job at Pac Bell that she risked getting transferred to the Sloth building. The employees called it the graveyard, where management sent operators when they wanted to get rid of them. It was south of San Francisco, near Candlestick Point on the last cable-car stop, an hour-and-a-half trek from her one-bedroom apartment on McColl Street. But losing her job didn't worry Desi very much.

Desi had felt the presence of Satan in her life. Maybe she wasn't quite with God now, but she had begun to submit to Him. In an immediate sense He felt safe to her, strong and stable, as her father Harold had been before he started drinking, beat down their door, and became wrenched with self-hate. More broadly, though, He felt like a manifestation of the truth that she had always sensed in her gut and felt she had been denied. Sure, she was still going out and partying; some might even say she was sinning. But she wasn't drinking or smoking, and she was dating Bob, a firefighter she'd met at the AA meetings. He gave her gifts, took her out, and she let him make love to her, even though the Bible said that she shouldn't have sexual relations outside marriage. Bob didn't hit her, unlike her father, who had beaten her mother, and the men who had hit Desi.

None of those things seemed connected to the letter from the blood bank that she held in her hands. It thanked her for donating at the Pac Bell blood drive but said that her sample had tested "false positive" for HIV, the virus that causes AIDS. Desi knew about AIDS. She'd heard about a co-worker, a gay guy, who had committed suicide after he'd been diagnosed. Even that didn't worry her, though; AIDS was a gay disease. The key word in *false positive* was probably *false*. Still, the letter said to call a number. So, not thinking much of it, she sat down on her living room carpet, leaned back against her couch, and picked up her phone.

The counselor who fielded the call didn't sound concerned when asking Desi a couple of routine questions. None of them particularly alarmed her. She didn't shoot heroin. She never wanted to be one of those nodding junkies with the purple holes in their arms. And she didn't sleep with bisexual men. Well, the counselor casually continued, it's probably nothing, but you really ought to come in and get tested anyway.

The "nothing" part was all that stuck with Desi, as she set down the receiver and discarded the letter. There had already been too much confusion, too much suffering, too much chaos in her life. At some points it was hard to tell if the drugs inflamed the rawness of that experience or shielded her from it. She just knew that now that she was clean, it was once more safe to feel. Even the simple details of Oakland—a city of lush green hills, turn-of-the-century Victorians, and long stretches of flat, crumbling black neighborhoods—seemed vivid again. Until recently feeling much of anything had been too dangerous.

Born in 1959, she was a member of the first generation of Americans to inherit the legacy of the great southern black migration and the civil rights movement. She wasn't politicized, educated in American racial or urban history, or even particularly self-conscious about her blackness. Still, she had been aware since childhood that there was something acutely wrong with her city, family, and life. Yet her mother and father, friends, and teachers had always implied to her that her American life was as it should be, that her parents' marriage was ordinary, and that the violence, poverty, alcoholism, and drugs that sporadically disrupted Oakland's black neighborhoods and homes were normal and to be endured.

The disconnect—between this internal sense that something felt profoundly off and the experience of being told in a thousand small ways that

it wasn't—seemed to translate for Desi into a searching and often directionless mass of anger, confusion, and pain. She rarely—if ever—indulged
in casting blame on the government, whites, blacks, or some vague notion
of the American system. To her there didn't seem to be any straight lines
between those increasingly abstract entities and the visceral mixture of
internal and external events that had shaped her experience. Often she'd
fallen back on a strong intuitive sense that the chaotic moments of her
life were related by a binding theme. Eventually, that position had become too difficult to hold. She was married to Philip then, and her sense
of what was normal and what was out of control had blurred.

———————

AT LEAST A DOZEN people were milling about Desi and Philip's two-
bedroom second-floor apartment overlooking Alice Street in Oakland, on
the night a couple of years earlier when she had thrown his stereo off the
balcony. Desi's sister Monique was there. So was her cousin Yolanda.
Desi was in the living room, anger coursing through her muscles. She
didn't know where it came from, just that it needed to be either extin-
guished or released. Maybe it was because Philip had been so rude to one
of her girlfriends. But that wasn't really the root of it. Her anger was older,
hotter, and more explosive than anything that had happened that night.
Little in her life had made easy sense. Not her explosive relationship with
Philip; not the murder of her cousin Crystal; not her father, Harold
Theus, and his drinking or her own drug use. Desi had everything she
needed—a home, a job, her sisters—and yet still something felt profoundly off center in her life.

Desi's son, Kentrell, would probably sleep with her mother, Wafer, tonight. Wafer Theus, whom everybody called Granna, had always ignored
Desi's drugs, even when they were right in front of her, and if she saw
Desi's pain, she said little about that either. Granna mostly stood strong
and quiet. Or maybe it was weak and quiet; it was hard sometimes for
those who met her to tell the difference. Ken would likely stay with
Granna tonight because it was the place he felt safe. He was small, in elementary school, and always frightened. Granna calmed him; she was
warm and soft and shielded him from Desi's occasionally erratic behavior.

Desi's anger flared again, and she walked past her friends, grabbed hold of Philip's stereo, and tore it from the wall. The music cut off. She strode out onto the balcony into the night and hurled it over the railing. The plastic and metal broke onto the pavement. Sometimes when she felt this explosive, she would hit Philip, and often he would beat her back. Most nights, though, they found themselves upstairs, sucking in the acrid smoke from a bit of rock cocaine, a small piece that would last her all night. She'd smoke it slowly until her heart started to race. Then she'd stop and wait for all the confusion and anger to dissolve into a numb world of nothingness.

She never smoked crack alone. She didn't know how to cook the rock herself. Usually she smoked late at night with Philip and an assortment of his and her family members who hung out at the house. They weren't what people would call crackheads, out on the street selling themselves for a hit. Neither were the other people they knew who smoked the cheap crystal form of cocaine. Philip was a contractor, and Desi worked full time for Pac Bell. They were people who liked to keep up appearances. Desi wore new dresses, kept her nails long, and made sure she didn't miss hair appointments. Occasionally, she might drive with Philip to buy fifteen or twenty rocks, but she'd never get out of the car. As soon as the dealer appeared, she'd scrunch down, hide below the dashboard, and wait for Philip to duck back behind the wheel.

She hadn't always been so secretive. The first time she smoked cocaine was shortly after she graduated high school, at her family's old three-story Victorian on Forty-sixth Street, near the MacArthur Freeway overpass. Her uncle owned the place, but she wouldn't have been surprised if their neighbors thought it was some kind of a house for women. Desi's grandmother, one of Desi's aunts, and her aunt's three girls lived on the bottom floor. Another aunt lived upstairs with her daughter Yolanda. Granna; Desi; her infant son, Ken; and Desi's four younger sisters—Chan, Gigi, Monique, and Simone—lived in the middle apartment. Thirteen women in one house. There was always somebody home, and kids from the neighborhood were constantly dropping by to hang out.

So no one thought much of it when one of the teenage boys who lived down the street showed up one afternoon wondering if anyone wanted to get high off a piece of rock cocaine. The drug was most likely freebase, a precursor to crack that had been circulating in Bay Area drug-using circles since the mid-1970s and operated in the body similarly to the way crack would. He wasn't a pusher, just a sweet kid, the kind of guy who'd never even jaywalked. Desi and one of her cousins said sure. It seemed like no big deal—as far as Desi was concerned, he might as well have brought over some Riunite box wine. They might have heard Wafer creaking about on the old floors of the flat below. If they did, they didn't worry about it. And why should they have? They'd never even heard of crack. *Just let me hit it* was all Desi was thinking. The rush felt better than the sparkly high of a first cigarette. But it wasn't any big deal, just a little fun—certainly not something she needed tomorrow, or that she needed to hide.

The paranoia came later with the addiction, which seemed to accelerate by itself after that unremarkable afternoon. It continued through five years of screaming, violent fights with Philip, unpaid bills, mornings late to work, and weeks when Ken would spend most nights with Granna. The strange thing was that Desi didn't even really like the high. She hated the way it made her breath come shallow and fast, as a sheen of feverish sweat broke out across her forehead and her heart beat like a drum. There was nothing euphoric about it, at least not in that crisp, C-note, razor blade, "the world is mine" way that people described cocaine. No, if anything, it was the emptiness of the high that she loved, and how the emptiness insulated her insides from all the jagged, illogical edges of her world.

Desi's mother, Wafer Theus, busied herself around the kids' bedroom one afternoon in the early 1970s, while her daughters played downstairs with their German shepherd, Missy. Wafer wasn't sure what she was going to do when her husband, Harold, came home. He'd been gone for a couple of days. She figured he was probably drinking Tanqueray and tonic at Dorsey's Locker. Wafer had decided to seek a divorce, a risky move since there were no guarantees that a housewife with few real skills could put food on the table in these hard times. Still, she didn't think things could possibly be worse without Harold. Something had changed in him after his basketball career faded out. Drinking and anger, anger and drinking, drinking and anger—they had twisted up inside him and turned him into a man who threatened her. She looked into his deep brown eyes now and couldn't find the shy star junior college basketball player who had spotted her darting around the badminton court at Oakland City College back in the mid-fifties.

He had been rail thin then, soft spoken but intelligent and most of all hopeful. Wafer had never had a man pursue her the way he did. He just seemed to believe—to know—that there were great things in his future. Pete Newell, the coach of the Cal basketball team, recruited Harold to Berkeley. Harold, though, like any American kid, wanted to go away to college, and he took a scholarship to play with the Utah State Aggies. Most guys who headed off to school on an athletic scholarship would have broken things off with their hometown girl, but Harold rode the bus to Oakland to see Wafer. On one of those visits he proposed, and they drove up to Reno and were married. Wafer joined Harold in Logan in 1958 and within a year gave birth to their first daughter, Desiree. Logan was rural and Mormon—so different from the industrial sprawl of Oakland. Sometimes Wafer felt as if they and their friends from the basketball team were the only blacks in town. As best she could tell, that never seemed to bother Harold.

They lived in Logan for two years, and by the time Harold finished with school, she was pregnant with their second daughter, Chan. Harold hadn't drawn much attention from the NBA, and they both longed to return to Oakland, so they moved back, and Harold got a job at the Continental Can Factory. Then he got word that Abe Saperstein, the owner of the Harlem Globetrotters, was putting together the American Basketball League, which he hoped would rival the NBA. Former USF coach Phil Woolpert had been lured out of retirement to coach San Francisco's charter team, the Saints. During the 1950s Woolpert had assembled arguably the first fully integrated Division 1A basketball team in the country. And in 1959 and 1960 he had guided a USF team laden with black stars like Bill Russell and K. C. Jones to back-to-back NCAA championships. Harold tried out and won a spot on the team.

Saperstein wasn't able to get stars like Russell to jump from the NBA, but he managed to bring in talented players like Dick Barnett, Kenny

Sears, and Brooklyn playground legend Connie Hawkins. Harold couldn't break the starting five for the Saints, but even playing off the bench in front of the crowds at the San Francisco Civic Auditorium seemed to enlarge his essential sense of optimism. Harold bought a new Thunderbird, which he named for his wife. Wafer told him that she was pregnant for the third time. Following a familiar story line that was repeating itself across the country, the job market was drying up in Oakland, and housing conditions were deteriorating as whites undertook a mass exodus to the suburbs. Neither Harold nor Wafer was worried, though—basketball had given Harold a free pass from the economic realities that were straining postwar black American urban life. He was making three times what his father had earned for a full year of work. Every now and then he'd blow off practice, and Wafer believed that was when he began to develop a fondness for alcohol. Then, midway through the Saints' season, he was cut from the team. Shortly afterward Saperstein abruptly folded the ABL. Harold, who had never been more than a bench player, had no chance of making the NBA. Suddenly he was in his early twenties, the father of three little girls, and out of a job.

Now, nearly ten years later, Harold had changed. It was hard for Wafer to get a feel for what exactly had perverted him from the hopeful quiet man she had married into an abusive husband who hit her in front of their baby daughters and gave out his home phone number to women he met at bars. She knew it was a hard time for blacks all over Oakland. Between 1950 and 1960 the city's black population had grown by more than 70 percent. During that same period nearly one-sixth of the city's whites had left for the suburbs. Oakland's manufacturing companies, the backbone of the local economy, had laid off workers. Many black families had been displaced from West Oakland, which had been the spiritual center of the black community, so the city could build a series of new freeways and the Bay Area Rapid Transit System (BART). By the late 1960s, unemployment had swollen to 7.7 percent, the highest rate of any comparably sized city in the nation. Yet still more blacks were moving to the city in waves.

It was hard for Wafer to draw a clear line from those trends to her husband's behavior. His childhood best friend, future congressman Ron Dellums, had hooked him up with promising city jobs. The government gigs weren't about to make them rich. They probably didn't even pay as well as the union jobs down on the docks. Even so, his salary paid for the Theuses' two-story white stucco home on Dover Street, which had a non-descript 1950s California Americanness to it that yawned middle-class comfort. And it would have been enough to cover the bills—if Harold hadn't drunk his paychecks at Dorsey's Locker.

A poisonous air of anger and disappointment was swirling through the city. Everyone could feel it, and it had a distinctly racial edge. Would-be black leaders were known to preach on street corners about the white necklace that was choking the black neck of Oakland. Black labor groups had protested the longshoremen's unions that were shutting blacks out from waterfront jobs. Huey Newton and Bobby Seale were presiding over meetings at Dorsey's Locker, splitting two beers among six people, and making talk about arming black men against the police, who were reportedly beating blacks indiscriminately across the city. A different kind of violent potential was germinating inside Harold. He had thought he would ascend, and for a while it seemed that he had. Now his demeanor seemed to reflect that of a man who was purposeless and stuck. But who was at fault? Wafer had never heard Harold throw blame at whites, cops, unions, or politicians. She believed that he knew his failure was his own. If anything, however, that self-knowledge just amplified Harold's anger and alcoholism. Wafer could see it written all over him. He messed around with women and threatened to hurt her. She harbored no love for him now. He had already hit her twice, just like her daddy had hit her mother. The second time he had gone at her, she hit him with a hammer on his hip. If he messed with her again, well, she was five foot ten and strong, and she'd hurt him.

She heard Harold enter the house. He walked up the stairs and started badgering her about his dinner. Wafer didn't care, she didn't owe him any dinner. He walked into the children's room in his boxer shorts. Wafer didn't turn around. Harold strode up and hit her from behind. She fell to her knees. He came at her again. Wafer reached back behind her head, grabbed at Harold's crotch, and twisted. He still didn't let go of her. She kicked him until his boxer shorts were wet with blood, and he released her.

The Heir

IT WASN'T SUPPOSED TO turn out this way: not for Harold, or for Wafer, or for any of the other children of the southern blacks who flocked to Oakland from the cotton fields and plantations of Mississippi, Alabama, and Texas after the Japanese bombed Pearl Harbor. Five-year-old Harold had arrived with his family in 1942. His father had worked in the paper mills outside Baton Rouge. In Oakland, he was hired as a longshoreman at Moore Shipyard. Harold's parents made a point of telling him about what it was like to be "niggers" with a white boot on their necks. No child of theirs, he was raised to believe, would ever peel their eyes wide like a fly and say "yes suh" and "no suh" to anybody. If the white man wanted something unreasonable, Harold could let him know that "bug dancing" was dead. It was a sentiment that reflected the broad optimism shared by blacks who had left the South during the war for cities across the rest of the country.

Oakland was one of several American cities that the Roosevelt administration targeted to become a hub for war production. At the end of the 1930s the city emerged as the Bay Area's industrial center. The transcontinental railroad flowed into its downtown, it was the end line for several trucking companies, Ford and General Motors had made it home to their West Coast headquarters, it had the San Francisco Bay's only deep-water access to the Pacific Ocean, its harbor was a major departure point for the South Pacific, and it boasted the country's first modern shipyard. In 1940 Oakland's shipbuilding and manufacturing companies won more than $125 million in defense contracts, and the federal government expanded the Oakland Naval Supply Depot, the Oakland Army Supply Base, and the Alameda Naval Air Station. But the city lacked the labor force to support this rapid growth. Ninety-five percent of Oaklanders were white, and many were middle class and already employed. So after Pearl Harbor, Oakland was promoted in an expansive labor-recruiting campaign launched across the South in an effort to assemble the nation's war machine. Between 1940 and 1946 600,000 people moved to the Bay Area. It was the largest population boom in the country. And the number of blacks in Oakland jumped from 8,462 to more than 45,000.

The rush of migrants transformed Oakland from a sleepy midsize town into a vibrant and racially diverse metropolis. Garages and furniture stores were converted into all-night movie houses where defense workers could catch the new James Cagney, Jimmy Stewart, and Katharine Hepburn films. Couples strolling through downtown on a Saturday night might hear the strains of Glenn Miller, Duke Ellington, and the Dorsey brothers spilling out of Sweets Ballroom and the Oakland Auditorium. On weeknights sweaty dancers jitterbugged in cramped, smoke-filled halls like McFadden's Ballroom, Melody Lane, and New Danceland. Bars were packed with servicemen throwing back drinks while they waited for orders to ship off to the South Pacific. And tent shows, carnivals, and boxing matches barnstormed through town.

Along with many of the other black migrants, Harold's family settled in West Oakland. In the most basic sense the war had remade Oakland into a city of financial promise for the poor. The cramped projects that sometimes housed three families to an apartment were like Gold Rush camps. Dockworkers still in hard hats could be found trying on furs in downtown department stores after work. Preachers opened Baptist, African Methodist Episcopal, and Pentecostal churches in their living rooms. The Pullman porters working the rails brought news from New Orleans, Chicago, and New York. Longshoremen bought sedans and drove them home to places like Monroeville, Vicksburg, and Baton Rouge. Their families followed them back to Oakland, so that at times it felt as though entire towns had arrived intact.

Then, almost as suddenly as the war had reinvented the city, the Japanese surrender tore the legs out from under its economy. The shipyard jobs rapidly dried up. Harold's father joined the merchant seamen and then uprooted his family and took them to Indiana. Soon after the move, though, Harold's mother returned to Oakland with her two youngest children, Harold and Sting. Certainly no suburban middle-class life awaited her in the East Bay. Dow Chemical, General Motors, and Shell Oil had left or were in the process of leaving Oakland for sites in Contra Costa County and elsewhere in Alameda County. Whites were moving to suburban towns like Hayward, Orlanda, and Walnut Creek. There was a severe shortage of low-income housing, and with a declining tax base, the city wasn't eager to stretch its budget to build new apartments for the poor.

West Oakland, though, still had a vital energy that invited comparisons to Harlem. But it wasn't saddled with the same history of political ambition, cultural wealth, segregation, and intractable poverty that had established and hardened the physical and cultural boundaries between the races in New York City. Oakland's historical whiteness, its absence of a racial past, and its essential nondescriptness—which had helped immortalize native daughter Gertrude Stein's line that "there was no there there"—seemed to imbue the city, for many southern blacks, with a lasting air of possibility. This promising, virginal quality was distinctly western and seemed to create space to reimagine what it was to be black. Perhaps that was what made it possible for the black nationalist and black power movements to blossom in Oakland during the 1960s. Most likely, it allowed Harold's mother to raise him to feel that he was not limited by his blackness, foreshadowing the promise of a post–civil rights black experience that was free from both the external circumstance and the interior psychology of racism and segregation.

———

DESI SEEMED to inherit her father's sense that she was not constrained by her blackness, and perhaps even more than he did, she felt the sense of possibility that is an essential ingredient of the American experience. But by the time she was in the eleventh grade in 1976, her life had been marked by enough physical and emotional disruptions that they threatened to rob her of the optimism that been characteristic of Harold as a young man. She wasn't, however, fluent in any racial, political, or psychological language that could help her delineate which parts of that experience were tied to being black and which parts were specific to the vagaries of her parents' relationship, or decide whether it was all simply the product of her father's battle with alcoholism. Often she'd lie alone out in her mother's backyard on Forty-sixth Street to get away from it all: her boyfriend James, Harold, her mother, the aftermath of their divorce, her sisters, everyone. It was one of the few places where she felt at ease.

The soft green blades of grass gently brushed the back of her neck. The fence to one side was chain link and, to the other, wood. Goldfish swam in the little pool that her uncle had built for Wafer's mother, Hattie. She liked to lie there and flick questions like rubber bands into the empty cobalt sky. She needed to make sense of why her father terrorized her mother. Why her cousin Crys had been murdered. Why she always saw things that others didn't. What kind of God would inflict this much pain? She didn't believe it could be God. No god could be capable of that kind of cruelty.

On the surface, Desi's and her sisters' lives had actually gotten easier after Harold moved out and their parents divorced. Wafer found a job in the library at Washington Elementary School, a few blocks from their house, and between work and welfare she was able to patch together enough income to put food on the table. She doted on her girls, walking them to school every morning, worrying relentlessly for their safety, and making sure they were always well dressed and clean. But there seemed to be more subtle and enduring signs that things weren't right. She was a woman who could seem distant, more a presence than a force in her daughters' lives.

Meanwhile, Harold broke boundaries. He sank into a drunken morass, and as he grew older, he developed the countenance of a starved man; shadows fell from the cliff of bones beneath his eyes, and his legs were so thin that when he walked it looked like his joints were grinding in on each other. Sometimes he'd stop by Wafer's house and plead with her to take him back. His sadness was palpable, but it was often undercut by a stony anger that occasionally exploded into violence, as on the day Wafer refused to let him into the house and he broke down her door. More often his fury seeped out in drunken rants aimed at his daughters.

Desi suffered all the usual symptoms one might expect children to endure when their parents separate: her grades fell, she had discipline problems, and in junior high she experimented with cigarettes, alcohol, and pot. More than that, she knew on a gut level that her childhood wasn't normal, or at least not what a childhood was supposed to be. It wasn't so much that she fantasized about living in a picturesque home on a fictional Elm Street in Kansas, where her father took snapshots of her boyfriend as he pinned a corsage to her prom dress and her mother made flapjacks and planted roses in the garden. It was just that everything around her felt too chaotic. At the same time, she couldn't recognize it as chaotic because it was all she knew. That strange concoction of knowing and not knowing shaped her into one of those children who seemed to inhabit a pointed innocence. Usually she would just rebel against discipline. Sometimes, though, she'd get a gut feeling that something terrible was about to take place or had already happened. She always felt that her parents and the people around her dismissed her intuitions. Don't tell us this stuff, Desi, they'd say to her. Sometimes in life you just got to let things happen. Everything is fine. Anger was the main way she knew how to get hold of the wild feelings that sparked inside her mind like a fallen electrical line and to connect it up to the outside world.

When the chaos of her own home was too much for Desi, she could always escape to her cousin Crystal's house in East Oakland. Crys was Harold's sister Sting's daughter. She was a few years older than Desi, and there was something about her life that was safer, more ordered, and more normal. Crys had recently separated from her husband, and she lived with Sting in a wealthier, more mixed neighborhood than the working-class, largely black streets where Desi had grown up. Maybe that was why the sheer arbitrariness and insanity of Crys's murder—more than Harold's bitter anger and disappointment, her parents' fighting, or Wafer's wounded distance—was what made Desi want to disappear from the world.

On an afternoon shortly before Desi graduated from high school, she was working at her job at the Census Bureau when she felt a compulsion to call Crys. The two girls had gone to the carnival the evening before. Sting had agreed to stay home and watch Crys's two children, and it had been one of those rare nights when Desi had her cousin all to herself. Desi had borrowed one of Crys's shirts at the end of the night, as she sometimes did, and worn it to work. When her break rolled around, Desi found a pay hone and dialed Crys's number.

Crys's stepbrother answered the phone. He had recently been released from a mental institution and was living at Sting's. Is Crys home? Desi asked. No, she isn't here, he replied. Desi got a strange feeling. She reluctantly laid the phone back on the receiver.

After work she rushed home. When she got to her street, she stepped over the markings on the sidewalk where she and her sisters had scrawled their names in the cement, and skipped up the first flight of stairs. There she ran into her grandmother Hattie.

He killed them, Hattie said.

What are you talking about? Desi asked.

That crazy fool killed them.

Killed who? Desi asked frantically.

He killed Crys and Sting, she said.

Crys had been home with her baby daughter when her stepbrother attacked her. He killed the child, raped Crys, and killed her. When Sting came home, he murdered her, too. Desi ran upstairs to the apartment she shared with her mother and sisters. Wafer, Chan, Gigi—everyone was gone, and the house was quiet in the fading afternoon light.

She went into her mother's bedroom, sat down on the floor, and leaned against the bed and looked down at Crys's black and orange blouse. Crys's murder didn't have anything to do with race in America, or Oakland, or poverty. It was the kind of capricious human tragedy that can strike any life. Maybe if Desi had lived in a stable environment, she would have integrated it as such. But in the context of a life that was chaotically and invisibly shaped by the legacy of race in America, the tragedy profoundly undermined her faith that life was governed by morality or reason. *God, do it over,* she prayed silently. *Reverse this thing. Something is wrong. The right person didn't go.* The words just tumbled out into her mind. *She got two kids, Lord. Let it be me! Take me! Lord, please do it over! Take me, Jesus! She got two kids!* And then everything went blank.

———

Do you use drugs, Mommy? Ken asked. It was 1985, and he was small for a seven-year-old. A few weeks earlier he had wandered into the bathroom and found Desi's base pipe at eye level, jammed up under the sink in their apartment on McColl Street. She had lied to him then—said it was meant for cleaning the toilet. Now she hesitated. Sometimes when Philip would go off to buy the drugs, she'd sit in their living room, clutch the Bible, and pray to God for Him to give her the strength not to use again. He never did. Desi had always taken care, though, not to smoke crack in Ken's presence. She could lie to him again; he was probably too young to know any better. But there was an innocence and a fearfulness to him that were unusual, even for a child. And she sensed that if she continued to lie to him, forcing him to choose between her word and his own instincts, she would cripple him.

Yes I do, Ken. They call us crackheads, Desi said. I'm a crackhead. That's what I do, Ken. I smoke crack.

Still, it hurt to tell him that she was a crackhead. It felt too much like the day she had to explain to him why his daddy didn't live in Oakland.

Ken's father, James, was Desi's first boyfriend. The summer after Crys's murder, he was caught participating in the robbery of a Baskin-Robbins and sent to prison for a few months. That semester Desi rarely attended school or even left her bedroom. When James got out, he found a job working at the General Motors plant, twenty minutes south of Oakland in Fremont, one of the few good industrial jobs left in the East Bay. Desi graduated in 1977 and within a few months was pregnant with Kentrell. Oakland didn't offer many options to a black mother with only a high school diploma. The city was 46 percent black and in an economic morass, and its problems reflected those in cities across the country. According a *Newsweek* article on black youth published in August 1978, American black teen unemployment was nearly 40 percent, half of all black children were born out of wedlock, and one in three were supported by welfare. Desi saw her options as either welfare, government work, Pacific Bell, or Pacific Gas and Electric. She had worked all through her teens to help Wafer with the bills and felt that welfare was too degrading. So she got a job at Pac Bell.

Desi wasn't in love with James anymore, nor was she ready to be a mother. Wafer would push through her door, kick past a pile of dirty clothes, ignore the marijuana seeds on the coffee table, and grab baby Ken from the bedroom. Desi would get off her shift and go to parties with her girlfriends. Sometimes she'd drink, other times she'd smoke pot, and by the time Ken was a few months old, she had experimented with cocaine-laced cigarettes. She met Philip at one of those parties. Desi was instantly drawn to the tall, muscular man. He was a mixture of black and Indian, with hair that ran down his back. Desi flirted with him all night, until she, Philip, and her cousin drove back to her apartment. Desi and Philip made love in the bedroom while her cousin kept watch for James.

In 1982 GM announced it was going to shut down its Fremont plant and offered James a job in Kansas City. Desi decided not to follow him. Within weeks after he left, she called Philip. They quickly fell in love and moved in together. For the first couple of years everything seemed okay. Philip was making good money, and they frequently moved to better apartments. Desi introduced Philip to crack. It was just one substance on a menu of drugs they used. Desi, Philip, and their friends would often sit up in the front room, smoke pot, drink beer, and get high while Ken and the kids played with Tonka toys in the back. Wafer was actually doing much of the work raising Ken.

Meanwhile, something explosive was happening between Desi and Philip. It was difficult to identify its cause. She loved him more than ever, but she just couldn't harness her anger. She'd lash out, then he'd beat her back. She felt out of control. In 1984 she told Philip that if he wanted her to stay in his life, they had to get married. Just like Wafer and Harold, they eloped to Reno. But things didn't get better. She baited him. She threw his stereo onto the street. Another evening she plunged her hands into the cool water of his fish tank, clenched his goldfish in her fingers, and flushed them down the garbage disposal.

Crack became part of their nightly ritual. They'd hole up in their apartment with a few other friends and smoke. She could make a rock last a whole night. The paranoia, though, was excruciating. They'd smoke upstairs, and she'd all but hear the boots of policemen coming up the steps, and men passing like shadows by her windows. She even briefly checked herself into rehab to give herself a break and remind herself that she was in control. And she was—maybe. But when Ken asked her if she used drugs, she knew something had to change.

Even so Desi, Philip, and maybe some friends or members of Philip's family still got high on most nights. And Desi and Philip tore even more deeply into each other. There was no going forward anymore. Desi finally realized it on the night of January 24, 1986, when Philip eased his Lincoln up in front of Wafer's house on Forty-first Street and Telegraph Avenue in Oakland. Desi was so high that she could barely feel her legs. They had broken up before, but this was it. Philip knew it, too. She sat beside him in the darkness, and they cried together. Philip pulled Desi close to him, until she disentangled herself from his arms, pushed out of the car into the dark, and steadied herself.

It was Wafer's fiftieth birthday. Desi was lucky she made it up the stairs to the door. She lingered there for a moment. *Lord,* Desi prayed, *if you clean me up to go in here and tell my mother happy birthday after everything she's done for me, after all the pain and problems that I've put her through, if just this one night you let me do that, I promise you I'll never touch any dope again.* She knocked. Wafer pulled back the door. "Happy birthday, Granna," she said, and hugged her mother.

———————

FOUR MONTHS LATER, the night before Easter Sunday, Kentrell sat on the couch next to Desi on McColl Street, and he was frightened. Desi was sweating. She had been sick for two days. Some sort of flu bug had taken over her body, and she looked cold. Desi's new boyfriend, Eddie McKnight, paced back and forth in front of them with a cigarette clenched between his fingers, poking it at Desi, threatening to burn her. He turned to Kentrell. "If someone did that to my mama," he slurred, "I'd do something about it."

Ken felt himself wrench up inside. He was only eight years old, but he was already intimate with this kind of cold shaking fear. He thought they'd gotten free of it when Desi left Philip. But now she was back with someone worse than Philip. Desi and Philip would violently light into each other, and Ken would hide in the corner of his bedroom. But Eddie scared Ken more than Philip. He had this way of dragging his words so that you weren't quite sure if they were aimed at you. And now he was challenging Ken. Tears welled up in Ken's eyes, even as he felt the desire to lash out and kill the tall leering man in the red flannel shirt.

Desi tried to fight through her feverish haze. She had been clean for nearly four months, and she had met Eddie through Yolanda's husband, Terry. Eddie had been in rehab for what she believed was crack at a place over in Richmond. He was tall, lanky, and dark-skinned with a Jheri curl. They'd been dating for a few weeks; she'd maybe slept with him a handful of times. She had thought he was trying to get himself right, too. But it hadn't taken her too long to figure out that there was something off about him. They'd only gone out a couple times when he jealously struck her with the back of his hand because she bought some McDonald's for her brother-in-law. She had forgiven him that, but when he sprained her arm just because she had been a little hesitant to file her divorce papers with Philip, that was too much.

Apparently he didn't take too kindly to rejection. He had come over tonight uninvited, and he was acting crazy. Maybe he was using again, which would explain his irrational behavior. Eddie didn't scare her; she'd seen her parents go through the same thing. But she hated that Ken had to see this.

Eddie walked into the bathroom and sat down on the closed toilet. His eyes looked to Desi like they had Satan in them.

What's wrong with you? she demanded. She had been sweating all night, hot and cold, hot and cold. Did you watch your mama go through this? Did your daddy do this to your mama? The words seemed to hit Eddie. He stood up, looked at her uneasily, reeled, and walked out the door.

About two months later Desi was startled out of sleep by the sound of glass shattering like ice onto her mother's driveway. *He went and done it,* she thought to herself, *he went on and done it.* She lay there silently in the dark. There was another smash, a third, then a fourth, and she figured all the windows of her car were now a thousand shards of glass scattered across the pavement.

Eddie had promised to get help after the incident at her apartment and had even checked himself back into rehab. Desi had tried to be supportive. But when he checked himself out a few days later, saying he'd been diagnosed with TB or some such nonsense, she'd broken it off. Eddie had grown furious and threatened to smash up her new Pontiac Firebird. Desi had called the Oakland police, only to be told that they couldn't arrest him until he actually committed a crime. And now the fool had done it. She didn't even have insurance on the car yet. Desi rolled over in the darkness and tried to go back to sleep.

The next day she called Eddie. He was sorry, he said. He didn't know what had gotten into him. He had already spoken to his mother, and she'd agreed to pay for the damage. So later that week after work Desi took BART over to Eddie's mother's house in East Oakland. She lived in a beautiful old neighborhood near Mills College. When Desi's parents were kids, whites wouldn't even rent homes to blacks there. So Desi wasn't overly worried for her safety. Even if Eddie was angry, most of his family would probably be at the house. Besides, if his pattern held true, he'd most likely be sobered up and sorry. Indeed, when she got to the house, Eddie's mom, his brother, and his sister were there, along with a few of his nieces. Desi asked where her money was. Eddie acted as if he didn't know what she was talking about. Desi felt a flash of anger, thinking this was probably just some ploy to get her over here.

Well, I need to get back to my son then, she said, backing away.

You're not going anywhere, Eddie said, and then he punched Desi in the face. She stumbled, and Eddie grabbed her arm. Desi looked frantically around the house. No one moved to help her as he dragged her through the kitchen and into a back bedroom.

He sat Desi down on the bed and began pulling off her jewelry. Take it, Desi said, you can have it. Just let me go. She peered at him through the darkness, and he looked crazed. All she could think was that she didn't want to get hit again.

He pushed her down on the bed and pulled off her clothes.

Desi said she wasn't going to have sex with him, but she didn't struggle. She knew she couldn't overpower him. *Where is his mama? His brother? His sister? Why isn't anybody helping me?* Eddie was up on top of her now. *This is no big deal,* she told herself. He tore her legs apart and pushed. *We've had sex before.* Eddie continued to push harder. *Just don't let him hit me again.* After he was finished, she lay there in the blackness.

"I killed you," Eddie whispered. "I got you."

She didn't know what he was talking about—he didn't have a gun or a knife. After a time she gathered her clothes and shoes. Eddie sat on the bed and searched the room with his eyes. Every now and then he'd point to a corner. Did you see that? he'd ask. Did you see that? There was noth-ing but darkness. She had to get out of there. But it was impossible to flee. The house was laid out railroad-style. Even if she made it out of the bedroom, he'd catch her in the kitchen or the living room. Dawn approached. Neither of them had slept. Desi's only hope was the bathroom. If she remembered right, it had a window that opened up onto the driveway.

She told Eddie she needed to use the toilet and walked to the bathroom. Her eye was turning black, and she was only half dressed. She yanked the window open as high as it would go. It was small, and she was at least 140 pounds. Quietly, she squeezed through the opening out onto the driveway. Sunlight was beginning to break over the horizon. She broke into a run down the hill. It'd be just a few seconds before he figured out she'd escaped. She glanced over her shoulder. The street was empty, awash in the predawn gray. A block up she saw a sign for a drugstore and a pay phone on the corner. And she knew she was safe. She picked up the receiver and frantically dialed Chan's number. She was angry now. But not with Eddie. Something was wrong with him. He needed help. She was furious at his family. They knew he was crazy. How could they do nothing to help her? God, they must be terrified of him, too. Chan answered the phone. Desi calmly explained to her younger sister what had happened. And Chan wept.

———

WE'VE BEEN TRYING to get in contact with you, the voice on the answering service said. We need you to come down to the clinic regarding the test you took. Desi set the phone down on the receiver. It was the end of 1990, two years since she had received the false positive. She looked around her mother's living room. It was modest, clean, comfortable, and familiar.

She walked upstairs and found Wafer. I took a test at the Berkeley Health Clinic, Granna, she told her, and they want me to come down to the clinic right away. It's about HIV.

I'm sure you'll be okay, Wafer answered calmly.

That was so Granna. Desi could say that she had just blown up the bank of Omaha, and Granna would say, Well, I'm sure you needed the money.

Desi grabbed her keys, went outside, ducked into her Firebird, and pulled out toward the clinic. She was frightened and confused. She had never bothered to follow up on that false positive. She'd agreed to take the AIDS test at the Berkeley free clinic a few months ago, when she'd gone there to get treatment for a yeast infection. But she knew now that she had it. It seemed so crazy that this should happen to her at this moment. She had lost her job at Pac Bell back in 1988. She could have gone on welfare or back to drugs, but instead she had enrolled in respiratory therapy school. She had finished the program two months ago and was now in the middle of studying for her licensing exam. She had also begun to deepen her relationship with God.

A few months earlier Desi's childhood friend Ada had been leaving all kinds of messages on her pager to come to services at Oakland Christian Center, a large church in Southwest Oakland. Desi had resisted at first. All the jumping up, whooping, and hollering at the Holiness and Baptist services of Desi's childhood had always felt a little artificial. Ada was persistent, though, and Desi had finally given in and agreed to attend an informal outdoor night service. She'd worn shorts, tennis shoes, and a black top. But when she arrived, the service had been moved inside the center, which resembled a warehouse. Confronted with the carefully dressed parishioners, she'd been embarrassed by the gum stuck to the back of her sweater, but she was struck by the straightforwardness of the service and had an instinct to stay. Oakland Christian Center was a Pentecostal church, which Desi called a "Word Church," meaning that Pastor Lester Hughes studied and taught the letter of the Bible without warping it with his personal interpretations or histrionics.

After the sermon the pastor's wife had asked if anyone wanted to come forward and receive salvation. Desi felt herself pulled out of her seat. Desi met her at the front of the sanctuary and was led into a private back room. "If you believe in your heart and confess with your mouth," Hughes's wife said, invoking Romans 10:9, the salvation prayer, "that God rose Jesus from the dead, then you will be saved." As Desi repeated the words, she realized that she was no longer working on her own anymore; she felt the Lord was in her. Do you want evidence of God, to be filled with the Holy Spirit, to speak in tongues? the woman asked, now referencing Corinthians 14:2, which says "For he that speaketh in unknown tongues speaketh not unto man but unto God." Mysterious words poured from Desi's mouth. They frightened her a little. But they were clear, and she knew at that moment that she would receive salvation.

She pulled into the parking lot of the Berkeley clinic on University Avenue. The lobby was small and spare. The receptionist led her down a hallway and opened a sterile white door onto a cubicle. A white woman with long blond hair was seated behind a desk, frantically sucking on a cigarette. A standing fan buzzed behind the desk, swirling the cold smoke through the fluorescent light. Your test came back positive, the woman said nervously. Desi looked at her blankly. You look like you already knew, the woman said, and Desi thought she looked scared. *I've seen my mama beaten by my daddy,* she thought to herself. *I've been addicted to alcohol and crack. This is just one more thing that I got to handle.*

CHAPTER FOUR

Fire

1988–1990

B EN BOWSER AND THE older local man from Bayview-Hunters Point hung back at a safe distance on a grassy embankment off the edge of the sidewalk, and took in the stream of brakelights that flashed red like warning signs in the San Francisco night. It was one-thirty A.M., in the winter of 1988. The gridlocked traffic inched its way toward a small clutch of young black men who had gathered in front of the projects on North Point Drive. They were kids, really; none could have been much older than eighteen or nineteen. Lean, muscular, and youthfully attractive, they had the untempered air of boys who have just grown into their shoulders and are a little drunk on their first dizzying taste of freedom. Maybe it was this fearless quality that emboldened them to sell crack openly on the street, like men working the pumps at a filling station.

Neighborhood people were frightened of these boys. Nobody wanted to witness a crack deal; people got shot for seeing. Stories of children toting semiautomatic rifles were starting to filter up from Los Angeles. The neighborhood seemed braced for bloodshed. Families had taken to shuttering their windows in the height of the afternoon sun. Parents hustled their children behind locked doors. Rusting swings hung silent and brown in the neighborhood's asphalt playgrounds.

But it wasn't just the threat of gunplay that worried Ben. He feared that these boys were unknowingly peddling a more insidious brand of death than murder. "I've caught several couples high on crack," the older man said to Ben, "doing it in the hallway of my building."

Ben asked if that was more common than before. The man was one of dozens of local informants he'd interviewed.

"Man, where you from?" the older gentleman answered, laughing. "These girls used to have boyfriends of sorts. Now, with this crack thing, they'll do anybody, anytime, anywhere. All they want is that dope and sex. Dope and sex."

Ben doubted this man had any idea of the public health implications of what he'd seen. But he figured it would scare Mindy Fullilove; the information he had unearthed implied that thousands of kids had been infected by HIV or stood to contract it. Now it was a question of whether there was anything they could do to save them, before AIDS shredded their immune systems and killed them just as they reached the threshold of adulthood. When Mindy had phoned him in the early fall, to see if he'd be interested in helping out with some AIDS research, Ben had certainly never expected to uncover a brewing crisis like this.

He was somewhat surprised she'd asked. Her husband, Bob, had helped him find his job on the faculty of Cal State Hayward's sociology department, but he didn't know her very well. He didn't even know much about AIDS, or public health for that matter. Body fluids, sex, IV drug use—he basically had a layman's understanding of the disease. His specialty was urban studies and racism, areas that allowed him to focus on what he considered to be more salient black problems like poverty, segregation, and education. Mindy, though, didn't want Ben for his epidemiological expertise. She had been operating MIRA out of the Bayview-Hunters Point Foundation for a year and wanted to ensure that AIDS didn't spiral out of the Castro into San Francisco's largest black neighborhood.

For that she needed someone to investigate Bayview-Hunters Point from the inside. Basically, she wanted an ethnography, which to Ben meant finding out everything he could about the people who lived there: where they were from; how they put food on the table; what their politics were; the root of the neighborhood's drug problem; where the junkies hung out to shoot up; and if they shared needles. By hiring him, he felt, Mindy was acknowledging that there were intergenerational and internal factors, melted into the racial and historical ore of the neighborhood, that made poor blacks vulnerable to heroin addiction. And buried in those factors were the keys to halting the epidemic.

Ben, though, had his own purposes for investigating Bayview that had nothing to do with AIDS. The neighborhood reminded him of Harlem, where he had grown up in a brick apartment building on the corner of 150th Street and Riverside Drive. During his teenage summers he'd obsessively pedaled his black British three-speed bicycle down every humid block of northern Manhattan. When he started high school, Harlem—with its startling collection of street-corner preachers, musicians, churches, and nightclubs—had had a carnival atmosphere. By the time he finished his undergraduate degree at Franklin and Marshall in 1969, it was unsafe to walk the streets above 126th Street alone. People still referred to Harlem as the spiritual center of black America. Perhaps all the romanticism of that phrase, though, overshadowed its darker modern implication. One could argue that with Harlem fractured and darkened—a forbidden land even to New Yorkers—the black community was losing its shape, identity, and place in the American imagination. This idea made Ben want to excavate the life history of a still-functioning black community like Bayview, in the hope that he might unearth some clues to help restore other midsize black ghettos across the country.

Ben knew how to gather that kind of information. He was a tall, muscular, molasses-colored man with a first-degree black belt in Okinawa Goju Ryu, an early Japanese martial art, who could slip easily between academese and street talk. His self-described "don't tread on me" attitude had alienated some members of the academy, but he felt confident that he could win information from black informants that his more circumspect colleagues could never hope to unearth in their surveys. Even so, he realized that if he asked questions about covert behaviors like sex and drugs in a proud, tight-knit neighborhood like Bayview, his attitude and appearance were only going to get him so far. The older residents, who had settled there in the 1940s to work in the shipyards, boasted the highest occupant home ownership rate in San Francisco, and the junkies were their children. He'd be tagged as an outsider, probing at issues that people understood to be private and perhaps reflective of their failures as parents, children, and citizens. So he got Shirley Gross, the director of the Bayview-Hunters Point Foundation, to hook him up with Lewis Whitely, a longtime local ex-addict, to serve as his guide.

During their first few weeks on the street, Lewis played the role of AIDS-prevention worker and Ben posed as his assistant. It wasn't much of a stretch for either of them. Lewis had a physique that reminded Ben of an aging boxer whose biceps and shoulders had been rounded by age, so that he wasn't exactly threatening but still commanded a certain street respect. Ben stood behind him offering condoms, and bleach for cleaning needles, in exchange for information.

The material they gathered told a familiar story. Bayview had prospered during World War II and the Korean War, and the older generation had made enough money working in the shipyards to buy up most of the modest green, yellow, and white single-story homes that lined the fog-shrouded streets off Third. But in the 1960s and 1970s the shipyards had gradually closed. Heroin had moved in on the heels of the failing economy and enticed the neighborhood's children. Ben had seen worse ghettos; parts of Oakland, another troubled city where he had gathered data, came to mind. Psychologically, though, Bayview felt like a bad slum. The optimism that had drawn southern blacks there in the 1940s had decayed into an air of hopelessness that, in his opinion, could ultimately inflict more lasting damage on the neighborhood than transitory economic trends. One addict he interviewed—sitting on the street underneath a help-wanted sign—told Ben that he would never be able to find a job in San Francisco. The residents seemed to have lost their sense of possibility. He suspected that that mind-set was exacerbating the heroin problem in the second-generation blacks. And it seemed likely that AIDS would gradually work its way into the neighborhood through them.

Ben's work for Mindy probably would have ended there, if Lewis hadn't asked him if he wanted to come back after dark and check out the drug traffic that jammed up the neighborhood every night. Crack was a relatively new fad, a crystallized brand of smokable cocaine that had started to get some media play in the past couple of years due to the rash of violence linked to the young dealers who peddled it. Snorted or smoked, cocaine couldn't transmit the AIDS virus. But Lewis kept bugging him, so Ben agreed to meet him one evening. The streets leading up to the projects were clogged with slow-moving cars. Ben was familiar with drug scourges. In the 1970s his mother, a secretary for the CDC, had informally counted the number of Harlem kids she knew—from her days on the PTA, as a Cub Scout den mother, and as a crossing guard—who'd become involved in heroin. She arrived at three hundred, which had seemed like a staggering number then. This was something entirely different. The lines of cars resembled a mall or a fast-food drive-through.

When Ben told Mindy, she instructed him to dig up all the information he could get his hands on. Ben started hanging around the trafficking sites, talking to residents and teens. The locals knew how the operation worked. The dealers had armies working out of the projects. Apartments were maintained as command and supply centers. There were "near-in lookouts" who served as sentinels watching for police, rip-offs, and rival gangs. Runners brought crack in from off-site locations. "Far-out guards" signaled in long-range warnings. The militant efficiency of the organization was unsettling, and he figured it would attract more kids, who could make an instant fortune dealing this stuff. The drug's euphoric high lasted only a few minutes, and then the junkie was ready for another rock. Moreover, it was cheap; at five dollars a dose, it didn't cost much more than lunch at McDonald's. Children could smoke their allowance. Women didn't even have to buy it—they were selling themselves for the drug. Meanwhile, it was withering the neighborhood. The trafficking areas looked bruised: apartment units near the crack houses were boarded up and littered with broken glass; dusty abandoned cars hugged the curbs; garbage bags were left uncollected; and the grass in front of the crack houses was scraggly and unkempt.

Amid this physical decay it was the dealers' fervor that made Ben uncomfortable. They seemed so ravenous for power that they had become oblivious to the fact that they were literally destroying their community to get a taste of it. The dealers were so numerous that they had spread out from the projects to other streets off Third. One evening Ben arrived around sunset. It was the best time to be out because business was still slow, and in the light there was less chance th... a gun on him. He was walking down one of the side s... ted a slightly older dealer, probably about twenty. Be... up as he approached the young man and started int... questions—Why are you doing this? Where are you fi...

vously listened for any kind of verbal clue that the guy was hiding a gun. Finally, he asked the young man why he might want to buy crack. The dealer looked at him oddly. "Besides getting your head bad," he said, "you'll want to fuck all night." Ben wondered how many of these children were going to die.

Mindy had completely overlooked crack. If heroin was a slow-burning log, fueling the outbreak of minority AIDS infections, then crack was the kerosene that could explode the epidemic into black America. Over the spring she searched for scientific literature on the drug—some sort of foundation on which to build an investigation. There was almost nothing. She was going to have to mobilize the scientific community herself. Ben's findings were too anecdotal for a major scientific journal. MIRA had begun publishing a quarterly AIDS newsletter with the latest research and news on the minority epidemic. She could fire a warning flare by publishing Ben's report there. Ultimately, though, she knew she had to prove a link between AIDS and crack.

The biology of AIDS made that difficult. Crack use had exploded only recently; crack wasn't a vessel for transmission; and AIDS was a retro-virus, meaning victims often weren't diagnosed until four years after they were infected. That meant the CDC's surveillance system wouldn't pick up the impact that crack was having on AIDS rates until the early 1990s. STD rates were probably the best real-time barometers for how crack was accelerating the spread of AIDS. Gonorrhea rates had recently spiked in the city's black community.

Meanwhile, across the country, clues hinted at a larger disaster. Some higher-ups at the CDC suspected that crack was driving a recent rise in syphilis infections. Nationally, syphilis rates had swollen 35 percent in the first nine months of 1987, but the vast majority of new cases were concen-trated in a few inner-city neighborhoods where crack had become endemic. In New York City syphilis rates had shot up a staggering 100 per-cent; they had increased 97 percent in Los Angeles County, and 86 per-cnt in South Florida. Penicillin-resistant cases of gonorrhea were also ⌐hing, and there had been a sharp rise in chancroid, a bacterial infec-⌐ich causes genital lesions and was suspected of propelling the spread of AIDS in Africa. Mindy had to fight off an instinct to drop every-thing and focus all her energy on crack.

Her colleagues didn't all agree with her that crack represented such an obvious threat. Steve Hulley, for one, had a lukewarm reaction to Ben's report. To him it didn't intuitively follow that a smoked substance could substantively increase AIDS rates. Furthermore, Ben's methods didn't mold to Steve's idea of science; the information was too anecdotal. Steve had a long-range vision for the AIDS research center. Under his leader-ship it had won a $7.1 million supplemental grant from the NIMH and the National Institute on Drug Abuse (NIDA). He had hit upon the name Center for AIDS Prevention Studies; everyone had already taken to call-ing it CAPS. It was getting national recognition. HIV incidence had been reduced to one percent in San Francisco's gay population. Now Steve was focusing much of his energy on Mindy's work at MIRA. For months he had been patiently mentoring her in the intricacies of quantitative survey methods, and together they had designed the country's first large-scale AIDS study to examine the minority epidemic. Over the next three years they planned to interview fifteen hundred men and women in the neigh-borhoods surrounding the Castro, draw their blood, and take their STD and substance abuse histories. If crack was as important as Ben seemed to think it was, Steve was confident that this study would bring it to the surface. So when Mindy came to him and said that they should launch research into this new drug scourge, he said, "I don't really see why you'd want to study it, but it's your budget."

Mindy was unsettled by Steve's reaction. She loved and respected the older white doctor from Iowa, and she trusted him as a mentor. But his failure to grasp that crack portended a public health emergency high-lighted his limitations. He seemed to view the world in quantitative terms. When they first opened CAPS, Steve had naïvely suggested that the quickest way to contain AIDS was to instruct the infected simply to tell their prospective lovers that they had been diagnosed with HIV. It didn't occur to him that gay men had a thousand painful reasons to keep that information secret. There were even fewer straight lines in the black neighborhoods Mindy was investigating—no hard rules, and few logical models upon which to base theory. The kind of chaos and pain that could drive thousands of inner-city girls to sell their bodies for a five-dollar hit

of crack was probably too far outside his experience for him to concep-
tualize.

This put Mindy in a complicated position. She had been brought on
partly for her academic pedigree but also because she was black. Clearly
her sensitivity to the realities of black life alerted her to the potential consequences of crack, but she wasn't a trained epidemiologist. For most of
her time at CAPS, she had been feigning expertise to her peers and training herself on the fly. There was no way she was prepared to put together
a scientifically sound study of crack and AIDS. No one else at MIRA was
qualified to do it, either. Ed Morales had left the center, and she and John
Peterson had utterly failed to entice any established black researchers to
join their team. Most of her staff were graduate students and volunteers.
The hard part was that she knew Steve would likely help her, if she asked.
But she feared that the kinds of questions she needed him to answer were
so rudimentary that they would expose her as a novice and undermine
what respect she had earned from him. The one person in her immediate
sphere whom she felt comfortable approaching to put a study like this
together was her husband, Bob, an administrator at UC Berkeley. He had
a doctorate in education, was an expert at survey research, and had
already done some statistical analysis for CAPS on a contract basis.

But she couldn't get Bob to help her, either. He was afraid she'd get
shot. A few months earlier a handyman had stepped off a bus on Third
Street into a crowd of teens high on crack. He had recently moved back
to the neighborhood, and the kids mistook him for a police narc. He managed to break free from them and ran through the night toward his sister's
apartment. The mob chased after him. One of the teens pulled a pistol
and shot him in the back. Worse, it wasn't even an isolated incident.
Crack dealers had pulled a series of "stagecoach" attacks on bus and muni
drivers in Bayview. Some cops suspected the attacks were revenge for the
city's stepped-up efforts to stop cocaine dealing.

Bob's concerns were deep seated. When he was down in Mississippi
in 1964, working for SNCC, he'd drawn a line against getting himself into
situations where he could get killed. Mindy, though, couldn't allow the
dangers posed by the research to deflect her. Crack was going to drive the
AIDS epidemic. She had to investigate it. And she needed Bob to help
her.

Bob had that rare ability to charge people with a sense that they had just been touched by someone important, without making them feel in any way smaller or less than he was. He had been raised to be something of a standard-bearer. His father, Robert Fullilove Jr., a urologist in Newark, used to sit Bob and his brothers down at their kitchen table and force them to enunciate their words until they were stripped of any black inflection. Bob's parents made him the first black student at Pingry, an elite prep school for boys, and they enrolled him in Jack and Jill, an etiquette program for upper-middle-class black children. During his sophomore year at Colgate University his father proudly handed him a thousand dollars to go down to Mississippi with Stokely Carmichael and register black voters.

The summer of 1964 in Mississippi was seminal for Bob. Soon after he arrived in the South, Michael Schwerner, Andrew Goodman, and James Chaney were kidnapped. The violent black-and-white documentary footage of dogs searching for the bodies of the missing volunteers and police spraying fire hoses on civil rights workers helped spark a turning point in the civil rights movement. But there is another picture from that summer, which reappeared in books and magazines, that better captured Bob's experience. It shows a group of black and white kids standing in front of a bus, singing "We Shall Overcome." Bob appears on the left, wearing black-framed glasses and a crisp white shirt, arms locked with a young white man.

Bob was twenty when he returned to Colgate, and he had grown into a man who could unify people with his expansive warmth and intelligence. But he had difficulty translating the intensity of his experience in Mississippi into a larger vision. He was successful by most conventional measures; he worked at SNCC for four years after college, went to Union Theological Seminary to avoid the draft, was married for a time during the 1960s and 1970s, had a son, Bobby, and earned his doctorate from Columbia. Somehow, though, his descriptions of that time made it sound relatively purposeless. It was as if he had been baptized into adulthood on the pinnacle of a mountain but could never figure out how to build on that moment. He wasn't alone in this experience. He could see that even his most successful friends from the movement—like Stokely and his mentor Ivanhoe Donaldson—had wrestled with similar demons.

His first marriage eventually fell apart under a variety of pressures. As he grew older, people continued to gravitate toward his energy and insight. In his public life he drew them around him like a protective blanket and was unfailingly generous with his time and energy. But beneath his garrulous veneer he had the subtle air of a loner. That alchemy of cynicism and warmth probably aided him in his career, but it seemed to amplify his chronic fear that he was not genuinely respected.

Bob's job at Berkeley seemed to promise to bring his ability as an integrator into line with his more internal battle to define his sense of purpose. He'd been brought to the university to run a program designed by Philip Treisman, a mathematician who had bet that he could help make black college science students academically successful by linking them to a network of peers and top faculty. Bob always felt that during his childhood he had thrived in white institutions because he was one of the rare black kids who knew how to talk white and had educated parents who ran in the right circles. Treisman's ideas excited him because they were based on the premise that what helped minorities succeed academically was not so much elite social skills and preparatory academic training as the fact that those abilities imbued them with the social confidence to reach out intellectually, and helped them forge personal connections with friends with whom they could study and mentors to train them.

The program got good results from the students—one of the girls even became Berkeley's first black Rhodes scholar. But the job, unfortunately, proved to be more contentious than Bob had anticipated. The politics at Berkeley were messy, and Bob felt that Treisman was a bad diplomat. The program had run a deficit under Bob's leadership, and lately he'd been working additional hours at CAPS and using the money he earned there to keep his program afloat. He enjoyed the attention he got at CAPS, flirting with both the men and the women, and he loved the moments when he surprised a researcher, who had mistaken him for "just Mindy's husband," with an incisive solution to some scientific problem. But such pleasures weren't enough to make him want to leave Berkeley to work full time for Mindy.

In fact, he was so worried that the administration was going to shut down Treisman's program that one morning in May 1988 he went in to work despite an excruciating pain that tore at his side when he faced the toilet. He felt as if he'd peed broken glass. He wasn't on campus long before he collapsed onto the floor of his office in Stevenson Hall. The doctor said he'd passed a kidney stone and was suffering from a severe urinary tract infection.

Back home in bed, Bob was at his wife's mercy. Have you had enough? she asked. This job is going to kill you. You don't have to put up with their shit anymore. She was speaking directly to his fears. This is a wake-up call, she continued firmly. You have a chance to do something that will change your life. Mindy was taking advantage now, employing her authority as mother, doctor, and psychiatrist all at once. As your doctor and your wife, she said, I'm telling you that you need to give this job up and come and do something that cannot possibly be as stressful, something that has some real possibility. Bob felt weak. His program was turning disadvantaged minority undergraduates into elite science students. Mindy was right. Those assholes at Berkeley hadn't given him enough respect.

All right, he consented. I'll draft my letter of resignation.

The summer of 1988 was at once frightening and exciting. In June Bob flew with Mindy and her daughter Molly to the International AIDS Conference in Stockholm. He quickly took stock of what kind of numbers they'd need to prove the link between crack and HIV. It was a daunting prospect. They didn't have either the time or the money to put together a large-scale survey like the one that Mindy was undertaking with Steve's help. He knew from Ben's report, the CDC's STD surveillance data, and the newspapers that it was mainly black kids who were smoking the drug. But he wasn't sure how to find them, get them to talk, or ensure the safety of the research team. Finally, it was unlikely that many of these teenage junkies had been tested or would agree to be tested for HIV.

When she and Bob returned from Sweden, Mindy got in touch with Dr. Gail Bolan at the San Francisco Department of Public Health. Bolan was the director of the STD prevention and control division and a veteran of CDC's Epidemiological Intelligence Service. Her small staff had been trying to get a handle on the gonorrhea epidemic that was rising among the city's black teenagers, and she'd recently called the CDC for reinforcements. Mindy and Gail decided to pool their resources and put together a joint study. The sexual risk factors for HIV and gonorrhea were nearly identical, and a gonorrhea diagnosis was a strong indicator of HIV risk. It was also relatively easy to find people who were infected with gonorrhea because the symptoms were painful urination and vaginal bleeding, and because the state and city were permitted to keep an active database of people diagnosed with STDs. If they could correlate risky sex and STD diagnoses with crack, then they could make a reasonable argument that the new drug scourge was fueling the AIDS epidemic, which would mobilize the public health service to take action.

Bob worked on the design of the study, and they used their contacts in the drug treatment community to find addicts. Gail looked at one group of teens in San Francisco. The MIRA team, meanwhile, decided to take two samples: one in Bayview and, at Ben's insistence, another in Oakland. Their information-gathering technique was simple. They placed young black research assistants on street corners to wait for dealers to offer them crack. Then the researchers identified themselves and asked the dealer if he used. If he did, the researchers paid him ten bucks for an interview. If he claimed to be clean, the researchers asked to be taken to the addicts. The researchers found that the kids wanted to talk, and over July and August they interviewed more than two hundred teen crack users. Kids were asked how often they used crack, if they had ever had sex while on crack, if they exchanged sexual favors for the drug, if they used condoms, and if they had ever been diagnosed with an STD.

Bob kept late nights analyzing the data. The results from a preliminary sample were ominous: 44 percent of the kids owned up to having sex on drugs; 30 percent reported that they had been diagnosed with an STD; 91 percent said their friends used drugs; and 61 percent said their relatives were users. The deeper they dug, the worse it looked. Heroin junkies were switching to crack because they thought it would protect them from AIDS. Crack addicts were taking heroin to blunt the pain of crashing from the cocaine high. That meant they were cross-contaminating. Further complicating the epidemic, crack was driving Oakland's and San Francisco's inner-city economies. It seemed as though every boy over twelve wanted a piece of the action. Selling heroin and powdered cocaine were also lucrative gigs, but the highs from those drugs lasted longer, and addicts could consume only so much before they either overdosed or their noses went numb. The crack high, by contrast, was short-lived, and it was hard to kill yourself from it. Consequently, there was no "dose" for crack. If a crackhead had a hundred bucks, he smoked a hundred bucks; if he had a thousand, he smoked a thousand. Crack use was so pervasive that, in the middle of the study, Bob and Mindy came to suspect that a counselor who was helping them recruit addicts stole the money they had given him to buy crack for himself. Bob and Mindy estimated conservatively that in the United States there were 330,000 black kids between the ages of fifteen and nineteen using and selling crack. The number they were all afraid to see was how many were already infected with HIV.

In September Mindy was scheduled to fly to Washington for the American Psychiatric Association's fall committee meetings. Bob hadn't yet completed their analysis of the crack data, but Mindy scheduled conferences at NIDA anyway. The data was strong and pointed in a clear direction. The Reagan administration hadn't dedicated the necessary resources to successfully address AIDS in the black community, but Mindy knew that the White House was disturbed by the nation's growing crack epidemic. As in the early days of heroin, the response had been largely punitive. Newly proposed federal laws stated that possession of five grams of crack carried a five-year minimum sentence. Now Mindy had evidence that drew a direct line between the drug and the raging AIDS epidemic. Thousands of kids might die. It was the kind of data that could reshape the nation's war on drugs and that should mobilize a full-bore public health campaign.

Mindy spent a week in Washington meeting with doctors and administrators. Her childhood experience of segregation had made her profoundly anxious about entering foreign spaces. She felt helpless against this consciousness and nearly suffocated in it as she walked the lengths of NIDA's windowless halls, trying to get its researchers to listen to her warning of how crack was going to sweep the AIDS epidemic into the bloodstream of America's black youth. She had seen the future, and it held intolerable suffering for black Americans. The meetings blended into one another in a wash of fluorescent light. One researcher listened to her placidly, sitting in his white public health service uniform. He seemed bored as he looked over her data. The government was supposed to act when confronted with something this potentially destructive, but Mindy couldn't get anyone to believe her.

———————

MINDY WASN'T the first scientist to warn the federal government about the public health implications of crack. In July 1979 Yale psychiatrist and pharmacologist Robert Byck appeared before the House Select Committee on Narcotics Abuse and Control to testify about America's growing fondness for snorting cocaine. The drug treatment, prevention, and law enforcement arms of the federal government had yet to launch an all-out campaign against the drug. Cocaine was popularly understood to be an expensive party toy for the rich, the beluga caviar of designer drugs. Drug experts were actually divided over whether it was addictive or even particularly harmful. As he waited his turn, Byck listened to a line of witnesses testify that cocaine would probably prove to be a minor public health threat. In a sense, Byck agreed with them. Cigarettes and alcohol posed a greater danger to Americans than snorting cocaine. But he wasn't there to talk about the powder hors d'oeuvres that movie executives were serving up on mirror platters for their guests in Beverly Hills. He had a more serious warning to deliver, and he was concerned about how the government would respond to it.

A year earlier Byck had sent David Paly, one of his graduate students, to Peru to gather blood samples from Indians who chewed coca leaves. In Lima Paly was introduced to Raul Jeri, a police psychiatrist, who regaled him with stories about research he had conducted on a cocaine epidemic that had hit Lima in 1974, torn through Peru's major cities, and then spread to Bolivia and Ecuador. The unique thing about this particular cocaine scourge was that the addicts were smoking a sticky paste called *basuco*, an intermediate substance produced in the process of refining powdered cocaine. They dried the *basuco,* crumbled it, and then rolled it into cigarettes. In his reports Jeri described the *basuco* addicts as pale, thin, and paranoid. They suffered from hallucinations and made terrified claims that they were being followed by apparitions and shadows that were trying to kill them. Some, Jeri wrote, had actually wounded themselves in desperate efforts to scratch apparitions out from beneath their skin. And when the level of cocaine in their blood dropped, they suffered from *angustia,* a consuming physical and emotional pain that drove them to steal and starve themselves so they could buy more of the drug.

Paly wasn't impressed with Jeri's studies. They were anecdotal and not very scientific. But then he began to hear about medical students—kids from strong families—who had dropped out of school and become consumed by addiction. Riding his motorcycle through Lima Paly noticed gaunt youths wandering the streets, and he could smell the sweet stench of *basuco* smoke. Jeri's far-fetched claims started to seem more plausible. Coca paste, Jeri wrote, "is the main drug reported by patients who are admitted to psychiatric hospitals or drug treatment centers in Lima. There is no zone of this city where youngsters do not get together to smoke coca paste, and where pushers do not sell the drug in their own homes or in the street. They even come to the school entrances to do their business." Paly called Byck and told him that if this stuff ever hit the United States, they'd be in serious trouble.

Cocaine aficionados in the United States were already smoking a form of the drug. In the early 1970s drug dealers in California had figured out how to transform powdered cocaine into a smokable crystal by heating it with baking soda and water. It became known as freebase. Chemically, *basuco,* freebase, and powdered cocaine were all essentially the same thing. What set *basuco* and freebase apart from powder was the way they were absorbed by the body. A person could sniff only so much cocaine powder. Nasal membranes absorb the drug slowly, and the nose eventually overloads and goes numb. The lungs, however, transmit the drug to the bloodstream more efficiently. When cocaine vapor hits their large surface area, it is metabolized almost instantly: the result is euphoria, and minutes later a crash—then the user needs another hit, and the lungs are ready.

In the 1970s *basuco* addicts had overwhelmed Peru's public health system. At the end of the decade, though, freebase was still relatively scarce in the United States. Most of the cocaine smuggled into America was in powdered form, and it had to be reverse-engineered in order to become smokable. That had kept the street price high. But it was just a matter of time before drug traffickers figured out how to cheaply produce smokable cocaine. Cocaine smoking, Byck told Congress that day in 1979, threatened to become one of the most severe drug scares in American history. There was still time, he testified, to prevent the epidemic. Then, using the basic tenets of public health, he laid out a plan of action for the government. "Number one," he said, "find out about it. Number two, establish some kind of collaboration with the media; and number three, show what happens when this drug is used, so that we don't get an epidemic."

———

NINE YEARS LATER, on October 10, 1988, Bob crowded into the observation room at the Bayview-Hunters Point Foundation, with a group that included Shirley Gross, Gail Bolan, Mindy, and their guest from the CDC, Dr. Sandy Schwarcz. The room was actually a converted kitchen that had been fitted with a two-way mirror that looked out onto a meeting space. Night had fallen, and on the other side of the mirror six teenage crack dealers were seated around a table flooded in white light. They were handsome and casually dressed; none probably had to shave more than once a week.

The MIRA team had interviewed hundreds of teen crack users over the summer, but this was the first time they'd formally spoken with dealers. The presence of the CDC officers made this focus group particularly significant to Bob. The CDC rarely dispatched investigators to monitor a study in progress, and he was eager to win their respect by showing them that a team of black researchers could put these kids behind a two-way mirror—a setting that looked vaguely like an interrogation room—and get them to describe frankly how crack was driving the AIDS and gonorrhea epidemics.

A slightly built black UCSF medical student had been tapped to question the boys. Bob wasn't precisely sure what they would tell him, though he figured they'd confess to all the risky sex that surrounded the crack trade and say selling rock was the only way to make money in the neigh-

borhood. The medical student began with basic questions. The boys'
answers came quickly, monosyllabic and predictable: they were from
Bayview and Oakland, came from broken families, and had been raised
by their grandmothers and mothers. Their idea of a good time? Toss, they
agreed, using the local slang for sex. The boys were asked about their girlfriends. All of them had "main girls." They kissed their main girls, maybe
bought them some dinner, then gave them a hit off the "henna rock" and
"fucked them." Then he asked them about "toss-ups," the girls that they
just used for sex. That was when the boys suddenly veered, dove below
the surface, and dragged Bob into a world that resembled a dream.

"Do you spend money on toss-ups?"

"Hell naw," came the first answer. "No can do," said another. "That's
why they're toss-ups," answered a third.

"Where do you usually have them?" the medical student pressed.
"Like at home, in cars, or what?"

"On the streets."

"In the park."

"At the house."

"Anywhere?"

"A toss-up don't care. Anywhere."

"And you don't take all your clothes off?"

"Just pull my dick out." The kid laughed.

Then a few minutes later: "When you are about to have a toss-up or
anyone else," the medical student started, "do you think about the fact
that she might get pregnant?"

"That's on the bitch."

Roughly ten minutes after that the boys all described being treated for
STDs.

"So what happened once you found out? Did you go back and tell the
girl? Did you know who gave it to you?"

"You didn't even talk to that bitch. You know who you fucked last."

"You dropped her."

"Tell her off."

"Beat her ass."

"Burned her."

"I punched the bitch out in the telephone booth and shit."

"Knocked her around a little bit. Told her she gave it to me."

"I couldn't find her."

"Downshift her ass."

A few minutes after that the medical student asked, "So you're saying you just don't want to use rubbers?"

"Man, fuck rubbers. If you don't want to fuck, just don't fuck. You might as well don't fuck at all. What the fuck you want rubbers for? Damn."

The interviewer looked small to Bob, who wondered if he was in danger. But the crack dealers' thoughts were focused outside the room.

"Y'all don't know where AIDS come from, y'all don't know how to get rid of it."

"You know where it come from. From them faggot motherfuckas. That's where it come from."

"I think God put a curse on us."

"You think God had something to do with it?"

"Yeah."

"Yeah."

"Yep."

"He say niggas doin' wrong."

"Niggas shouldn't be fuckin' niggas."

"Yep. That's why they gave bitches pussies."

Minutes later the discussion turned back to women: "Some black bitches are just dumb."

"Yep. Dumb as fuck!"

"The whole meaning of dumb. I mean dumb, man. You got to be slappin' them bitches. All in the head, man. Some hos like getting beat up. I tell you."

"They like it?"

"They like it, and you just fuck 'em after you beat 'em! They be lovin' that shit."

"I tell you they just be talkin' that shit so you can beat 'em."

"Once you beat a ho, you gon keep beatin' that bitch."

"Hell yeah."

And then it was over. Bob could tell they weren't bragging; their tone was too matter-of-fact. The words they chose and the actions they described were brutal, but the strange thing was that these boys didn't seem angry, hateful, or even cornered and frightened. And they didn't strike him as evil or naïve. They had chosen a life that would get them murdered, land them in prison, or perhaps lead them to AIDS, and yet their voices were clear and palpably strong. They appeared to have no sense of the immorality of their actions. They were amoral, and that made them dangerous—not just in a physical sense, but to the cause and authority of the black community as a whole.

Bob's parents had raised him to be a standard-bearer partially because they wanted him to realize the full promise of postwar America, but also because they wanted him to help close the cultural gulf between the races by engaging intellectually, socially, and politically with white America. For much of his adult life Bob had been ambivalent about their methods and fervor. Clearly, he had achieved a level of professional, academic, and social success that transcended the color of his skin. But he continued to encounter the racial gulf, whether in the negotiation between Sala Udin and the CAPS administration, or in the discussions with Mindy and Steve Hulley over the appropriate response to the crack data, or even in the UC Berkeley administration's failure to appreciate the value of the program he'd run for Treisman. On a certain level, encounters with the gulf were to be expected; Bob and his peers were the first generation to mature in an America where both public policy and sentiment dictated that the races commingle on an equal footing, and that process was bound to be complicated. It was equally reasonable, though, to expect that each successive generation would find it easier to engage in a richer, more honest, and ultimately successful exchange. These boys, though, were alien and asocial, not just to the white audience Bob, Mindy, and Gail had assembled on the other side of the two-way mirror but also to Bob himself. In that sense, their testimony seemed to embody the failure of black America, which made Bob and Mindy's job infinitely more complicated.

Bob could see that Mindy was shaken. It was close to nine-thirty. Bob felt conscious of the doctors from the CDC. This wasn't about science anymore. They had exposed their own entrails in the most graphic, visceral, and disgusting form to these white people. And Bob didn't know how to handle it. The researchers filed into an empty meeting room for a debriefing session. Dr. Schwarcz was eager to discuss the remarkable testimony. Gail Bolan felt embarrassed, as if she had accidentally walked in on a parent getting cussed out by their child. Mindy stood up and delivered what amounted to a stiff half-apology for these boys and for her race. Then, to Bob's relief, she suggested that they all go home.

―――――――

"'THE CRACK HOUSE of today has become what the gay bathhouse was yesterday with regard to all sexually transmitted diseases,' says the Centers for Disease Control's Director of the Division of Sexually Transmitted Diseases, Willard Cates, Jr., speaking at the 1988 STD National Conference in Boston.'"

Mindy held the quotation in her hands. It was the lead sentence to a one-page article titled "Sex Tied to Drugs = STD Spread" in a section of the *Journal of the American Medical Association* called Medical News and Perspectives. Mindy took it as a validation of their summer partnership with Gail. "Crack," Cates was quoted as saying, "is spreading whatever STD seems to be prevalent in the core group even more widely into the lowest-income communities." He then went on to lay out a blueprint for how to halt this inner-city bushfire: rope "nondisease" government programs like family planning, drug treatment, mental health, and child welfare into the STD prevention campaign; fund more methadone clinics; mobilize the private medical community; and employ behavioral change strategies— the ones that had been so effective in helping gay men modify their sexual habits—in the inner city. It was unlikely that Cates's plan would ever be funded. The Reagan administration had announced cutbacks in federal funding for all STD-prevention programs except AIDS. From a public health perspective, they were making a largely artificial distinction: syphilis, gonorrhea, chlamydia, and HIV were all spread through unprotected sex. STD programs, though, were concentrated in the inner city.

It was November 1988, a month after the focus group with the teen crack dealers. Steve had recently moved all five components of CAPS onto the fifth floor of a skyscraper on New Montgomery Street in downtown San Francisco. Mindy had been conflicted about leaving Bayview. She shared her father's conviction that she should stay rooted in the ghetto. At the same time she felt that the MIRA team needed to mingle with the other members of CAPS if they were ever going to be respected as equals. Ultimately, the new building with its marble foyer, brass-gilded elevators, on-site library, corner offices, networked Macintosh computer system, and collegial atmosphere had proved too seductive to resist. Now she wondered if she had made a mistake. The behavioral prevention strategy promoted by Tom Coates and Steve Hulley was working in the gay white community. Tom, Steve, and others in the field had bet that the AIDS epidemic didn't reflect fundamental flaws with the homosexual lifestyle as a whole. Rather, they figured that if they focused on personal responsibility by simply educating gay men about AIDS in a respectful and culturally appropriate manner, then they, as individuals, would change their behavior. Mindy didn't believe that this strategy would work in black America. Individual decision-making, it seemed to her, was profoundly compromised in the chaotic context of the ghetto.

Her appraisal seemed to make intuitive sense. A crack addict, physically shaking with the desire to get high and fighting off the ghosts of childhood trauma, was unlikely to stop using because a prevention campaign—even one that was culturally sensitive—warned her that she might end up having risky sex while intoxicated. An eighteen-year-old crack-dealing high school dropout, who had seen his father broken by unemployment and his mother suffer the indignity of welfare, wasn't going to turn down a multithousand-dollar-a-month gig dealing crack because some poster said that it was up to him to prevent AIDS from spreading through the neighborhood. And what black teenage girl was going to risk having her boyfriend knock out her front teeth by "responsibly disclosing her sero-status"? These kids didn't live in a cohesive, upwardly mobile, and fastidious world. In the late 1960s Senator Daniel Patrick Moynihan was accused by the left of playing into the hands of racists for saying that the black family was in crisis, but conditions had only deteriorated since then. In 1960 78 percent of black families were headed by married couples. That figure had fallen to 40 percent by 1985. Young blacks seemed to be dealing with issues that felt more immediate than AIDS, a disease that apparently they didn't even believe threatened them. "It ain't that many niggas fuckin' [niggas]," one of the teenage crack dealers in the focus group had commented. "If they is, then they got a fucked-up mind." Then he had laughed. "If they do, the white boys influenced them into that shit."

Yet even as the proportion of infected blacks continued to swell, Mindy's colleagues at CAPS were canonizing their prevention strategy, making it the normative approach for fighting AIDS. Even CDC heavyweights like Willard Cates believed in it. To Mindy, they were acknowledging that it was logical that blacks should be disproportionately infected with AIDS. She found herself sensitive to offhand comments like: AIDS is a sexually transmitted disease, isn't it? Don't blacks have all that syphilis? All that gonorrhea? All that chlamydia? And isn't it about drug use? Don't blacks have all that drug use? While some black communities did indeed suffer disproportionately from these health problems, Mindy objected to the implication that race was a cause of AIDS—that the disease and the behaviors that led to its transmission were somehow endemic to being black—and that therefore they should not expect better results from their prevention efforts among blacks. Viruses, she was well aware, did not discriminate. If the prevention model that was working in the gay community was failing with African Americans, then she felt they needed to fundamentally reexamine their methods.

But she didn't have a language to make her colleagues understand what she felt were the dangerous implications of their position, and when she tried to express her position, she would get angry or else cautious. She didn't really believe that Steve and Tom were calculating racists, disdainfully dismissing blacks as beasts who lacked the civilized will to control their sexual urges. After all, Steve wanted to nurture and mentor her as a scientist. He had striven to build CAPS into a space where scientists had overhead, support, and freedom to pursue their interests. And she understood that he believed that scientific methods remained strong across populations.

When confronted with their reasoning, though, Mindy had difficulty transcending the rhetoric of racism. But did that matter? She believed racism was a systemic force that shaped all issues. Wasn't it racist of them to fail to question how racism was influencing their analysis? She was sure of herself there. But this kind of thinking inevitably led her to the weakest ledge of her mind. She felt outnumbered and increasingly entrenched at New Montgomery. It even seemed that she couldn't hold on to her young research assistants, whom she saw as ready to abandon her in their hunger to work with the established white scientists. She felt she was fighting a rearguard action. Instead of having room to creatively solve this difficult public health crisis, she could barely hear herself think.

During the winter of 1989, Mindy and Bob worked to refine their crack data in an effort to get it into shape to present at the next International AIDS Conference, to be held that year in June in Montreal. More immediately, though, Mindy seemed to be in a racial corner. She had all these descriptive facts that explained why AIDS was floating through the veins of black America. But they all blew out to seemingly intractable problems—crack, heroin, family breakdown, poverty, homophobia—that each in its own way pointed the blame back at her own race.

There was no shying away from the truth that something had gone wrong in urban black America. It was impossible to soften the testimony of the teenage crack dealers. The neighborhoods Mindy was investigating simply didn't feel right—it was hard to find a bank, a grocery store, or a restaurant in Bayview. And on the East Coast, where the epidemic had taken even deeper root, black neighborhoods resembled postwar zones. In 1986 Mindy and Bob had flown to Newark, New Jersey, to spend Christmas with his mother. They rented a car and drove through the city, revisiting childhood haunts. Snowflakes flitted through the air, blanketing the streetscape, which looked to Mindy almost as if it had been bombed out. Bob's childhood home was a vacant lot, the house torn down years ago for a freeway project that had never been completed. Their favorite department store stood empty and dark. Bob's mother's mansion was surrounded by collapsing buildings, and the sidewalk outside was populated by homeless men, drinking from paper bags in the winter cold. Once they got out of the car and went inside the mansion and were safely behind locked doors, the car was stolen from out front. Bob had grown up well off, the son of a prominent doctor. Now his mother's neighborhood looked diseased. Mindy believed that there was a connection between this communal decay and the AIDS epidemic. But she needed a new way of conceptualizing the problem.

The first clue came to her when she read an article titled "A Synergism of Plagues: 'Planned Shrinkage,' Contagious Housing Destruction, and AIDS in the Bronx," published in an obscure journal called *Environmental Research* by Dr. Rod Wallace, a white physicist at the New York State Psychiatric Institute. The South Bronx was the epicenter of the AIDS epidemic in black America. There were credible estimates that as many as one in five black men between the ages of eighteen and forty-four were infected there. These extraordinary rates had always been attributed to the borough's heroin problem. Wallace hadn't accepted that as a complete explanation and had dug deeper. Using methods from epidemiology, quantitative geography, and community ecology in a series of articles, he postulated that the raging AIDS epidemic in the Bronx was tied to a process he called "contagious housing destruction."

Contagious housing destruction, Wallace argued, had been set off by the rash of fires that burned through New York City's minority neighborhoods from the late 1960s to the early 1980s. Initially, the city responded to the blazes by opening a series of new fire companies in the most vulnerable communities. The policy was successful, and fire damage gradually decreased. Then between 1972 and 1976 the city disbanded fifty firefighting units in some of its most densely populated, high-fire-incidence, minority neighborhoods. The companies that remained suffered staffing cuts of 20 to 25 percent. First response to fires was reduced from five to four—and then eventually to three—fire companies. The fires returned, concentrated in the heavily black sections of the South Bronx, Brownsville, and East New York. According to Wallace's research, fires destroyed half the housing in some areas of the South Bronx—a level of destruction, he noted, that had previously been seen in modern industrial nations only during wartime.

This burnout, Wallace argued, spawned an epidemic of contagious urban decay. The symptoms spread in the predictable pattern of a disease. Housing stock in the South Bronx during the late 1960s and early 1970s became dangerously overcrowded; buildings rapidly deteriorated, then often caught fire; apartments near the fire zones were abandoned by residents and landlords, and they too eventually burned. The fires, Wallace said, displaced blacks and Latinos, who migrated en masse to the West and North Bronx. It was difficult to quantify how this phenomenon impacted families and individual lives, but the economic numbers suggested devastation. Thousands of middle-class New Yorkers fled the borough. And the West Bronx deteriorated from a working-class neighborhood into one of the worst poverty areas of the city. Now it too was severely overcrowded.

The fires, Wallace said, dramatically inflamed the AIDS epidemic in the Bronx. The geography of AIDS in New York City was largely the geography of heroin abuse. Intravenous drug use, it turned out, was highly correlated with overcrowded housing. During the early 1970s the Bronx's heroin problem was primarily confined to the spine of poverty that ran through the south-central section of the borough. The fires, Wallace wrote, had a twofold effect on heroin. Many of the burned-out and abandoned buildings became shooting galleries. More significantly, the fires drove intravenous drug abusers from their relatively well-defined center in the South Central Bronx and effectively blew heroin into a borough-wide problem.

The most dramatic accusation leveled by Wallace was that the city had deliberately cut back public services—including fire departments—in anticipation of the fires. According to Wallace's research, the New York City Planning Commission predicted in 1969 with almost perfect precision that fire rates in New York's poorest minority neighborhoods would increase and become "a cause as well as a symptom of urban decay." Seven years later New York City housing commissioner Roger Starr was quoted on the front page of the *New York Times* as saying that the city was considering policies that would accelerate the depopulation of slum areas. The city would then let the land stand vacant until new uses for it presented themselves. Finally, Wallace noted, in 1978 Perry Duryea, the Republican leader of the New York State Assembly and also a volunteer firefighter, published a report in which he cited evidence linking the fire department cutbacks to the policies of planned shrinkage.

It would have been easy for Mindy to feel that she had found the racist cause of the AIDS epidemic. Wallace's analysis was certainly inflammatory enough. But it was actually more interesting as a case study. Much of her frustration had been fueled by her colleagues' apparent willingness to settle for prevention strategies that weren't working, a willingness that seemed to be based on an assumption that black communities existed in a natural state of "dis-ease." It was that same mind-set, in her view, that made it possible for New York City planners to presumptively determine that "slum areas" should be "depopulated." Wallace's study of the Bronx didn't uncover the cause of the AIDS epidemic in black America. But by stepping outside the bounds of traditional epidemiology, he had demonstrated that the devastating conditions that had left blacks vulnerable to AIDS were not endemic to being black. Rather, they were fomented by policies rooted in the belief that black communities did not deserve the investment of public resources necessary to sustain their functionality on even the most basic level.

Bob could see that Mindy was wrestling with how to get her colleagues at CAPS to understand her position. Part of the problem was that she was challenging traditional scientific methods by advocating for a more interdisciplinary and qualitative approach that drew conclusions from focus groups and subject interviews. But on a certain level, he believed that the gulf between the races was always fundamentally one of communication. To that end he was proud of his ability to fluently slip between what he called "the king's English" and street dialect. Normally, he might have been able to mediate the situation at CAPS, but he had his own problems with the leadership team at the center that seemed to underscore his confusing relationship to race in a way that arrested his willingness to commit completely to their research. He chronically struggled with his concern that he was not respected. And he was beginning not to feel respected by Coates and Hulley. MIRA was founded on the premise that its research team's blackness qualified them to investigate AIDS in minority communities. Despite his graduate training in statistics, Bob was not a public health expert. He felt he had proved himself with the crack research, yet he had not been offered a faculty position, and Steve at one point had even asked him if his Ed.D. was a real Ph.D.

If Mindy had a tendency to retreat inward when she felt confronted with her deepest anxieties about her ability as a scientist or race warrior,

Bob withdrew by looking outward. He had moved twenty-nine times in twenty-six years. Although he hadn't decided to leave CAPS, he had already turned his mind away from that work and increasingly devoted his attention to a new love affair with the French language. He studied it with an almost monastic fervor. During the congested morning commute over the Bay Bridge, Mindy and Bob used to discuss their work. Now he listened to French. He immersed himself in grammar exercises, French television, articles, and books. So much so that, in a sense, he began to inhabit the language.

He viewed the International AIDS Conference in Montreal—scheduled to take place during the first week of June 1989—as both an opportunity to warn the public health establishment about the implications of crack and a place where MIRA's work might finally be recognized. The week-long conference was intended to draw international attention to the rapidly growing global AIDS pandemic. The organizers had flown in re-searchers from Europe, Africa, and South America and wired the whole thing for closed-circuit television. It was supposed to garner front-page headlines in papers like the *Times* of London, the *Washington Post,* and *Le Monde,* but the protests in Tiananmen Square, which exploded that same week, dominated the news instead. Even so, it was still a coming-out party for the MIRA team. They had feverishly prepared a dozen posters, many dramatically displaying their crack data. Doctors, epidemi-ologists, and academic researchers crowded around their table in the hangarlike conference hall. Mindy gave one of the conference's first oral presentations based on qualitative data. Bob joined Jim Curran, the CDC's celebrity AIDS doctor, on a television show and solidified warm connections with other top officials from the agency.

One evening he and Mindy dined with Anke Ehrhardt, the director of the new NIMH HIV center at Columbia University, at a French restau-rant in the old quarter of Montreal. Bob had met Anke at other AIDS meetings, and she'd consistently expressed an interest in their work. Your ideas will be welcomed at Columbia, she said, wooing them to join her staff. New York is the center of the epidemic; we believe in what you're doing, and there'll be a faculty position for you, Bob. Her words were intoxicating. She understood that the epidemic was intrinsically linked to community disintegration. And she was right: he and Mindy were both graduates of Columbia—joining her team would be a homecoming. She'd furnish them with staff. Their offices at Columbia's north campus would be in Harlem. New York was the fallen capital of black America and the epicenter of the epidemic. He knew that they had officially arrived.

In October they decided to accept the offer.

CHAPTER FIVE

Invisible

1989–1992

Laura Hall's hands started itching Thursday night, December 15, 1989, on the drive from her family's home in Huntsville, Alabama, to South Carolina. She was at the wheel of her 1989 Dodge Dynasty, and her teenage daughter Janeka was in the car with her. Laura usually loved their annual Christmas trip to visit her parents in Pendleton, a one-stoplight town at the foot of the Blue Ridge Mountains. There was something calming about the way the last blush of autumn bathed the Tennessee Valley in red, orange, and brown. But it was one o'clock in the morning, and the colors were lost in the darkness. A few hours earlier her cousin Valeria had phoned her in Huntsville to tell her that they had to make the trip home that night if she wanted to see her father, Eleziah, alive again. She hated driving in the dark. Even on weekends she liked to be asleep by ten. She'd left a hurried message with the assistant principal at the high school where she taught, with instructions for a substitute teacher. She'd definitely miss finals. He'd surely understand.

She hoped they would make it in time. At least she knew Eleziah wasn't alone. He was pastor of Smith Chapel Fire Baptized and Holiness Church. Laura had converted to Catholicism when she married John, but she still sometimes missed the warmth and energy of the Pentecostal faith. In that world there was always a line of volunteers ready to cook a meal or to stand vigil at a hospital bed. Her brother and sister, cousins, aunts, and neighbors would be at his side. They would help her through this ordeal. She just wanted to hold her father's hand and pray with him one more time before he passed. Her mind turned to her twenty-three-year-old son, Ato—who would be driving to Pendleton with John the next day. She wondered what his grandfather's death would mean to him, especially with everything that was going on.

On the surface it seemed odd that Ato and her father were close, because they were so different. Eleziah was a strict and taciturn man, whereas Ato—whose name meant "brilliant" in Swahili—was naturally playful and lighthearted. Seen through a longer-range lens, though, the connection between them was more obvious. Eleziah was born at the turn of the century, into the Jim Crow South. He and Laura's mother, Elizabeth, both left school before the eighth grade to help their parents sharecrop. When the civil rights movement swept through South Carolina in the 1950s, he was one of many blacks who chose not to march, drink out of white fountains, or engage with the element of the white southern world that was intent on dehumanizing African Americans by casting them as rapists, sexual beasts, lazy degenerates, and intellectual children. Rather, he elevated himself to a purer moral plane. He often worked as a manual laborer, freely gave money to needy black townspeople, did not complain about his own poverty, and spoke righteously about God, virtue, and sin. Even after World War II and then the Civil Rights Act raised the expectations of blacks across the country, Laura still never heard him raise his voice in accusation. He pushed Laura through college and then graduate school, and when Ato and his sister, Janeka, were born into a warm, wall-to-wall-carpeted, garbage-disposal-in-the-kitchen, suburban childhood, their comfort seemed to affirm his faith in the Christian values that, as far as Laura could see, he had always believed would ultimately redeem both America and blacks from the legacy of slavery.

Ato, Laura thought, was going to need Eleziah now. Right around then, she noticed the itching. She had never felt anything like it before. It felt unbearable and foreign. Fighting the impulse to rake her skin, she pulled off in Garnerville and found an all-night pharmacy. Inside she showed her hands to the man at the counter. There was no rash.

"Have you been under any unusual stress?" he asked.

"Not really," Laura answered.

Eleziah died the day after they arrived in Pendleton. She spent the weekend preparing for the funeral. On Monday John took Ato to the doctor to pick up some test results. Laura had wanted to go with them, but she hadn't felt strong enough to face the potential news. She'd started to worry about Ato over Thanksgiving. The whole family had driven up to Pendleton to spend the holiday with her parents. Everyone had been preoccupied with Eleziah, who was in the final throes of leukemia. Ato, though, coughed violently over the weekend. He'd been fighting a recurrent case of walking pneumonia, but she thought he'd beaten it off. The Friday after Thanksgiving, on the drive back to Huntsville, John and Laura had taken Ato to the doctor. Ato himself had suggested a health clinic in Atlanta. Laura and fifteen-year-old Janeka sat in metal chairs in the waiting room, while Ato and John met with the clinician. The minutes dragged into a half-hour. After an hour John and Ato emerged from the clinician's office. John's eyes were cloudy. Ato was silent. Laura and John followed their children out into the parking lot.

"Is it what I thought it was?" Laura asked softly.

"The doctor thinks so," John answered. "But he's got to wait for the test results to come back from California to be sure."

It seemed unfair that they were scheduled to pick up the results the day of her father's funeral. The wheels of John's car crackled over the driveway. She knew what he was going to tell her, but she tried to shove the thought aside. John pushed through the trailer door first. His ashen face and the tired way he carried himself told Laura enough. Ato was close behind, sullen and gaunt. She tried to fight back the tears. *This can't be happening now,* she thought to herself. They were supposed to attend her father's wake in an hour. Ato and John sat down next to her. I don't want you to tell anyone, Ato said. And if you do, I won't talk to you.

———

LIKE MOST YOUNG MEN, Ato had kept secrets from his family before. A few years earlier after, his sophomore year at Benedict College in South Carolina, he had rented a car and driven to Atlanta. His parents didn't hear from him for months, and the car was eventually found on the side of the road. Perhaps he was wrestling with his sexuality, perhaps the drugs he had experimented with in college had begun to consume him, or maybe he was simply struggling with teenage angst. Laura didn't know, because when he returned to Huntsville, he kept to himself whatever demons had inspired him to suddenly abandon his promising college career. AIDS, though, robbed him of the luxury of discretion. It no longer mattered if he was really a homosexual or an addict. The virus physically tainted him with these sins. His face would soon be covered with lesions, and his clothes would hang limply from his bony frame. Then he would die disfigured. That was an inevitable truth that he could not change. By choosing to die in secrecy, he could protect his family—and to a certain extent probably himself—from confronting the moral and spiritual challenges presented by his infection. That decision, though, at once severed his richest bloodline to the black community and seemed to underscore some of the ways in which his interior experience was still informed by the politics of race that had defined much of the southern cultural landscape before civil rights.

Although Ato had grown up in Huntsville, his roots were still in Pendleton. When he was a baby, Eleziah and Elizabeth had cared for him there, while John taught during the day in nearby Greenville, and Laura studied for her master's degree in Atlanta. Even after the Halls moved to Columbus, Ohio, and then to Huntsville, they celebrated most holidays with the sprawling clan of Vandivers in Pendleton, and they turned to the Vandivers whenever they needed support.

Eleziah was a Pentecostal minister in the neighboring town of Pickens, and as a kid Ato—who was raised in John's Catholic faith—liked to attend services with his grandfather. The parishioners who crowded into the small sanctuary every Sunday to celebrate their love of God and cleanse themselves of Satan had a joyous energy. Eleziah played the guitar during the service, while aging men in suits and their wives in blue and yellow dresses leaped from their seats crying out hymns and testifying to Christ. Ato's grandmother Elizabeth and the rest of the Vandivers were members of the African Methodist Episcopal church. They liked to say that service was the writ they paid to God for the gift of life. Certainly the web of black country churches seemed to knit the black community in Anderson County together. In that respect Anderson resembled rural counties across the South, where, during slavery and Jim Crow, the church was the black community's spiritual, political, and often material anchor. Blacks across the South still looked to their churches for food and clothes; the church was where they gathered money to help congregants pay for doctors' bills; family fights, mental illness, death, and birth fell under its roof. Ato was a middle-class kid and certainly didn't need material help from the church. But as he descended into AIDS, he could have leaned on the community's spiritual and emotional support, which had helped sustain African Americans through slavery, segregation, and racism. At the same time, though, his sensitivity to the moral standards that were hardwired into that culture seemed to amplify his shame about his infection and prevented him from seeking not just their help but the support of many who loved him.

Ato tried to live at home after he was diagnosed, with the understanding that his parents would keep his secret. John, a clinical psychiatrist, badly wanted to care for his son and insisted that Ato move into his apartment in College Park, and shortly after that into his new condo in Smyrna, a wealthy Atlanta suburb where he worked during the week. The arrangement seemed to work out for the first few months. Ato had to adhere to a medication regimen that required him to take AZT every four hours, and caused his entire body to itch. John would rouse himself in the middle of the night, plod down the carpeted hall, gently shake his son, and hand him a glass of water and a fistful of pills. He paid for Ato's doctor visits, gave him spending money, and boiled him oatmeal with raisins, the way he'd liked it when he was a small boy.

For a while Ato clung to the hope that he would survive. He endured the side effects from the AZT and was obsessed with alternative therapies. Once he even asked his father to sign him up for a dangerous experimental procedure to have all of his blood replaced through transfusion. But his health inexorably deteriorated. His eyes became sunken, and weight slipped off his 160-pound frame. He found a job at a restaurant, but it was everything he could do to stop himself from clawing at his skin in front of his co-workers. Visits to the doctor devolved into harrowing confrontations with death, as his T-cell count ticked slowly down to zero. He began to skip appointments and stopped taking AZT. In the summer of 1990 he drove to a Vandiver reunion in Pendleton. During the family softball game he sat on the edge of the field, sweating in the stifling heat in white athletic socks that he had self-consciously pulled high over his knees to hide the knot of black lesions creeping over his spindly legs.

The pressure to hide and the specter of death seemed overwhelming to him. Sometimes he'd drive from Smyrna to Atlanta and search for crack cocaine. He had experimented with drugs when he was in college. Now crack was the most effective medication he could find. A part of him felt safer in the ghetto than in the suburbs—the streets and projects were swollen with addicts like him, who didn't seem to care if he had AIDS. By the winter of 1990 he was spending more time in the slums of Atlanta. He'd tell John he was running to the corner store and would disappear for three days or maybe a week. John often cruised through the neighborhood in the cherry-red Pontiac Grand Am he had bought for Ato. Sometimes he would pull up to the corner where a skein of young girls had gathered in the artificial street light. Most times they recognized him, and instead of offering him sex, they'd amble up to his window and beg him for some food money. John might pull out a five-dollar bill, tacitly accepting that it was for crack, and ask if any of them knew where to find his son. When Ato had smoked away all of his money, he'd call home and beg his father to pick him up. Some nights John would tell him in his quiet pained way that he wouldn't rescue him again. But Ato knew that his father would never abandon him.

In May 1991 Ato told his father that he was stepping out to meet a girl he had been seeing, and he never returned. He almost wavered once, while staying at one of his informal crash pads. Bill Cosby was on the television doing a show on AIDS. Ato badly wanted to call Laura, but he couldn't bring himself to phone collect. So he curled up alone and cried. When he ran out of money, and the drug dealers, prostitutes, and junkies stopped caring for him, he still couldn't bring himself to leave the ghetto. Perhaps he fantasized that his secret would die safely with him, if he could disappear into death. Perhaps he didn't want to burden his parents. Or perhaps it was simply easier to die openly there than to live in hiding at home.

It was October now as he made his way up the sidewalk. Something had broken in him. He'd been sleeping on the streets and was near death. He wanted to be home, in his own bed, listening to music, near his father and mother. B. J. Baxter's shop came into view. Baxter was an old family friend from the Vandivers' religious community who owned a garage on the outskirts of the ghetto. It was nearly one in the afternoon when Ato walked into his office.

B.J. was startled at the young man's appearance. John had told him that he was having problems with drugs. Ato, though, looked like he was starving to death.

Do you want to lie down here in the office? B.J. asked.

Three hours later John pulled into B.J.'s parking lot. This time he was driving his own car, a black 1964 Chrysler. He cut the engine, stepped out into the late afternoon light, and strode toward the garage. Ato was asleep in the front seat of a powder-blue 1960s Cadillac that B.J. had been restoring. He had gathered a ratty blue blanket up around his shoulders. The failing light pulled Ato's diseased features into relief, and he looked thin and small to John in his dirty dungarees and red-striped sweatshirt. Beneath the decay, though, John still saw his son, and he felt a pure rush of joy and relief. He opened the Cadillac's door and shook him awake. Ato opened his eyes, eased out of the front seat, and wrapped his arms around his father. John held his son and cried. Then he said, "Let's go home."

Laura felt as if she had been awakened from a dream, as she drove from Huntsville to Atlanta that weekend to meet her son. She had been waiting for some policeman to call and inform her that Ato's body had been found on a street corner or in some crack house. Not knowing had been almost worse than watching him die. When she arrived at John's apartment, she didn't press Ato to explain why he had left—she wanted only to be in his delicate presence. Over the following weeks, Laura cared for Ato, and gradually his cheeks grew fuller, and he began to resemble himself. At Thanksgiving, Laura, John, and Ato drove up to Pendleton. It felt reassuring to be near her family, even if she still couldn't tell them that Ato was dying. John, though, had begun to worry that Ato would disappear again and asked Laura to move him back to Huntsville with her.

Laura hesitated. Like any mother, she wanted to care for her son, but she felt an instinct to say no. What was wrong with her? She told herself it was because she was worried that he wouldn't get the best medical attention in Huntsville. They'd heard of only one doctor in town who took

AIDS patients. Where would she take him if he stopped breathing or if they had to rush him to the hospital? But she knew there was more to it than that. She didn't want people to find out he had AIDS. Despite all her sorrow that he was so isolated, she had never wrapped her arms around her son, comforted him like a child, and reassured him that he should feel no shame, that he should trust in the people who loved him.

She had tried to tell herself that she kept quiet out of respect for Ato. Privately, though, she was relieved that he'd decided not to tell anyone. She told only her priest, Bruce Greening, a family friend, who lived in Washington, D.C., and was bound by the priesthood to be discreet. She had even taken risks with Ato's health to keep his infection secret. In May 1990 her health insurance company had dropped Ato because he was officially too old to remain on her coverage. Laura figured that they were legally obligated to let him roll over onto his own plan. But they informed her that if he reapplied, they would treat him like a new applicant and reject him on the grounds that his AIDS infection was a preexisting condition. Laura easily could have tried to fight their claim. As a teacher, all she had to do was put in a call to the teachers' union representative. He was a friend and would have taken care of it. But she didn't. What cruel thoughts would he have had about her son? Was he gay? An addict? And what might he say about her? Instead, she decided it was better to pay $1,000 a month out of pocket for Ato's AZT. John eventually found a pharmacy in Atlanta that bought the drug in bulk and sold it for $162 a week. By that time, though, Ato had stopped taking his medication regularly. Soon afterward he disappeared.

Now John wanted her to take Ato back to Huntsville. Secrets have a way of working their way through small southern cities, and Laura didn't know if she could keep this one contained behind the walls of her house. She was a well-known high school teacher and active in the Democratic Party. John had taught at Alabama A&M, and it seemed as if every school principal in Huntsville had been a student of his at one time or another. They were both prominent in the Catholic Church. Ato had been an altar boy. Anyone who saw his hollow cheeks and rheumy eyes would be able to tell that something was dreadfully wrong with him. Of course, no one would say anything directly—this was the South. There would be whispers and glances. Every missed handshake or greeting would feel like a rejection or a judgment. Colleagues in the cafeteria, friends at church would politely say nothing but would wonder to themselves if she had shared a glass with her son, kissed him on the cheek, or held him after he had coughed through the night.

Laura hated herself for having these fears. Ultimately she managed to swallow them, and Ato returned to Huntsville in late November 1991. Ato spent his days alone on his water bed, listening to his headphones amid piles of clothes, CDs, and books. He grew thinner, and Laura felt as if she could see her son disappearing toward death. They had always been alike: indomitable, quick to laugh, mischievous, and disorganized. Now he seemed confined by his shame, an experience that seemed to capture in reverse everything that Eleziah—and in turn, Laura—had hoped for Ato to achieve in post–civil rights America.

Laura's ambitions for her children were in many ways tied to her relationship to her father. He had expected her to break free from a two-hundred-year cycle of family poverty. It was difficult for her to tell how much of the pressure that he exacted on her was born from his experience of being a black southern man. His spiritual calling was so encompassing that Laura had always found it hard to penetrate his interior hope, pain, guilt, anger, or disappointment. When Laura was nine years old, he took her to a Pentecostal revival at St. Luke's Fire and Baptized Holiness Church, and she watched as he was saved. He often preached from the Book of Revelation, spoke openly of hell, and sternly instilled in her a sense that she had an obligation to achieve.

His desire for her success fit with her own hunger for middle-class comfort. Seven of them were crowded into two rooms. Laura hated having to pick cotton in the summer heat so that her family could pay their bills, and in the mornings, as she searched for her worn school shoes amid the clutter of her sisters' clothes, she'd think to herself that there had to be another way to live. She became a disciplined student and eventually attended Morris College, a black university run by the Baptist Educational and Missionary Convention in Sumter, South Carolina. But as she grew older, she began to resent her father's righteousness. When she married John, her willingness to convert to Catholicism was motivated, at least in part, by a need to escape Eleziah's proselytizing.

Laura was able to impart a fuller sense of freedom to her son than men like her father had given to her generation. She and John organized holidays and family vacations around Ato's favorite activities, lavished him with unconditional love, and gave him free rein and financial support to pursue his interests. For most of his life, it seemed that she had succeeded. Ato was a child who laughed freely, sang with confidence, and excelled in school.

Now, as she watched him slowly be devoured by this disease, Laura was angry with God. She admired people like her father who could accept the Lord's will, even when it seemed to impart unbearable suffering. To her they possessed the true spirit of Christ. Her faith, though, wasn't that strong. She had lived by strong Christian and American values. She was a good teacher, and John worked with underprivileged children. What, she wanted to know, had they done wrong to deserve this?

Ato had excelled in Benedict College at first. But during his sophomore year his grades plummeted. Laura hadn't pressured him for an explanation. Even when he left school, she thought he would be fine. Maybe that was when she started to lose him. He seemed directionless and somehow lonely. While Laura held no illusions that it had suddenly become simple to be a young black man, the questions that confronted Ato in the late 1980s were different, somehow more amorphous, than the ones she had faced in the 1960s, as a standard-bearer for her family. Still, she continued to give him space to float, space to come to her, space to find his own purpose. He considered the military and even went to bartending school. But rather than being empowered by his freedom, here he was now, dying in his childhood bedroom, in a sense farther away from her than ever.

By mid-December 1991 Ato was having difficulty walking, and Laura recognized that she needed help. She found an agency in the yellow pages called the AIDS Action Coalition. Not knowing what else to do, she drove him to the coalition's small office suite. Always sensitive to the racial makeup of a situation, she noticed that all the employees were white. Still, she appreciated how tender the social worker, Diane, was with Ato. Diane asked if they had tried to get him on disability. After two years of carefully avoiding any discussion of Ato's infection, Laura didn't know that her son qualified. Diane patiently filled out the paperwork, gave Laura the name of a black doctor, and urged them to come to a support group.

Laura knew Ato needed some kind of emotional support. Certainly, she needed it. So they returned at night for the group. Once again she was sensitive to the fact that the room was a ring of white faces, and emotionally she shrank back. She felt as if she couldn't talk to these people— the gulf, to her, between black and white still loomed large enough that it seemed impossible that they could empathize with her experience. She and Ato cautiously joined the circle and listened quietly. Gradually, Laura began to relax. There was something, she would later think, reassuring about the racial divide. She wasn't particularly worried that Ato's disease—with its implications of perverted sexuality, drug use, and moral corruption—tarnished her family or community in white people's eyes by confirming some kind of racist stereotype about blacks. Her shame, it turned out, really had more to do with how other blacks might judge Ato's AIDS infection: as a failure to meet the strict moral standards set by African Americans like her father before civil rights. The anonymity of being an outsider, she found, actually helped her bridge the racial gap. For the first time she was publicly at ease with Ato's illness, which helped her stop focusing on the whiteness of the faces, and the unlikelihood that they might understand her, and instead see mothers like herself, with boys dying of AIDS. As for Ato, perhaps the shame he carried was too deep to overcome in the company of anyone, or perhaps he didn't feel yet that he could share his story with Laura. In any case, he barely spoke.

At the end of January Ato began having seizures. Laura and John moved him back to Atlanta so that he could be near the AIDS clinic at Grady Memorial Hospital if and when he needed it. Laura took a leave of absence from work so that she could nurse him through the day. It was strange in Atlanta: the three of them were together, but to Laura they seemed somehow more separate from one another than ever before. John felt as if his insides were crumpling, and Ato was gently withdrawing into death. It was as if they were underwater watching one another drown and couldn't break through to the surface. In February Ato had surgery to remove boils from his face. After the operation Laura returned to Huntsville for a few days to see Janeka and deal with some business at school. The next day John called and said that Ato was having seizures that made his face freeze up as he tried to eat his oatmeal.

When Laura got back to Atlanta, they took Ato to Grady Hospital. Laura and John met with Gail, the nurse practitioner, in the waiting room. "There's nothing there," Gail said, crying. "He could go at any time." Take him home, she said, and try to make him happy. The words hit John in the gut. Laura, though, couldn't absorb them.

The next morning John left early for work. Laura dressed and went next door to Ato's room. It was her habit now to make him breakfast and get him out of bed. He was curled up under the covers.

"It's time to get up," Laura said.

There was no response.

She walked over to his bed. He was very gaunt now. There were small scabs around his eyes where the doctors had cauterized the boils.

She nudged him. No response. She tried again. "It's time for breakfast."

"Uh, uh," he mumbled.

She shook him again, and he wouldn't open his eyes.

She grabbed the phone from the night table and dialed the infectious disease center at Grady Hospital. The receptionist on the other end said the doctor wasn't in. Laura asked for Gail, the nurse practitioner. She waited a few anxious moments, and then Gail picked up. Laura told her that she couldn't rouse Ato.

"Mrs. Hall, we're probably in the very last stages of his illness," Gail said gently, "and you will find, at times, he will go into these deep sleeps when it will be difficult to rouse him. Sometimes he may come out of it and sometimes he may not. It depends on the individual. But I would like to advise you that if you haven't made any plans, you need to make some."

Laura felt as if a weight were crushing down on her chest. *Oh my God, this cannot happen,* she thought to herself. *It just can't happen.* "I don't think I can handle this right now" was all she managed to say.

"I hate to say this," Gail said, "but I'm just trying to get you prepared for what might be happening."

"Okay," Laura answered.

"Some funeral homes won't accept his body," Gail said. "If you'd like, I can give you some numbers to call."

"Thank you, no," Laura said, "that won't be necessary."

She hung up the phone, found her address book, and dialed Charles Ray, the director of a black funeral home in Huntsville who been an active philanthropist in the education community. When he picked up, she didn't know what to say.

"Do you take the bodies of individuals who have AIDS?" Laura asked cautiously.

"Sure," Ray answered.

"It's Ato," Laura said simply. "I need to start to make some arrangements, because he's very sick."

Ray said he was sorry to hear that but reassured her she could call anytime. Then he added that it wasn't necessary for her to make arrangements over the phone. She could simply stop by when she returned to Huntsville. And if she needed help before then, he would drive out to Atlanta himself.

Ato still hadn't moved. He was dying right there in front of her. Then her faith in God began to slip. She needed someone to help her understand what was happening, to help her accept it, and to tell her that she could survive. She picked up the receiver again and dialed Father Bruce Greening, the priest in Washington, D.C., who was one of the only friends she'd confided in.

"Ato has been pretty sick over the last couple of days." Laura started. "We went to the doctor yesterday. Today it's been hard to wake him. I called the nurse practitioner, and she said to me that we need to start making arrangements. I'm not able to wake him up. You've got to do something! You have to help me!"

"Calm down," Father Greening said, "and take a deep breath. I know what his situation is, and you know what his situation is. But always remember that even in one's sickest hour, there is always healing." *Right,* Laura thought to herself. *This child is going to die. How can you tell me there is some healing in that?* "I'll tell you what," Father Greening continued. "There are some things that I have to clear out this evening, and I'll catch the next flight out to see you tomorrow."

"If you're coming, I'll call in to see what kind of flight arrangements I can make."

"Yeah, that's something to keep you busy. Why don't you do that," he said. And then he prayed: "Lord, give her the strength to accept whatever your will is. Give her the strength to accept it."

Laura felt calmer after Father Greening hung up. She called John at work. No, she told him, you don't need to rush home, Ato's only sleeping. Then she phoned the airlines and found a Wednesday flight for Father Greening. Ato woke up in the afternoon. He was groggy and didn't eat anything but did manage to shower.

That night Laura met with John in the living room. Ato was asleep again. It was time for Mama to know, she said. Now that she had accepted that Ato was going to die, she felt there was nothing her family could to do to hurt him anymore. But still she needed to steel herself against their judgment. What if they didn't want to be part of Ato's death? What truth would that reveal about her family? About herself? How could she forgive them? Laura gathered herself, walked into the kitchen, and dialed her uncle Eathren's number. He was the best person to drive Elizabeth to Smyrna. He was Eleziah's closest brother, had sixteen children, and was a father figure to all the Vandivers. When he answered the phone, Laura hesitated, then said, "Ato's real sick, and I think you need to bring Mama down." Eathren didn't press her for specifics. He just said they'd be there in the morning. *Well,* she thought to herself, *this time tomorrow we'll know.*

John wasn't surprised when Eathren called at ten the next morning and said they were lost—the Vandivers had never been great with directions. He grabbed his keys and told Laura he'd go find them. For weeks now he'd felt a darkness growing inside him as he waited for Ato to die, knowing that he had nothing to give that could save his life. When Ato was in the hospital, he'd slipped John a card. "I never thought that anyone could love me," it read, "as much as you love me." John promised him that he would be with him when he took his last breath. "You'll be okay," Ato had tried to reassure him. But John knew that he would never really be okay again. They had endured for so long alone. Now that Ato's death was near, he wished the Vandivers would stay away. He knew it was selfish, but he wanted his son all to himself.

John spotted Eathren's car on the shoulder of the road and pulled in behind it. Elizabeth was in the front seat. Two other figures were in the back. It was Eleziah's sister Lois, a Fire and Holiness minister, and her brother Thomas. The Vandivers always came out in droves if someone in the family was sick. It might worry Laura to have them all there, but to him it didn't really matter anymore. John told Eathren to follow him back to the condo.

Laura greeted them at the door. What a pleasant surprise, she said, when she saw that Eathren had gathered the family elders. She led everyone into the living room. Eathren and the two women sat on the couch. Thomas sat himself in a nearby chair. Laura and John stood.

The day after Daddy died we found out that Ato had AIDS, Laura said calmly. John had always known her to be skilled at masking her emotions. Her voice, though, seemed genuinely warm and steady. Ato, she continued, didn't want anybody to know. He had seen how other people with AIDS were treated, and he had no idea how people would respond to him. His T-cells are very low now, and the doctors have pretty much given up hope.

The room was silent for a second. Then to John it seemed as though Elizabeth and Lois exploded into tears. I just hate the fact that it has taken you so long to tell us, Eathren said. We are family. If families aren't there when you need them, then they're not family. That's how your father would have felt. John didn't pay close attention to the rest of what he said. The three elderly Vandivers stood up and embraced Laura. They were quiet, but John could see that in their own way they were telling her not to worry; whatever she needed, they would be there.

Let's have a word of prayer, said Lois.

John joined hands with them to pray for Ato. Then Laura led them toward the darkened bedroom. Ato was propped up on his pillows. He looked thin, as they had hardly been able to get him to eat anything for days, but he was smiling openly, and John could see that he had heard everything from the living room. They gathered around his bed, and Lois prayed that he would find eternal rest.

That night Laura slept easily for the first time in months. Ato often played music until three or four in the morning, and John lay awake in the dark, listening, in case his son fell on his way to the bathroom.

At around midnight John thought he heard Ato's voice, coming from down the hall. He shook Laura awake. She followed John to Ato's bedroom. His light was on, and he was in bed.

"I'm hungry," Ato said.

Laura felt like crying. He hadn't wanted food in weeks. John went into the kitchen and pulled chicken and cucumbers out of the refrigerator. Laura thought of Father Bruce Greening and wondered if this was what he meant when he said that even in sickness there was healing.

When Laura got home from work, she set down her keys and headed straight upstairs toward Ato's room. It was March 1992, and a month had passed since they told the family. Physically he was still deteriorating—he weighed less than a hundred pounds now—but somehow it seemed that he was alive again. Childhood friends, neighbors, and a steady stream of cousins, aunts, and uncles from Pendleton were constantly at his bedside. They didn't ask questions or look at him sideways: they just enveloped him. Laura felt that she could finally touch, listen, and talk to her son again. That Sunday she and Ato had attended services at an AME church. The pastor, in preparation for Easter, spoke about Christ's willingness to give his life for man's sins. On the drive home Ato had turned to her and said, "I am not afraid to die."

Today Laura found him lying across his water bed in a gray polyester warm-up suit. The place was in its typically disastrous state: clothes falling out of drawers, and wires from a Nintendo set crawling across the floor. But the blinds were open, and the room was bright with afternoon sun. Everything was so perfectly normal that it almost seemed as if nothing were wrong. She walked over and sat down on the edge of the bed.

"Guess what I did today?" Ato asked calmly. "I took care of what I wanted said at the services."

"You did?" she asked cautiously.

"Yeah. You're going to love the one part, though. I've got some song requests."

"Oh." She knew that he liked rap and was thinking that they couldn't be playing that at a church.

"No, it's not rap," Ato said knowingly. "One of them is Patti LaBelle, the one that she does about telling your family that you love them. Another one is Kenny G's 'I'm Going Home,' and the last one is 'I'm Not Afraid To Die' by Reverend Bronson."

He's a lot better at this than I am, Laura thought to herself, *but we're not going to need this for a while.*

Ato looked her steadily in the eye. His gaze wasn't confrontational or falsely brave. "I want people to know what I had when I die. You know those triangle things, those things that say 'Fight AIDS, not people with AIDS'? I want you to make sure that's on my lapel. And I want you to have the casket open. I know y'all are not going to want to do that, but I want it open. I want people to see this face, and I want people to see this statement and this pin, and hopefully that message will start people to talk, and they will not suffer in the silence that I've suffered in."

"Okay, if that's what you want," Laura answered carefully.

"The other thing is that I want you to make sure you get people to donate," Ato said. "Get people to give at the service."

"Okay," Laura said, trying to hold back her tears, "if that's what you want."

"Y'all are going to have to take care of buying the casket," Ato continued evenly. "I'm not going to be able to do that for you."

"The Lord is in charge. You are not in charge," Laura said, not ready for either of them to surrender to the inevitability that he was going to die.

"I know," Ato said. "But the Lord is asking me to do this."

———

FOUR MONTHS LATER Laura gripped the handle of her grandson Darren's stroller in her black hands and pushed him past the line of blue police blockades, out of Times Square, back toward her hotel. It was July 14, 1992. Her fifteen-year-old cousin, Dawn, walked quietly beside her. Thousands of AIDS activists, their pink cheeks flushed from the sun, still choked the streets of midtown Manhattan. Laura had marched with them from Columbus Circle to Forty-second Street, to challenge America's next president to declare a war on AIDS, build a national health care program, double the budget for medical AIDS research, make HIV prevention a top federal priority, and pledge to protect the infected from hatred and discrimination. She stood out in this crowd of largely gay white men and their lovers, sisters, mothers, and friends. Yet she felt an intimacy with each of them, a sense of safety, as though she could collapse in their embrace. And in a sense she had. She had let journalists from around the world photograph her. And when Catherine Manegold of the *New York Times* spotted her in the crowd and asked why a high school science teacher from Huntsville, Alabama—who had come to New York to serve as a delegate at the Democratic National Convention—was protesting, Laura told her, "My son died of AIDS six weeks ago. I made a commitment to him that I would get involved and try to work, particularly in the black community."

Now, as Laura made her way back up Broadway, her high faded, and the summer air felt heavy against her skin. The crowd slowly dispersed, and as they let their hand-painted signs fall to their sides, they resembled revelers making their way home from a summer parade. To Laura they seemed to be withdrawing, losing themselves in private reflection, and for the first time she gave her thoughts permission to wander back over her own ordeal. She had had many painful moments she could draw from: lying in bed at home in Huntsville, late at night, under the sheets, trying to force away terrified thoughts of Ato dead in some crack house; John's swollen red eyes the afternoon the doctor told them that Ato had AIDS; and Ato, begging for change on the streets of Atlanta. Some memories came back, some remained buried.

She wondered at her fellow marchers. Where were all the black people? And why did she trust these white strangers more deeply than she had trusted her own family? She felt a pang of anger, and then the tears began to stream down her cheeks.

"Are you all right, Laura?" Dawn asked. She had accompanied Laura and John to the convention to help take care of Darren.

"You take the stroller," Laura said, seeing the helpless look on her young cousin's face. "Push him and let me walk on a while."

Falling back into the thinning crowd, Laura wept for the first time since Ato's death. The tears felt cleansing. But even as she cried, she wondered what would have happened if she had told her family at the outset that Ato was ill with AIDS. Ato's shame, and their fear of the Vandivers' judgment, had seemed so well founded, and yet it had proved to be a phantom threat. That disconnect had nearly driven her middle-class son to die in the streets. She couldn't yet unpack what that said about Ato, her family, and the ways the legacy of the American story of race continued to inform the black experience. But she was painfully aware now of how the forces at play had created a culture of silence that had nearly ruined her family, and she sensed that those forces had much to do with why just a handful of blacks had joined her to demand resources for an epidemic that was killing thousands of African Americans. Even so, she believed that the Democratic Party would hold true to its tradition of fighting for the neediest African Americans and would make addressing the epidemic a priority. Her faith had been reinforced the night before, during the opening of the convention at Madison Square Garden, when New York's mayor, David Dinkins, in a keynote address, implored the delegates to "walk the streets of this city and feel the pain of an entire nation. Feel the pain of families where three generations are ravaged by AIDS. Of tiny babies who crave deadly crack cocaine the way other babies crave their mother's breast."

CHAPTER SIX

Fractured

1992–1996

As Laura Hall listened to David Dinkins from the Garden floor on July 13, 1992, Mario Cooper, a fellow black Alabamian concerned about the AIDS epidemic, was up on the stage sitting in a control booth beneath a fifty-foot projection of the mayor that flashed across a luminescent bank of television monitors. He watched with a mixture of satisfaction, calculation, and hope as Dinkins punctuated his remarks by raising his right arm in silhouette and pointing victoriously to the oscillating sea of red, white, and blue placards. "Our streets sizzle and scream out with an anger and fury," Dinkins declared, "not seen or heard since the early days of the Depression."

To Mario, the night felt historic, but not so much because the first black mayor of New York had just delivered a line reminiscent of Bobby Seale in a keynote address to the Democratic National Convention. Mario saw Dinkins largely as a token black face who had been drafted to keep the party's liberal base in the fold during a campaign squarely aimed at Reagan Democrats. His sense of the evening had more do with the significance that he, his mentor Ron Brown, and his childhood friend Alexis Herman were the first black team to orchestrate a presidential convention. They were going to deliver the presidency to Bill Clinton. And that, Mario believed, was the last best hope for his two crumbling worlds: black America and the gay community.

Ron Brown, chair of the Democratic National Committee, had asked Mario to manage the convention in 1990. After the Dukakis debacle, Brown was under intense pressure to position the Democrats for the

White House. He wanted to assemble a small, trustworthy team to put on the convention, the centerpiece of the fall campaign and the platform from which the Democratic Party would define itself to America.

Mario was well spoken and comfortable in the fraternal culture of national Democratic politics. And he was that rare political junkie who wasn't driven by ego or a thirst for fame. A veteran of Democratic politics, he belonged to a small clique of elite black political operatives. At seventeen he had worked on Marion Barry's first political campaign in 1971; the next year he helped his older brother Jay become a member of the first class of black southern mayors; at twenty-two he worked for Sargent Shriver's 1976 Democratic presidential primary campaign; at twenty-four he was an advance scout for Jimmy Carter; and then in the early 1980s he worked on and off under Ivanhoe Donaldson in Barry's mayoral administration.

He liked pulling the ropes and moving the props behind the curtain. It wasn't so much that he was meek as that he had decided early on in his career that negotiating the line between his sense of idealism and the realities of political compromise would be easier if he stayed off the stage. It had been a thrilling position to play in the 1970s, when the party had leaders who inspired him. But as the party lost focus during the Reagan and Bush 1980s, and its candidates grew increasingly unwilling or unable to offer up anything more than canned solutions to the country's most enduring and divisive social problems, it began to feel more like drudgery. He earned a law degree from Georgetown in the mid-1980s, mostly because he had observed that people paid attention to lawyers whether or not they knew what they were talking about, and parlayed the degree into a job as a lobbyist in the Washington office of the *über*-corporate firm of Finley, Kumble, Wagner, Heine, Underberg, Manley, Myerson, and Casey just before it fell into bankruptcy. It was an admittedly lucrative and cynical move, but he also felt there were more immediate and personal ways to work politically than as an agent in the Democratic Party.

Mario lived in Cleveland Park, just outside Dupont Circle, Washington's gay, largely white, gentrified ghetto. If sex and gay pride drove politics in the Castro, Dupont Circle was a more mainstream, politically ambitious community where politics sometimes led to sex. AIDS had devastated the neighborhood. As best Mario could tell, many of the infected people working on the Hill were hiding their illness and trying to subtly affect the policies being advocated by the more radical gay activists in New York and San Francisco. Mario joined the board of the Whitman-Walker Clinic, D.C.'s politically powerful AIDS agency, in 1990, and soon afterward he became a board member of the AIDS Action Council, perhaps the most powerful lobbying consortium of AIDS organizations in the country. Meanwhile, the epidemic was growing: more than 34,000 Americans were diagnosed with AIDS in 1989; 42,000 in 1990; and 44,000 in 1991. Mario was lucky to still be HIV-negative. By the time of the convention he was being tested roughly every six months. He knew that he was staving off the inevitable, however, and that like so many of the gay men he knew, he'd likely slip up.

Mario still wasn't thinking of the epidemic in racial terms. On its face, that seemed like a strange oversight for a gay black man who had spent much of his adult life enmeshed in both black politics and gay culture. But those two worlds rarely overlapped. When it came to dating, sex, gay politics, and AIDS, Mario's points of reference were mostly white. Homosexuality wasn't as taboo in his elite black circle as it was among what some of his peers considered to be lower-class black church folk. At the same time, though, it didn't have much of a place within the culture. Consequently, he and most of his black friends were far more focused on the arrests, violent deaths, poverty, and drug use that were splintering their community. Most of the black families Mario knew had been touched by one of these crises. In his case, all he had to do was close his eyes and summon the hazy police surveillance footage of his hero Marion Barry standing in a hotel room, dressed in slacks and suspenders, hands raised to his mouth, sucking on a crack pipe.

The primary characteristic his two worlds had in common was that they were both marginal groups that pinned their hopes on the capacity of the Democratic Party to produce a victorious presidential candidate. Ironically, he knew, the path to victory would require the party to publicly disentangle itself from its less mainstream constituencies. Shortly after Mario had agreed to manage the convention, Don Fowler, the chief executive officer of the 1988 convention, sent a memo to him and Ron in which he indicated that their main failure that year had been giving the liberal arm of the party too much national exposure. "Frankly," Fowler wrote, "the Democratic Party continues to be seen by many as a collection of fringe elements and not representing the broad middle of America's population." Identifying the party's message, he also said, was "**NOT** [emphasis his] a process of letting all of the voices in the Democratic Party speak."

Bill Clinton was, of course, the ideal candidate to employ that strategy. He had been chair of the Democratic Leadership Council (DLC), a nonprofit group made up of young, mostly southern and western Democrats, founded by former Carter White House aide and party insider Al From to reorganize the party around issues like economic growth, personal responsibility, and national service. Jesse Jackson called the DLC "the Democratic leisure class." To Mario, though, Clinton had done a balletic job of quietly reassuring blacks that there would be plenty of face positions for minorities in his administration, and he figured that even Jackson would eventually fall into line. Sure, Jackson had held back his endorsement and vented to Tom Brokaw and Tim Russert about feeling isolated by Clinton in an NBC men's room after a taping of *Meet the Press*. But Mario knew that Jackson's public equivocations about Clinton were just examples of Jesse being Jesse, holding out for perks and power. From Mario's position at the Democratic National Committee, it seemed clear that the black leadership was on board. Even Mario, who was primarily responsible for the logistics of the convention, had done his part by helping to convince gay leaders that it was in their best interests to march to Times Square rather than attempt to disrupt the convention itself.

One could argue, however, that Clinton was striking a deal with the American public that ultimately could prove troublesome for black or gay America. By casting himself as a middle-of-the-road moderate, he was potentially ceding the political leverage he might need to persuade the public to make the necessary investment to solve the black and gay communities' most enduring and divisive problems. At the same time, to Mario and many others, the stakes seemed to warrant taking the risk. If Clinton won, and if he granted gay and black leaders public access to the White House, then his presidency held the potential to bring each of them back from their respective abysses and reinvent them as members of his mainstream America. So as Mario walked back to his apartment on Fifth Avenue and Twelfth Street after that first night of the convention, replaying in his head how the keynote speakers—David Dinkins, Bill Bradley, and Zell Miller—had followed the script to perfection, his reservations about the integrity of the party, his nagging distrust of Clinton, and the increasingly compromised nature of presidential politics felt distant. If the sweltering New York streets were choked with the pain of families ravaged by AIDS and crack-addicted babies, then Mario didn't feel it. He was too overcome with the ecstasy of impending victory.

In the first months after the November election, Mario stayed on the DNC payroll and lost himself in the intoxicating victory celebrations. There were parties studded with political luminaries like Janet Reno and Donna Shalala where he spotted celebrities like R.E.M.'s Michael Stipe, moments of casual flirtation, and even some sex. By this point in the epidemic, it was not uncommon to see young men in gay enclaves like Dupont Circle, Chelsea, and the Castro gingerly walking the streets with canes to support their atrophying bodies. Yet most of the gay men he knew still slept around. The scene had a discernibly tragic quality. They knew their behavior would eventually infect them and that they would suffer excruciating deaths. And yet out of some irrepressible human need for intimacy, they continued to cruise bars, sex clubs, parties, and parks. They were usually careful, but many would, inevitably, lose themselves in some unself-conscious moment of attraction, avoid tainting it by bringing up the sobering topic of sero-status, and enjoy the naked pleasure of another body. And then they would hope they'd been lucky and hadn't either become infected or infected the other person. Mario was no different, except that by his nature he was probably more fatalistic than most. He continued to be tested regularly and never swallowed semen, and when he let a man sleep with him, he insisted with an almost fervent religiosity on using a condom. In the months after Clinton's victory, though, he felt a palpable sense of optimism and possibility. It wasn't so much that he particularly trusted the new president. It was more that after years of being on the outside, Mario had faith in the people who'd have access to Clinton.

Friends and people he admired like Alexis Herman, Ron Brown, and Harold Ickes gained prominent jobs in the administration. They hinted that there was a comfortable spot for Mario as well, and the *Washington Post* even published a rumor that he was on the short list to be named chief of protocol. He was flattered but not particularly interested. Taking a White House job required submerging one's own values to achieve the broader political agenda of the president. While he had always been more of a political pragmatist than an activist, something raw and unself-conscious in the way Clinton had loosely played politics with his convictions, and in the way they all had gone along with him at the DNC in their hunger for the White House, made Mario uncomfortable. So in early spring he moved into an apartment in Dupont Circle and began looking for a job in public relations. More significantly, he decided to focus his political energy on the AIDS epidemic.

For the first time in a couple of years, he had time to cruise the bars and every couple of weeks or so take someone home for the night. One evening he had smoked a little pot, and was maybe a bit drunk, when he eyed a young man at a club a few blocks from his apartment. Washington, D.C., was a khaki-pants, sport-coat, and button-down-collar town, so this guy stood out with his long dark hair, heavy work boots, and earrings. Mario danced with him for a while and then led him out of the bar, through the darkened streets of Washington, to his apartment. The rooms were spare, furnished only to serve as a temporary landing place until he found an apartment to buy. He led the young man into the bedroom, kissing him, pulled off his clothes, and tossed them to the floor. The windows were open, and the soft spring air mingled with his lingering high. Soon he was naked, and the man was behind him. Mario knew he'd never see him again, that his name would fade in his memory, but nothing about that diminished the wonder of the moment.

To Mario, the entire gay community was losing itself in its optimism over Clinton's victory. Some who met the new president felt he projected a tone of comfort, even casual flirtation, that felt genuinely human. In March 1993 Mario helped organize a meeting between Clinton and a group of national gay and lesbian leaders at the White House. And in April hundreds of thousands streamed through Washington to rally for gay and lesbian rights. Although Clinton didn't address the crowd in person, the gay community felt that he was with them and that they were significantly responsible for his victory over Bush. With a friendly president in the White House, the shriller voices in the AIDS activist community were receding into the background, and a group of leaders were emerging who could mix more easily with the administration. During the election some in ACT UP had viewed Mario as a mole within the Democratic Party, useful mainly in brokering access to the Clinton campaign; he was now poised to take a more central position in the AIDS movement. AIDS Action Council was prepared to throw its weight behind health care reform, but the most critical piece of legislation in front of it was arguably the reauthorization of the Ryan White CARE Act.

The CARE Act, named for the teenage hemophiliac from Indiana who had died of AIDS, was originally conceived as a temporary emergency program designed to provide stopgap money for the dying who were falling through holes in their private insurance plans and the nation's medical and social welfare system. While it had indisputably helped thousands and was generally considered by public health experts and local activists to be a success, the architecture of its funding lines set a risky public health precedent. When the bill was first drafted in 1989 and 1990, AIDS activists successfully argued that state and city health departments could not be trusted to look out for the welfare of a despised minority and that therefore federal dollars should largely bypass the country's public health apparatus and be funneled directly into the hands of the affected and infected. That group was generally understood to be the gay men who ran most of the country's roughly eighteen thousand local AIDS organizations. The money dispersed through Ryan White had helped transform AIDS advocacy from a grassroots effort into a multimillion-dollar nonprofit industry and an inside-the-Beltway lobbying force. With no vaccine, cure, or even effective treatment for the virus on the horizon, those funding lines remained critical to the hundreds of thousands of Americans living with AIDS.

The key to getting the CARE Act renewed, Mario calculated, would be for the national AIDS community to present a united front on Capitol Hill. That would be difficult, as the first few years of the program had been marked by bitter squabbles over how the money was divvied up. The bulk of the Ryan White appropriation was distributed from the Treasury through HHS to the states and cities, which were then required to convene local planning boards. They, in turn, developed funding priorities, which states and cities were obligated to follow when they handed out contracts. Initially, the planning boards were largely populated by gay white men; their lovers, friends, and families; and their political and medical allies. Naturally, many had rewarded their own agencies with contracts. As the epidemic continued to spread, though, and as people anxiously realized that they were competing over a finite well of funds, accusations of favoritism, homophobia, and racism were traded between cities and planning boards, blacks and whites, the large agencies and their smaller community-based counterparts. Mario thought that AIDS Action Council—with a core membership that included the "big six" AIDS organizations in San Francisco, New York, Boston, Miami, Los Angeles, and Washington, D.C., in addition to more than one thousand smaller agencies—was poised to emerge as the leading voice in the reauthorization process. The council's strategic planning committee was scheduled to meet in June 1993, and Mario wanted them to determine, for internal purposes at least, whose interests they represented.

A few days before the meeting he was hit with a fever at work. Every muscle and bone in his body felt rusted. He left early and canceled plans for the evening. Night came, and his temperature shot up. His head felt as if it were going to split open. He managed to fall asleep, but only for a few hours, then woke up soaked in a sweat. Cramps gripped his gut. He stumbled toward the bathroom and tried to vomit. Nothing. He made his way back to bed. The sheets and blankets were filmy and damp. He'd never perspired like this from the flu. The fever continued to rack his body for the next two days. He canceled the strategic planning committee meeting. On the fourth day his fever broke. He called his doctor, Michael Pistoli, who encouraged him to come in for a quick checkup.

Pistoli's office was only a few blocks away, near George Washington University. Mario was feeling better, and after so many days holed up in his little apartment the spring walk sounded good. Pistoli, who was openly gay, greeted Mario with his customary kiss and listened calmly to his symptoms. Mario thought he looked drained, as though the past few years had worn him down.

"Well," Pistoli said, "we just tested you a few weeks ago. But maybe we should do another, just to be sure."

"Oh, ah, yeah, yeah, sure," Mario stuttered. He hadn't really thought of AIDS, but it made sense. Fever, night sweats—those were textbook symptoms of sero-conversion. Of course, they also solidly described the flu. He held out his arm, felt the prick of the needle, and calmly watched Pistoli draw a vial of his blood. It wasn't until he got outside under the expansive June sky that he thought of the young long-haired man and remembered that he'd never asked for a condom. A hard metallic pang of fear coursed through his body. *God,* he thought, *how could I have been so stupid?*

Three weeks later the test came back positive. Mario digested the diagnosis quietly. It was the kind of news that changes everything and nothing at all. He was conscious now of this microscopic monster breeding in his veins, a presence that put him in a silent brotherhood with hundreds of thousands of other infected Americans. And yet he still felt hunger, desire, and the long clean strength of his legs and back. The HIV infection might have receded from his imagination then; he might have continued with his public relations work, focusing on AIDS on the side, until the virus had hollowed out his immune system and left his body bare for a fungus or pneumonia to ravage it.

But on some level Mario was different from most of the others he knew who carried this thing: he felt no compulsion to conceal it. Perhaps that was purely a function of wealth, education, or his secularity. Or perhaps those things naturally distanced him from most of black America, while at the same time his blackness distanced him from the white world he inhabited, so that in an essential sense he was alone, and that aloneness granted him a certain freedom of openness. He called his family with the news, and at the September AIDS Action Council board meeting, he announced he'd sero-converted. In December they elected him to be both the first black and the first openly infected chair of their board.

That same month the CDC compiled its year-end surveillance reports. The disease had become the number-one killer of black men and the second leading killer of black women between the ages of twenty-five and forty-four. Their plight had received minimal popular attention. Mario firmly believed that through the AIDS Action Council he could bring them into the fold and work to politically unify the American AIDS community.

· · ·

The first serious blow to that vision came in the spring of 1994 as the debate over the reauthorization of the Ryan White CARE Act began to develop. In May Doug Nelson, the chair of the council's public policy committee, who was also the director of the AIDS Resource Center of Wisconsin in Milwaukee, flew to Washington for a meeting of the Four Title Coalition, an alliance of AIDS organizations from across the country who received Ryan White money. He intended to alert them to some flaws he'd discovered in the program's funding formula. Nelson's Milwaukee center had been flooded with more patients than it could handle. He'd made some phone calls to other AIDS workers in the Midwest and discovered that they were scuffling, too. That had prompted him to take a closer look at the fine print in Ryan White. The CARE Act was divided into a series of titles. Title I, the largest block of money, was specifically targeted at the epidemic's urban epicenters. Title II, a smaller general fund, was distributed more broadly to every state for statewide distribution. They were followed by two much smaller titles: Title III aimed at early intervention, and Title IV targeted pediatric AIDS cases. When the CARE Act was written, Titles I and II ensured that cities like San Francisco, Los Angeles, and New York, whose public health systems had been overloaded by a crush of dying young men, received immediate financial relief, while regions of the country that hadn't been so heavily taxed by the epidemic were still supported.

The epidemic, however, was now beginning to filter through the center of the country and down into the South, a process that had created serious inequities in care. Milwaukee, for instance, was not a Title I city and therefore was completely dependent on the smaller stream of Title II money. That meant, according to Doug's calculations, that San Francisco got roughly $5,000 of federal money per AIDS patient while Milwaukee received only $1,000. So while San Francisco could offer its dying Chinese acupuncture and home-delivered meals, Milwaukee had to struggle just to get fundamental services like health care and housing.

Other differences in the funding formula between the two titles presaged potentially even more serious inequities. HHS distributed Title II money through a fairly straightforward formula based on the number of people living with AIDS in a region. The Title I formula, though, was based on the cumulative number of all AIDS cases that a city could claim since the beginning of the epidemic. In other words, it let those cities count the dead. That meant that every AIDS patient in San Francisco could recover and transmission rates could drop to zero, but because those cities had been hit hardest early in the epidemic, they would still receive a large share of funding. When Doug shared these numbers with the Four Title Coalition and tried to enlist support in changing the formula in the reauthorized version of the CARE Act, the representatives from the Title I cities, who were the most powerful AIDS activists in the country and had their own lobbying group called Cities Advocating for Emergency AIDS Relief (commonly called the CAEAR Coalition), flatly told him that the funding formula was not on the table.

Mario believed Doug was right: distilling the CARE Act into separate titles and then distributing the bulk of its appropriation through a formula that lagged behind the epidemic had produced an unevenly governed system that was at best sensitive to the gay urban communities hit by the epidemic and at worst easy to manipulate and inherently unfair. The evidence seemed to support his contention. If, for instance, AIDS moved into a place like Mario's home state of Alabama, where the epidemic was emerging and which had no Title I city and no substantive network of AIDS agencies, people there would die of AIDS with little or no medical support. A deeper subtext was developing as well, one that few were talking about: AIDS was taking deeper root in impoverished minority communities. Mario believed a reauthorization of the current system could give organizations founded in gay white neighborhoods a stranglehold on Ryan White funds into the next millennium, inevitably pitting blacks and whites against one another in the fight over resources.

For Mario, the trick was figuring out how to support Doug. Logically, the strategy seemed simple: point out the problems to Ryan White's original congressional sponsors—Ted Kennedy and Orrin Hatch in the Senate and Henry Waxman in the House—and get them to collapse the titles and implement a per capita funding formula similar to the one used for Title II. The problem with this strategy was that, like black leaders, the AIDS establishment had been particularly savvy at casting itself to the federal government as a persecuted minority. In the politically correct climate of the early 1990s, the congressional sponsors of the legislation had given the gay community latitude to draft many of the culturally sensitive specifics of the bill. Presumably, Mario was in a position to help arbitrate the problem through the AIDS Action Council, which claimed to speak for all four titles. But in reality he had to appear somewhat neutral because many of the full-member organizations on his board (the ones that paid a minimum of $50,000 in annual fees) were the same Title I organizations that were opposed to changing the funding formula.

Meanwhile Doug was garnering support from the members of Congress who represented the thirty-two states that didn't have a Title I city. In June 1994 he hand-delivered a letter describing the system's inequities to more than sixty congressional and senate offices. Ted Kennedy's office warned the CAEAR Coalition's lobbyist that Doug's insurgency was threatening the chances for an early reauthorization of the CARE Act—which could prove disastrous if the Republicans retook control of the House in the November elections and tried to substantively change the bill. Mario threw his weight behind a board vote for the AIDS Action Council to mediate the conflict. It barely passed.

AIDS Action hired a professional negotiator and invited representatives from all four titles to a meeting. Doug made his pitch for equitable funding. He was told that AIDS wasn't as complicated in the Midwest and that he just didn't understand how much more difficult things were in Los Angeles. He countered that Title II cities weren't the only ones that would benefit from a straight per capita formula. Title I cities like Detroit, St. Louis, and Chicago—which were getting 30 to 45 cents per AIDS patient for every dollar going to San Francisco—would get relief, too. Those cities, though, were represented in this negotiation by San Francisco, L.A., and New York. A representative from San Francisco raised the point that cities that had been burdened with AIDS for years needed the extra money guaranteed by the old formula to sustain their effort. Doug pointed out that the places where the epidemic was spreading vitally needed that money to build AIDS networks from nothing. The argument continued back and forth. The CAEAR Coalition was willing to tinker with the formula but refused to advocate per capita equity.

On the second day of the meeting negotiations collapsed, and Doug returned to Milwaukee with only minor concessions. Over the next few weeks AIDS advocates across the country accused him of playing into Republican hands, threatening the prospects for early reauthorization, and being roundly ignorant of policy. AIDS Action tried to mediate again. Finally, Doug surrendered and agreed to a compromise that added some funding to Title II and reduced the number of deceased AIDS patients Title I cities could count toward their caseload total. The congressional session, though, was drawing to a close, and any new AIDS bill would have to wait until after the election.

In September Mario flew to Los Angeles for an AIDS Action Council board-member retreat hosted by AIDS Project Los Angeles (APLA). APLA often played the extravagant host, providing tony dinners and catered lunches and putting up the board members at swank hotels. The debate over funding equity, though, had so fractured the council that some members were threatening to resign. The representatives from New York were open to negotiating the funding formula, but APLA seemed reticent, and Pat Christen, director of the San Francisco AIDS Foundation and a major player in the CAEAR Coalition, was adamantly opposed to the concept. First, she felt it was ethically wrong to take money away from one group of infected Americans to pay for services and medications for another. Collapsing the titles into something that resembled a block grant, she also believed, would make it easier for opponents of Ryan White to chip away at its funding stream as AIDS gradually receded from the public consciousness. Furthermore, she thought many of the Title II states that were advocating for a new formula would be better served by following the model established by AIDS advocates in cities like San Francisco and New York and lobbying their state legislatures to improve their social entitlement programs. Finally, she believed that Doug's campaign would alienate Title I cities from Title II states, a strategy that would ultimately fracture the national AIDS community. The best solution, she believed, was to maintain the current system and advocate for a greater funding stream that would allow places like Wisconsin and Alabama to build AIDS services comparable to the ones that were functioning in San Francisco.

On a certain level, Christen's position made sense. Every dinner the San Francisco AIDS Foundation delivered, every support group it ran, every visit it subsidized to a specialist for a twenty-five-year-old man facing death felt true and right. The notion that the foundation should support a resolution that tore funding out from under itself just as it was cementing a stable foundation to support these men seemed intuitively wrong.

But the hard truth of Ryan White was that it didn't provide permanent solutions to the systemic holes in Medicaid and Medicare, or create a national health care system that guaranteed full coverage for everyone who needed medical care. Rather, it was a parallel program that provided limited emergency funds to allow affected communities to take care of themselves. Ryan White had allowed some gay organizations to provide an impressive roster of services for the infected while the virus was concentrated in a few urban centers.

The epidemic, though, was like a large weather system, and as it shifted and became more diffuse, the money had to be spread more thinly, among communities that were historically segregated from one another. Perhaps a better means to determine which groups and regions needed funding was the CDC's surveillance of AIDS-related opportunistic infections (AIDS-OI), like pneumonia. Those numbers suggested that the Americans sickest from AIDS no longer lived solely in the gay enclaves that were commonly associated with the epidemic. Between 1992 and 1994 AIDS-OI incidence shot up 17 percent among blacks, and regionally, the South saw the nation's biggest rise in AIDS-OI incidence, 13 percent. There were few—if any—AIDS organizations in these states that could rival the San Francisco AIDS Foundation's multimillion-dollar budget.

Most of these numbers were buried in CDC reports that Mario hadn't yet seen. He had, however, reexamined the epidemiology and discovered that infection rates had actually been proportionally higher among blacks than among whites since the beginning of the epidemic. He was no expert in public health, but wasn't the CDC supposed to have response teams that warned Americans about viruses and stopped epidemics? He had privately asked Helene Gayle, the black head of the CDC's HIV/AIDS prevention division, why more radical measures weren't being taken to stop the epidemic in black communities. She had explained that the agency was staffed by deeply caring doctors, but the science of public health in America had become entangled with politics. The CDC was ultimately beholden to Congress for its appropriations, meaning that it was in the delicate position of having to craft a prevention platform that satisfied the various constituencies lobbying around the epidemic. It wasn't difficult for Mario to read between the lines of Gayle's comments. On AIDS prevention, the Republicans deferred to the Christian Right, and the Democrats bowed to the gay community. When the CDC tried to talk frankly about sex or employ more aggressive surveillance and prevention methods to track new HIV infections, it was either undercut by Jesse Helms or pressured by gay white men to protect people's privacy.

Mario knew that while the debate over Ryan White was not overtly about race, it had everything to do with inclusion. The title system and its funding formula drove artificial wedges between different groups of infected people. Now the epidemic was tipping. Any move to reauthorize the program in its current form promised to pit these groups against one another, precisely at a moment when—Mario believed—it was crucial for blacks that the national AIDS community unify.

Ironically, the Republican sweep in the November 1994 elections gave Doug a new opening to demand equity in funding because the Republicans were less beholden than the Democrats to the AIDS lobby. Mark Barnes, the executive director of AIDS Action who ran the group's day-to-day operation, declared that the council supported Doug's single-appropriation plan. The backlash was immediate and severe and did not come solely from white gay groups. Black AIDS leaders like Cornelius Baker at the National Association of People with AIDS, along with organizations like the National Minority AIDS Council, who were already sensitive to the fact that black urban AIDS agencies had struggled to compete with gay-white-run organizations for Title I funds, claimed that redirecting money to small cities and rural America would weaken their effort to provide for minorities in urban centers. Their argument, in Mario's opinion, was shortsighted. While it was true that the majority of black AIDS infections were still concentrated in cities, 49 percent of Alabama's cumulative AIDS cases were black. So were 34 percent of AIDS cases in Tennessee, another state without a Title I city.

In his quiet and analytical way, Mario began to break the problem down in political terms. If the Ryan White program and the CDC strategy, and indeed public health in general, were steered by the politics of appropria-

tion, then the black elite must exerci
sible measure was taken to protect b
called Mark Smith, one of the first bla
who now worked for the Kaiser Family
if Kaiser could help him put together a
ica. Smith thought he could get the fo
small sum for a mass prevention effort
a few newspapers, but Mario figured th
ficient to grab the attention of the rela
opinion makers.

Meanwhile, Dr. Rick Marlink at the Harvard AIDS Institute had asked Mario to join the institute's board. Mario mentioned that he was considering holding an emergency meeting on the epidemic in black America. Marlink said he thought he could get Harvard to host it.

Even as the Leading for Life Conference came together in Mario's head, though, he began to feel unsure that the AIDS Action Council was behind him. Indeed, he wondered, could the gay white AIDS community be trusted to shepherd the epidemic as it became increasingly black? Was it even their responsibility to do so? The council was already under attack for championing Doug's single-appropriation plan. In June 1995 Pat Christen wrote to Mario that she was resigning from the AIDS Action Council board and withdrawing the San Francisco AIDS Foundation's $70,000 in annual dues. In a litany of criticisms she specifically warned that collapsing the titles would directly injure the urban poor, people of color, and immigrants. Mario's reply was short and blistering, closing with "as an African American, HIV-positive person, who grew up in the South, and whose family spent decades in the battle for civil rights, I know racism when I see it. Your attempt to inject that issue into this debate is both mistaken and misguided."

Still, Mario did actually think racism, or some twisted version of it, might be at play. He sensed resistance in the AIDS community to talking about the changing color of the epidemic. In one AIDS Action Council committee meeting, a member wondered aloud if they should downplay the epidemiology that clearly showed that AIDS was becoming a minority disease, because the information could threaten funding. Mario didn't know if that remark reflected the perfectly justified paranoia of a gay

been conditioned to believe that wealthy philan-
federal government were both unlikely to devote
minorities, or if it was a dangerous revelation of latent
erhaps—no, most certainly, Mario thought—this man believed
the interests of minorities at heart, but his intentions were irrele-
nt. Hiding the fact that a preventable disease like AIDS was spreading
through black neighborhoods virtually guaranteed that it would continue
to tear through black America. That oversight, it seemed to him, was a
brand of racism. Yet he understood that accusing his colleagues of racism
would be both counterproductive and broadly understood to be inaccurate. But he didn't have a language to express his frustration.

In its absence, Mario withdrew from his white colleagues at AIDS
Action and grew increasingly sensitive to indications that they were unin-
terested in his campaign to partner with the black elite. To his dismay,
staff at AIDS Action soon began to ask him if he could realistically pull off
the Leading for Life Conference. And he heard, or maybe he just thought
he heard, suggestions that a campaign in the African American community fell outside of the council's policy-driven purview. In November he
decided not to seek reelection as council chair. In his letter of resignation
he implored the board to remember its responsibility as a "NATIONAL"
organization and to "err on the side of inclusion," a comment that was
meant to be a slap at the large AIDS organizations over the Ryan White
reauthorization process for their failure to advocate for a system that
would support resource-poor neighborhoods and regions of the country
where the epidemic was emerging.

Maybe his warning came too late. In May 1996 President Clinton
signed into law a five-year reauthorization of the Ryan White CARE Act.
Doug, with the support of a few Republican senators like Nancy Kasse-
baum, had managed to win some concessions in the funding formula.
Significantly more money was allocated for Title II, and the new Title I
formula was based on the cumulative number of AIDS cases over the previous ten, as opposed to fifteen, years. The new bill, however, did not
repair many of the inequities previously built into Ryan White. A "hold
harmless" provision buffered cities against the effects of the new formula.
This meant that San Francisco, for instance, would still receive almost
twice as many Title I dollars per AIDS patient as Oakland, which sat fif-

teen minutes across the bay. The new version also maintained the division between the titles, which meant that states where the infections
were concentrated in Title I cities would receive 40 percent more money
per AIDS patient than the twenty-eight states without a Title I city. This
provision would prove to be particularly troublesome for southern states
where the emerging epidemic was largely black and little AIDS infrastructure was in place. Similarly, Title I cities could double-count their
AIDS patients—first for Title I dollars, which primarily went to services
for the infected, and then for Title II dollars, a portion of which helped
pay for medications. Finally, 50 percent of Title I funds would still be distributed on a competitive basis, a process that many black AIDS advocates felt powerfully favored gay white organizations. Not all these
provisions specifically set black against white. AIDS organizations that
had been founded by gay white men in urban centers increasingly
recruited black executives, opened satellite clinics in impoverished
neighborhoods, and worked to serve minority clients with great sensitivity. Taken cumulatively, however, the reauthorized version of Ryan White
cemented funding inequities for AIDS care and fractured the national
AIDS community into groups—black versus white, rural versus urban,
and gay versus straight—who often viewed each other as fighting over a
finite pie.

If anything, it reinforced Mario's growing belief that the only group
that was going to look out for blacks was the black elite. So he called the
black psychologist Alvin Poussaint, who also sat on the Harvard AIDS
Institute's board, and Henry Louis Gates Jr., who offered to cosponsor
the conference through Harvard's W. E. B. Du Bois Institute for Afro-
American Research and scheduled the Leading for Life conference for
the end of October 1996.

Pouissant had been worried about AIDS for some time. Privately,
though, he had reason to be less optimistic than Mario that the old guard
of civil rights leaders would easily embrace the notion that AIDS was
becoming a black epidemic. Even in his intellectual black circles he'd
noticed a complex psychology about AIDS. At first blacks denied that
they were afflicted by this gay white disease. Then, when scientists traced
the virus to Africa, many had assumed a rote defensive position that the
government was attempting to blame them for it.

These broader concerns didn't discourage Mario, who was beginning to think of the effort as a political campaign and the conference as a convention of sorts. He'd gather the most influential names in black politics, academia, social advocacy, and public health; shock them with the epidemiology; arm them with social marketing and prevention strategies that they could take to their constituencies; draft a black AIDS Marshall Plan; and then unveil it to the national press.

Mario put out invitations to leadership at the CDC, the National Urban League, the NAACP, the Children's Defense Fund, the White House, the leadership of the Congressional Black Caucus, and HHS. Then he called his press contacts at the *Washington Post, New York Times, Boston Globe, New York Daily News, Village Voice,* and every significant black newspaper and magazine in his database and peppered them with statistics.

In 1995 the epidemic had officially tipped: for the first time there were as many black Americans diagnosed with AIDS as white, despite the fact that blacks made up only 12 percent of the population. Mario expected his aging civil rights heroes to respond with anger, righteousness, and calls to arms. AIDS, after all, was the ultimate manifestation of the crises they had been fighting against for forty years. Mostly, however, he was met with awkward silence. The Urban League had done little about AIDS. The NAACP had five hundred youth councils and 250 college chapters, but it hadn't made any concerted effort to educate young people about the epidemic. The Southern Christian Leadership Conference (SCLC) maintained that abstinence was the best mode of prevention. One prominent journalist, after examining the list of statistics that Mario had gathered together, said to him, "There ain't nothing we can do for these kids, 'cause they'll do what they want to do."

Occasionally, Mario thought, he himself was the problem; he didn't have the charisma to move out from behind closed doors and galvanize the public. He was tall, lean, and light skinned, with a delicate jaw—handsome, but not a man who made a striking impression. His tone was lilting and modest but also distant, so that at times he managed to come across as both aloof and unassuming, the consummate insider but somehow also deeply alone. At other times he would think that it was the government's and the media's fault that blacks weren't rallying to fight the epidemic. This argument made more sense. As many black AIDS activists wanted to know, where were the billboards in black neighborhoods warning in block letters that 40 percent of new AIDS diagnoses were among blacks? That AIDS had eclipsed homicide as the number-one killer of young black men and the second leading killer of black women in America? Why had Jonathan Demme been compelled to cast Tom Hanks as the victim in his AIDS film *Philadelphia* and Denzel Washington as his reticent family-man lawyer, when the epidemiology clearly showed that AIDS was becoming a minority, and more specifically a black, disease?

Still, Mario knew in his gut that it was too easy to deflect blame onto the government, the media, or even himself. Blacks knew about AIDS, or they should have. David Satcher, the director of the CDC, was black, and so was Helene Gayle. He began to think it was the black elite who'd lost their way. A few weeks before the summit Mario broke down and wept. What, he asked himself, had been the point of all the political striving, the elected offices, the White House appointments, and the national recognition if the upper echelons of black America weren't going to stand up for the broadest segment of the black community?

On October 22, 1996, Henry Louis Gates Jr. addressed the Leading for Life Conference. Mario stood in his customary position off to the side and surveyed the room. About fifty people were present. David Satcher and Helene Gayle had flown in from the CDC. Alexis Herman represented the White House. Patsy Fleming, Clinton's AIDS czar, was there from the Office of National AIDS Policy. Eric Goosby, the black doctor who oversaw the HIV/AIDS programs for HHS, had come. So had Pernessa Seele, the founder of the Harlem Black Church Week of Prayer for the Healing of AIDS, who'd brought in some members of the clergy. And there was a strong presence of black AIDS activists. But the only major civil rights leader who'd flown to Cambridge was Marian Wright Edelman, of the Children's Defense Fund. Kweisi Mfume of the NAACP had inexplicably sent an underling. Hugh Price of the National Urban League wasn't there. Nor was Jesse Jackson. Not a single member of the Congressional Black Caucus had responded to the invitation.

Gates looked out at the group and said, "In part because of the traditional homophobic tendency in our culture, in part because of ignorant stereotypes of HIV and AIDS, our people, our leaders, our culture have long been in denial about AIDS in the black community."

CHAPTER SEVEN

Surfacing

1990–1996

Desiree Rushing saw the sign for the church car wash on Mac-Donald Avenue in Richmond, California, and pulled her car into the parking lot. It was the spring of 1995, four and a half years after she had been diagnosed, and she was with her friend Edwin White. They'd met at Faith Full Gospel Church on nearby Rumrill Boulevard. Her younger sister Monique was dying, and she felt vaguely attracted to the comfort of his company. Still, she didn't think the relationship would go very far, since she'd been trying to steer away from men. It wasn't so much because she was frightened to tell them that she was infected. Her ex-boyfriend Bob was one of the first people she'd called with the news that she had HIV; he'd tested negative and was still after her, along with a few other black men whom she'd told about her diagnosis. Rather, her decision to stay single had been driven much more by her desire to live by the word of the Bible, which made clear that sex outside marriage was sinful. It may have been hard to be a thirty-six-year-old black mother with no man in her life—hard to be alone and hard to forgo sexual pleasure. But she had to live by God's will. She believed that He had a purpose for her and that He had promised to keep her alive so she could fulfull it.

Desi had matured in an increasingly chaotic black urban world, where she and many of the people around her seemed to persevere only by inuring themselves to the events that disrupted their lives, to the point that at times they seemed to be blind to them. Desi's diagnosis in 1990, though, had been incontrovertible, a truth she spoke with confidence, and she had told everyone about it. The day the social worker informed her that she was HIV-positive, Desi went back to her apartment on Alcatraz Avenue in Oakland and waited for Ken. He was twelve. When he came home from school, she looked into his open face and said, I have something to tell you. He stood there quietly. I have AIDS, she said. She told her sisters, Wafer, and her best friend, Ada Pierson, as well as the men she had slept with.

She wasn't sure how she expected them to react. She simply felt that the truth had to be told, and she wanted to give them a choice that she had never been given by the man who infected her: to stay with her, or get away. But what she got in response was almost nothing. Ken was quiet and kept his fear to himself. A few weeks afterward he went to Chucky Cheese Pizza for his cousin Dominique's birthday. It was a children's party heaven, with bowling lanes, prizes, and Chucky the giant rat mascot. He wandered off into the men's room, pushed into an empty stall, and cried alone. Wafer was calm as always. You're gonna be all right, she said. Only Desi's sister Monique was openly devastated by the news—and she seemed convinced that Desi going to die.

In a way it seemed as if her words, the information—her impending death—had sunk into the same ocean of silence and denial that Desi had spent her whole life trying not to drown in. Even Desi had refused to become overwhelmed by the news. But she still seemed to need to make sense of it. To Desi the Holy Spirit—and the tongues she had spoken—were irrefutable evidence of God's existence. She believed that her salvation would be eternal and that she would pass on to heaven. Why then, a part of her needed to know, had God allowed her to contract this disease?

A few weeks after her diagnosis she attended an all-night prayer meeting with Ada at Oakland Christian Center. They spoke in tongues. Dawn broke, and Desi still wasn't tired. She asked Ada if she could go over to her house with her. Something was going on. She felt as if God were tugging at her. Ada's apartment was small. Desi sat down at the kitchen table by herself. *Lord,* she prayed, *if your word said that Satan came to kill, steal, and destroy, and you came so we could have life, why do I have AIDS?*

Then she believed she heard God respond: *How dare you suggest that I gave you this disease? You haven't been sick. You didn't even know that you had this disease until I told you.* The voice wasn't magical or overpowering. It was much like her own, and it seemed to penetrate her soul. *I will keep you,* He said, *if you tell people that I am real.*

"Ada," Desi called out, "I'm going to be all right."

"Yeah," Ada cried back from the living room, "I got it, too. God said you're going be healed."

Desi believed that Ada was wrong—he had promised not to heal her but to "keep her," meaning that the virus would stay alive in her bloodstream. She believed that He was calling on her to find others who were suffering and tell them that they did not have to fear Him, that He did not hate them, and that He could protect them—so long as they lived by His word. Her enduring good health would be her proof.

Nearly five years later, she sat in the church parking lot with Edwin White waiting for her car to be washed. And a part of Desi knew that she was failing to fulfill God's bidding.

Desi looked up. The man washing her car was speaking to her.

The Lord is not pleased with you.

Do I know you? Desi asked. It wasn't unusual in black Christian circles for even strangers to advise one another on their relationship with God.

No, the man answered. But God has got a calling on your life. And you need to do what He told you to do.

Thank you, Jesus, Desi started reflexively.

No, no, no, it's deeper than all that, he said. I don't know what it is. But you're supposed to be dead.

———

FOR NEARLY a year after He spoke to her in Ada's kitchen, Desi did not fully embrace God's call to seek out the suffering and the faithless. Maybe that was because she hadn't wanted people thinking that she was crazy; maybe it was too difficult for her to be near others in pain and to sense, touch, and inhabit their suffering; or maybe she felt that she needed comfort herself. Whatever the reason, she immersed herself in the safety of the Oakland Christian Center. Pastor Hughes made sure that she sat up near the front of the church. She attended Bible study and prayer groups, and testified that she was infected and saved in front of the large Sunday morning congregation.

At the end of 1991, after the incident in Ada's kitchen, she moved to the neighboring city of Richmond. Desi's youngest sister, Simone, encouraged her to join a local congregation, Faith Full Gospel, a few blocks from her new home. Desi attended a couple of services but had no intention of leaving the Oakland Christian Center for this plain church that looked more like a storefront than a place of worship. In the equally spare interior chairs were set up in a windowless room no bigger than a kitchen. Pastor George Robinson, not much more than five and a half feet tall, preached the word to his wife, their two children, maybe a friend or two, and Desi and Simone.

She didn't go back, but then a week or two later she woke up in the middle of the night with the words *tend thee to thy own backyard* running through her head. Perhaps, she thought, it was the remnant of a bad dream brought on by all the drug- and gang-related violence that had helped cement Richmond's reputation as Oakland's ghetto. But the phrase lingered with her, so she asked God to show her what He meant. Then she was awakened again with the same words—*tend thee to thy own backyard*—floating through her mind. She shook it off. A few days later, after working the night shift, she stopped off at the twenty-four-hour grocery store near her house and picked up a frozen dinner. As she pulled out of the parking lot onto the street, a young man stepped off the sidewalk in front of her headlights. It was nearly two in the morning. Desi pressed on the brake. To his right were a group of teenagers. *Hoodlums,* she thought. The man pulled out a gun and aimed at the kids. Desi fumbled for the window handle, but her hand found only the side of the door. She screamed through the glass. The man fired a single shot into the crowd, and the kids scattered.

Suddenly she found herself sitting alone, bathed in the light of the streetlamps, with only the patter of soft rain disturbing the silence. Shaken, she eased her car into gear and drove home. She made it into her house, set down her purse, and then caught herself. *Oh Lord,* she thought, *I got to go back.* By the time she returned to the grocery store, the parking lot was quiet. She drove slowly through the dark streets and was about to give up when she noticed a group of kids walking through the rain. She pulled up beside them.

What you doin' out so late? she asked.

Oh woman, said an older boy, perhaps sixteen, this ain't none of your business. You don't have to worry about us. She could tell he was trying to make like a man.

Then another one pushed through the group and up to the side of her car. Lady, I been shot, he said, pulling up his shirt to reveal a torn streak of skin where the bullet had grazed his side. He looked frightened. These children struck her as lost and leaderless. She killed the motor and stepped out into the night.

Can I pray for you? she asked.

They gathered around her and clasped hands. The hardened masks of anger and defiance slipped from their faces to betray a group of tear-streaked children. *There is a Lord,* she thought, as they prayed in the rain. *There is a comforter.*

Where do y'all live? she asked.

On South Tenth Street, said one.

Her house was on South Eleventh. They were literally in her backyard.

The next morning she woke up, reached for her phone, and called Pastor Hughes at the Oakland Christian Center. She started to cry. She had to leave his congregation, she said. The Lord, she explained, had given her a sign. Pastor Hughes asked her if she was sure, but she simply thanked him through her tears and placed the phone down on the receiver.

She joined Faith Full Gospel and walked door to door through the chewed-up streets of Richmond telling people that God could reinstill a sense of purpose in their lives. She could feel God's power building in her. But it was hard work, and it seemed to her that God kept confronting her with people who were suffering. One afternoon she was working her shift at the hospital when she passed by a quadriplegic patient's room and heard God say that the man was going to be part of her life. Days later she walked by his door again and heard God say, *Go in his room and tell him that I'm with him and he's not going to die.*

She stopped. *I ain't gonna go in there and tell him God spoke to me,* she thought to herself. *He's going to think that I'm crazy. I ain't doing it.* Over the next month, though, she stopped in on him a few times. His name was Keith, and he told her that he had asked God for a sign that he was going to be all right. I need to apologize to you, Desi said. He asked me to tell you that you would be fine, and I didn't. I need to apologize to you, and I need to apologize to God.

After Keith was discharged, Desi ministered to him at his East Bay home. He had spent years alone in bed while his mother worked during the day. The black skin on his back had turned white from lying in his own urine. Desi learned how to turn and clean him. She put on gloves, reached up his anus, and loosened his bowels. She brought him to Faith Full Gospel. They watched the Christian Channel together. She brought social services in on his case. And she helped him get physical therapy, psychotherapy, and a new wheelchair. Why, his mother asked, would you come here and give of yourself like this? What do you want? And all Desi could think was that she was doing it for the Lord.

Gradually Desi helped build the congregation at Faith, and in time her HIV infection seemed to become incidental to her larger faith in God. She had one AIDS book, which the social worker had given her, a thin paperback titled *HIV: From A to Z,* published by the Sacramento AIDS Foundation, that had chapters like "Inner-health" and "Dealing with an HIV-diagnosis" and "HIV Relationships: Loving Yourself, Others, and Your Community." She studied it from cover to cover, but her faith was so strong that she didn't fear people's prejudice or need an AIDS support group. In her mind she had confessed her faith, and she believed that God was going to keep her so long as she followed His call.

Then in 1993 Wafer called and told her that her sister Monique had gone in for a routine physical, and they had given her an HIV test. The results hadn't simply come back HIV-positive. Her T-cell count, the number of disease-fighting white cells in a sample of her blood, was less than twenty. A healthy person had thousands. Monique had AIDS.

Desi was strong for Monique. She promised to find her the best doctor and tried to nurse her. But it was spiritually, emotionally, and physically devastating to watch Monique die. Over the two-year course of Monique's illness, Desi increasingly immersed herself in the comfort of the ministry. In fact, it was Monique's illness that drew Desi to Edwin: Desi didn't want to be alone when her time came. Then she was confronted by the man at the car wash, and a few months later, in July 1995,

Monique fell into a coma and was rushed to Alta Bates Summit Medical Center. Her doctor gathered the family and said there was nothing more they could do. Desi asked for a cot and sat up through the night next to her dying sister.

They had always looked remarkably alike—tall like Wafer, with high foreheads, mahogany skin, circular cheekbones, and sparkly brown eyes that pulled down into the shape of playful half almonds when they smiled. Monique, though, had been rounder and more corpulent than Desi. Now Monique was vanishing before her eyes. She had dropped from 300 pounds to 280, then 220, then 185; she passed Desi at 160 and then fell to 140, 120, 110, 98. Her mind was disappearing, too. More than once Desi had found her sitting in her little red car in front of Wafer's house staring off into space as if in a trance. Even her place in the world seemed to be fading. She had hidden her infection from her boss at the Berkeley Sanitation Department and had been asked to quit for missing too many shifts. She'd been evicted from her apartment because she couldn't pay the rent. Her skin hung loosely from the bones of her face, and much of her hair had fallen out. And as she lay there at Alta Bates Summit Medical Center in the oceanic depths of a coma, somewhere between life and death, her spirit felt unknowable to Desi.

To some, it might have been difficult to understand why God had chosen to keep Desi alive and allowed her sister to swiftly waste away. Monique was good, a single mother of two children. She had taken maybe two lovers in the last ten years. She rarely drank, never did drugs, and was quiet and unassuming, the kind of sister who cut school to look after Ken so that Desi could run the streets. It was Desi who'd had sex with men while her friends kept lookout for her boyfriend; it was she who had had to draw hot baths in the middle of the night to ease off her crack high, who had hit her husband, and who had let herself get beaten while her son hid in his bedroom closet. She was the sinner, not Monique.

Even as the question, twisted with guilt and fear, hovered over her, there was an answer that Desi, her mother, and her sisters could find in their faith: this wasn't the Lord's world; humans lived in it, but they weren't of it. Eddie on top of her, Philip's flying fists, Crys raped and shot dead, Desi's infection, none of them was His doing. He was the comforter. This world belonged to Satan. Satan made you doubt. He disrupted your essential faith. He surrounded you with suffering and then made you believe you had to anesthetize yourself. That was impossible. Sure there had been times when Desi had been able to dampen suffering's flame with crack and liquor and pot. But the pain had always come back hotter, stronger, wilder, and more destructive than ever. Only her relationship to God had been able to protect her from it. Monique wasn't with God; she hadn't been saved; she hadn't accepted Christ into her life. That had left her vulnerable to the ravages of this disease. Now Desi needed God to keep Monique alive.

Desi leaned over her sister, let the Holy Spirit course through her, and spoke to God in His language of tongues. The night bled into early morning. Desi wasn't sure if she had drifted off or was still awake. Suddenly she was aware that her sister had opened her eyes.

"Monique."

"Huh."

"Does God want you?"

One mile south of Monique's hospital room, early morning darkness swept through Wafer Theus's apartment, mixing with the quiet anxiety of death. Monique's children, Dominique and Christopher, were asleep. So was Wafer's youngest daughter, Simone. Wafer lay alone in her bed by the phone, waiting for it to ring. Until recently she had never deeply considered the possibility that AIDS would kill Monique. The day Monique burst into her apartment, screaming that she had AIDS, she had been calm. We'll work through this, she'd said. It'll be okay; they have medication; you're going to be all right; you're going to be strong. No, I'm not, Monique had repeatedly cried, no, I'm not. You'll be fine, you'll be fine, Wafer had gently repeated. And Wafer had believed that she would be, the same way she had faith that Desi would be all right when she had announced in that determined "I just quit my job" tone that she'd contracted HIV. Wafer's confidence could partly be explained by the fact that she didn't know much about the disease. Still, she knew it was deadly. Perhaps her stoic faith had more to do with the fact that Wafer had seen firsthand a long time ago that the specter of death could sometimes be more deadly than the agent of death itself.

When Wafer was four, her mother, Hattie, had piled her, her two brothers, and her sister onto a train in Kilgore, Texas, bound for Oakland, where their father had gone on ahead a year earlier to find work. Her most striking memory from the trip was of the train's conductor. He gave them a smoking car to play in. And he looked at Hattie and said, "Lady, if you make it to California, I hope you don't have a nervous breakdown." Hattie's marriage didn't last more than a year after she arrived in Oakland. She moved Wafer and the children into a large Victorian with a towering palm tree in the front yard in West Oakland and managed to pay the bills with welfare and the bit of money she could scrape together from a series of boarders.

But at the end of the war Hattie's sanity crumbled. She didn't leave her bed for nearly a year. Maybe it was the strain of raising four kids alone, or the move from Kilgore to Oakland, or maybe it had to do with those times she was beaten by her husband.

Wafer never let herself be broken in the same way. She fought Harold when he first started drinking, seeing other women, and burning through jobs. But as it became clear to her that he was lost, she disengaged. Even when he beat her, she was coolly prepared to kill him. After they were divorced, she worried about her daughters' safety and health, cooked, and cleaned. But she didn't let herself be overcome by the uncertainty of the city around her. She didn't balk when Desi decided to stay home from school for six months after Crys's murder; she often acted as though she didn't see Desi's drug use; she didn't fall apart when Harold haunted and harassed her; she didn't disintegrate when her older sister died of lupus, or when her developmentally disabled brother passed.

At times that calmness may have made her seem distant, accepting of the small and large tragedies that unfolded around her. And perhaps in some ways she was. But she didn't run from them. She was still in the center of a world marked by moments of threat. And that stoicism, which may have been what caused Desi to feel that there was a distance between the events that she experienced and how they were interpreted, also made Wafer the anchor of the family, the presence in which everything became quiet and perhaps, even for a moment, normal.

So Wafer didn't shrink from Desi's and then Monique's announcements that they were HIV-positive, and she didn't try to hide their diagnosis or fear retribution from her friends. But at the same time it seemed somehow unreal to her that either of her daughters would die. Desi looked so healthy. She believed that was because Desi was with Christ. Monique, though, had descended into a physical hell on the black leather couch in her living room. Wafer cleaned her after she used the toilet and held her steady when she vomited up the seemingly useless medications. Black sores spread like mold across her arms and breasts. Her legs swelled to a point that she would scream out if her children even brushed against her feet. Her lungs got so clogged with mucus that she could barely breathe without coughing.

After a while Wafer couldn't get her to take her pills and often found them hidden under her pillow. Monique stopped eating. She acted like she was dangerous to the people around her. Wash that out, she'd yell when Wafer picked up her water glass. Use sterile gloves, she'd demand when Wafer cleaned her. To Wafer, there seemed to be a haze of hopelessness about her, an emptiness; she had no faith.

Now the doctors had told Wafer that Monique wasn't going to come out of the hospital, and she finally had to face the truth that her daughter was going to die. She had spent a night praying with Pastor Robinson and nearly twenty parishioners from Faith Full Gospel for God to take away Monique's pain. Maybe the merciful thing to do now was to ask for death. Certainly, Wafer couldn't stand to see her daughter tortured any longer. But if Monique died now, before she found Jesus, Wafer believed that she would burn in hell for eternity.

The ringing telephone jarred Wafer awake. She knew it was Desi, and that Monique was dead.

"Granna," Desi said on the other end, "do you want to talk to Monique?"

"Don't play with me."

"Monique came out of her coma."

Then Monique was on the other end. "I love you, Granna, and I want to see you and the kids."

Wafer drove Monique's children to Alta Bates. When they found Monique lying awake in her room with Desi, there was a calmness about her, as if she had been freed from the anger, bitterness, and fear that had consumed her for the past few months. Christopher and Dominique wrapped themselves around their mother. The doctors discharged her from the hospital. Her father, Harold, came by the house; he found a wheelchair, took her to the mall, and bought her diamond earrings. On Sunday Monique told Wafer that she wanted to go to church one more time. Wafer helped her into a pink dress and brown shoes. Wafer, Desi, and Simone drove Monique to Faith Full Gospel's small sanctuary on Rumrill and sat near the back with her. At the end of the service Pastor Robinson asked if anyone wanted to come forward and receive Jesus.

Monique tapped Wafer on the shoulder. "I feel the spirit, Granna," she said. Wafer gently helped her daughter from her wheelchair, being careful not to disturb her shunt—the tube the doctors had attached to her to help her blood flow—and walked her slowly to the pulpit. She held Monique steady while Pastor Robinson laid his hands on her. The pain Monique had felt for months in her legs, feet, veins, throat, and lungs dissolved. She wept, shouted out in joy, and prayed. Then she began to jump and shake. In Wafer's eyes, Monique was feeling the presence of the Lord; she had accepted Christ and was saved.

A couple of weeks later Desi pulled up in front of Wafer's apartment building, one of dozens of characterless boxes that had been built during the housing shortage of the 1960s and 1970s. Wafer had called and said Monique was breathing funny. Desi followed the narrow alleyway along the side of the building toward Wafer's front door. Through the walls she heard a low and raspy groan, almost like the sound of the rolling ocean: the death rattle, as she knew from her shifts in the hospital. Desi pushed through the front door into the darkened living room and found her sister gasping for air. "Granna," Desi said strongly, "call nine-one-one."

Desi didn't feel frightened anymore. The medics packed Monique into the ambulance and rushed her to Alta Bates, where she fell into another coma. Desi asked for a cot, determined not to let God take her sister. The hours turned into days. Desi's sisters wandered in and out of the room. But Desi felt that she was with Monique, standing in the gap between life and death. When Monique felt pain, Desi felt it, too, and she screamed for morphine. When blood leaked from the tubes coming out of her sister's mouth and nose, Desi cleaned them. She was asking God to let Monique stay. She knew it was selfish: Monique was suffering, and He was ready to usher her into heaven. But she believed the Lord wouldn't take Monique in her presence. I haven't been a good person as a child or as an adult, Desi told her sister, but I promise to make you proud. When Wafer came again, Desi told her, "It's okay, Granna, you can let her go." Yet even as she gave Wafer permission to release Monique, Desi still wasn't ready to do it herself.

When August 17, 1995, dawned, Desi had been at Monique's side for nearly seventy-two hours. Wafer, Gigi, Monique's friend Sean, and Mary, a friend from Faith, joined Desi in the room. "Go on, Desi, and get some rest," Wafer said. Desi refused. But they insisted that she go home, if just for a few hours. *She's going to die,* Desi believed. *The Lord said He would take her if I leave.* But she was exhausted from trying to will Monique to live. Okay, she agreed, she would just go home for an hour.

She gathered her things, made her way to the parking lot, where she found her Firebird, and in a daze pulled out onto Ashby Avenue. She crossed Telegraph and then Shattuck Avenues. Gradually the Victorians—standing tall, wooden, and quiet like sentries on the corner of streets like Regent—became single-story black homes, with chain-link fences.

Meanwhile, at the hospital, Wafer looked at Monique, her teeth cracked from the seizures, holding a stuffed bear that Desi had won for her at a fair, and waited for her daughter to die.

Desi pulled up in front of her house. Edwin wasn't there. She didn't really care. She didn't love him. All she needed was God and the truth now.

At the hospital Mary went to Monique's side and began adjusting the bedclothes. Monique was very still. "She's stopped breathing," Mary said.

Wafer's face ran with tears. "She's out of her misery," she said. "No more pain and suffering."

Desi walked into her apartment, peeled off her clothes, slipped into her pajamas, pulled back the bedclothes, crawled under the covers, and let her head fall on the pillow. Then the phone rang, and she knew immediately that her sister was dead. She pulled herself out of bed, climbed back in her car, and drove to Alta Bates. When she saw Monique, the tension was gone from her face.

Eventually they drove back to Wafer's apartment, where Dominique answered the door. She was ten years old and thin like Desi. Her father had disappeared years ago, and so had Christopher's. Dominique had music playing. In that way that children try to control the uncontrollable by controlling the little things, she had cleaned the entire apartment. Desi told her and Christopher that their mother was dead. Christopher, who had clung to his mother over the final weeks, took the news silently, but Dominique screamed and ran across the small living room, up the stairwell, and into the bathroom. She stopped in front of the toilet, the back of which was an altar of medications. She raised her arm and swept the bottles onto the floor.

"None of them worked!" she screamed. "None of them worked!"

Pastor George Robinson felt a responsibility to help the Theus family make sense of Monique's death, so he insisted that he preside over her funeral at Faith Full Gospel Church. He had always felt that one of the most misread lines of the Bible was "The Lord giveth and He taketh way. Blessed be the name of the Lord," from the Book of Job. Too many people, he felt, understood it to mean that the Lord struck down their loved ones to punish them for their sins. This vision of a vengeful and punitive God was arguably troublesome because disease, violence, drugs, and prison had hit black families all over Richmond. Too many of them, even in his own congregation, had come to accept these tragedies as both deserved and natural. That perception had bred a culture of defeat, which, he thought, was why the members of his city and congregation, the children of the last great black migration from the South, seemed blind to how deeply their city had rotted; why they complacently received their checks from the government; why they let trash pile up on the streets, set cars up on cinder blocks in their front yards, and passively waited for landlords to fix houses that had fallen into disrepair. Nobody could stand to live like that for long, and it wasn't surprising that people were turning to sin for comfort. Kids were running unpunished with guns and drugs. Armed robbery, domestic abuse, alcoholism, and drugs were everywhere. He didn't believe his role was to condemn them for their sins. He felt he needed to show them that God loved them and that they could rediscover purpose, power, and hope through His word.

Pastor Robinson, then, never fixated on how Monique had contracted the disease. Instead, he focused on her lack of peace, the way she gingerly walked like an arthritic old woman, and how her skin hung slackly from the bones of her face. In her he saw a pain so deep that it had taken over her body and was sucking the life right out of her. Maybe there were medicines that could help her, but he wasn't interested in the mechanics of the disease. Only God had the ultimate power to help her in this world and the next. So in the final weeks of her life he prayed with the family for her to find Jesus. That day in church, when the Holy Spirit overcame her and he laid his hands on her, he had felt life flowing through her frail body.

Now, a couple of weeks later, on the afternoon of the funeral, Pastor Robinson pulled on a crimson robe. The sanctuary was nearly filled as he made his way past the mourners to a spot off to the side of the podium. Black church funerals were traditionally elaborate affairs. Even the poorest families often spent entire life insurance policies on motorcades, flowers, food, and caskets. The Theus women, though, seemed lost. They didn't rent cars or buy dresses. Pastor Robinson's wife had hastily oiled the pews and stapled fabric over the worn chairs in the windowless and carpeted sanctuary in an effort to make it at least presentable. Harold and Wafer were in the front row, stone-faced, with Dominique and Christopher, Desi, Simone, Gigi, and Chan. One of their teenage cousins walked up to the front of the sanctuary and stood next to a picture of Monique that Desi had found from before her illness.

He pulled out a sheet of paper and read a poem about a rose blossom that sheds its petals in the winter to make room for new buds. The words seemed to suggest that Monique's death was a natural part of an organic cycle of birth and life. But wasn't she the victim of an epidemic that was slowly seeping through the East Bay? And wasn't it true that there were no cures, no magic bullets—that once the virus spread through her body, she was as good as dead? And wasn't her death unjust? Shouldn't the government, the city, and the health department have done more to stop this disease before it ever reached her bloodstream? Those questions, and more like them, hung over Pastor Robinson as he gathered himself to address the Theus family. But for him, they were immaterial to the larger question of what role the Lord had played in Monique's death. Because if it was the Lord who took this woman, or if her death indicated the absence of God, then how could any of them move forward?

So before he stepped behind the lectern to deliver the eulogy, he hadn't bothered to research the disease that killed Monique; he didn't know that in 1995 40 percent of the Americans who had been struck by the disease were black. And when he spoke, he didn't tell the family that there was nothing they could have done. He didn't talk about the threat AIDS was posing to all the children in the room, or how the congregation needed to mobilize their elected officials, doctors, and clergy to protect the community against this plague. He didn't preach on sin, or address Monique's culpability in her own death. He didn't even say the word *AIDS*. Rather, he recounted the story of how Monique found God.

Slowly, the family rose from the pews and shuffled out of the sanctuary. Wafer, though, collapsed before the photograph of her daughter. "It's my fault!" she screamed. "I could have done more! It's my fault! I could have done more!"

Sometimes during a funeral there is a moment when the truth of death cuts so deeply that someone will suddenly let out a piercing wail of grief. The sound is so natural, human, and pure that most people simply accept it. When friends try to control the husband's or mother's or wife's or sister's sorrow, they usually fail, because it is a crushing pain, one so potentially overwhelming that it feels close to death itself and in that sense can be dangerous.

Desi hardly cried at Monique's funeral, and she hardly cried in the weeks that followed. She felt numb, as though wrapped in a muffling fog. This disconnected sense of nothingness permeated every area of her consciousness. She was, in a sense, only half alive. She asked her doctor to put her on disability. When he determined that her infection hadn't progressed enough to justify a state-sponsored paycheck, she found another doctor who thought it had. But she didn't seek psychotherapy or ask Pastor Robinson for spiritual counsel. She just attended church and prayed to God.

Fall blended into winter, gradually the fog receded, and Desi began to feel the edges of the world again. She had emerged from similar crises before—when Crys was murdered, after Ken's father went to prison, and after her parents were divorced—and she had met her pain with a rebellious, searching fire. Perhaps that had been a sign of life, a refusal to succumb, a radical rejection of those events. This time, though, her anger didn't surface. Desi had been reborn through her spiritual awakening, though not in the largely vacant sense of an epiphanic conversion to Christianity. It had been a more gradual and perhaps complete process of renewal that began with her HIV diagnosis. She had come to understand that diagnosis as a blessing from God: proof that He existed; proof that He loved her in spite of her sins; proof that this was Satan's world; and proof that she was not of Satan's world.

Discovering the comfort of God had been only the beginning of her rebirth. She didn't believe that God had healed her. She believed that God's gift to her had always been to see pain and feel compassion. Those "gut feelings" she'd had when she was a kid weren't just feelings, she'd come to believe that they were God showing her suffering. In that sense, she seemed to experience the comfort she found in her relationship to Him less as an anesthetic than as a way to linger with the chaos that had marked her life and the lives around her. She believed that God continued to put suffering before her—Keith, the children of Richmond, and then Monique—so she could bring them to Him. It had been taxing work. Monique's illness and death had taken Desi to the edge of her own life.

Now, as she emerged from her grief, she knew that she could continue to confront the painful realities of this world. She threw Edwin out of the house and began spending time at Tranquillium Center, a Richmond AIDS agency. Technically she was a client, but she spent most of her time counseling other patients. In 1996 the head of Tranquillium sent Desi to meet Rebecca Denison, the director of an Oakland AIDS agency called Women Organized to Respond to Life Threatening Disease (WORLD). Rebecca, an HIV-infected white mother of two, had recently organized a series of classes for other infected women under the name "HIV University" and had also started an HIV newsletter in which she published profiles of women living with AIDS. In the summer of 1996 they met in Rebecca's office.

Rebecca Denison immediately noticed Desi's directness—Desi wanted her story published. When she told it to Rebecca, her words seemed forceful and uncompromised, in a way that was different from the words of many of the infected black women Rebecca had interviewed. Desi fled through the landscape of her life. There was Eddie bashing out her windows, Harold drinking, little Ken brandishing her crack pipe, the pastor at the car wash telling her that she was supposed to be dead, her sense that she had been lied to growing up, Monique dead at Alta Bates, and surrounding it all, God.

Rebecca didn't question Desi about how any of these things were related to AIDS. The two women were sitting maybe four feet apart; they had lived in the same city for nearly ten years, probably at times within a couple miles of each other; and they were both infected with HIV. But Desi existed in a place where the rules were different, a place that Rebecca couldn't see. In that sense, she was like a woman standing in the center of a tornado trying to describe the wind. That frightened Rebecca, because there were thousands of black American women in Desi's storm, and in the absence of any organized effort to understand their needs, history, or faith, it had somehow fallen to her to link them together.

Rebecca felt that she shouldn't still have been there in her drab Oakland office, fifteen years after the first case of AIDS was reported, trying to map out Desi's life. She should never have been there at all. She had been twenty-eight, recently graduated from UC Santa Cruz, just married to her husband Dan, and looking forward to starting at Hastings Law School, when she was diagnosed with HIV in June 1990. She had decided to take an HIV test only as a show of support for her girlfriend Susana, whose sister Becky had been diagnosed with AIDS. They went in for the results on a Saturday. On the way to the clinic they stopped for ice cream and lingered at a yard sale in the Castro, where Rebecca bought a bundt pan. In the waiting room Susana was nervous. "If I'm positive," Rebecca joked, "I'll kill the guy who infected me." She wasn't worried about her own test. She was from Corvallis, a small Oregon town, and had slept with only four men in her life. And Dan—well, he was just a sweetheart of an elementary school teacher from an Irish Catholic family in San Jose, whom she'd met in an "intro to feminist thought" class in college.

Rebecca walked up to the counter and handed her paperwork to the receptionist, who introduced her to a counselor. Just then the receptionist hesitated and said, "Wait a minute. No. Never mind." Then the counselor led Rebecca down a hallway to a small cell. "Would you like to tell me why you got tested?" she asked Rebecca, flipping through her file. "Well, I'm going to law school, and my best friend's sister is positive," Rebecca began, and she started to feel rather sick. *What sort of question was that?* she thought. "Your test came back positive," the woman said coolly. Rebecca felt as if an invisible train had shot across the room and hit her in the chest. *Oh God, Oh God, Oh God, I'm never going to have children* were her first thoughts. *Oh God, Dan. If I've got it, I've probably given it to Dan.* And then *How am I going to tell my parents?* That's when the tears came.

The counselor handed her a stack of pamphlets with phone numbers for gay male support groups. "What about children?" Rebecca asked, repulsed by the woman's bloodless manner. Women give it to their babies 30 percent of the time, the counselor said. Then she started laying out the rules of safe sex. *What is this woman talking about? I'm never going to have sex again. I'm dead.* Careful who you tell, the counselor warned—you could lose your job and your health insurance. And then she asked if there was anyone Rebecca could confide in. Rebecca glanced toward Susana, who had been summoned to the office to check on Rebecca and was grinning with relief from her own negative result.

Dan flew back from Guatemala, where he'd been enrolled in a Spanish-language program, a few days later. He tested negative. On Fourth of July weekend Rebecca and Dan drove up to Oregon and told her parents. Her father, a mycologist, told her he could get rare medicinal herbs from around the world. Rebecca and her mother told the local paper, which published a front-page story on her infection. Back in San Francisco she withdrew from Hastings, and the law firm she worked for promised to keep her position so that she could maintain her health insurance. Rebecca began absorbing every piece of extant AIDS literature she could decipher. Gradually she realized that she was an anomaly. AIDS was predominantly a black and, to a lesser degree, Latino epidemic, especially among women.

By the spring of 1991 she was heavily involved in the women's arm of ACT UP Golden Gate, which along with other ACT UP chapters was driving negotiations with the government over everything from the speed of drug development to prevention policy to medical care. In March the women's caucus of ACT UP voted to cut off all dialogue with the government. ACT UP members—who Rebecca noticed were mostly white, lesbian, and HIV-negative—could attend hearings, conferences, and scientific meetings but only to listen. That month Rebecca traveled to Washington, D.C., where the AIDS Clinical Trial Group of the National Institute of Allergy and Infectious Diseases was holding a public forum at which there was to be a discussion of a controversial new drug that was supposed to prevent pregnant women from transmitting the virus to their babies but that had also been known to cause reproductive abnormalities in lab animals. The meeting was chaotic, with protesters blowing foghorns during the scientific panels. In response, the scientists shut down the meeting and took the discussion behind closed doors.

On the second night of the conference, Rebecca wandered the halls, worried that ACT UP's confrontational strategy was going to limit her access to the latest research. She stumbled across a long narrow room packed with activists who were hotly debating whether they had made the right move by disrupting the panel, and if now they should enter into any kind of dialogue with the scientists over the new drug. There was one other positive woman in the room, and she was arguing to shut down debate. The whole scene felt off to Rebecca. She could be dead in six months, and these people, most of whom weren't infected, were making unilateral decisions that directly affected her access to information, maybe even her ability to have children. What, she wondered, was she doing here with these other white women, arguing behind closed doors, as though they somehow represented the victims of the epidemic? Who was she to speak for blacks and Latinos?

When Rebecca returned to the Bay Area, she was invited to speak at a private memorial for her friend Becky, who had finally succumbed to the virus. As Rebecca sat in her apartment mulling over what to say, Dan called her over to the computer and surprised her with a mockup of an

AIDS newsletter on his monitor. The memorial was held on a bluff near Stinson Beach in Marin, overlooking the ocean. When it was Rebecca's turn to speak, she stood up and announced that she was starting a newsletter for women infected with HIV.

The first issue of *World* was published in the spring of 1991, and it featured the story of an infected immigrant named Alba. The *San Francisco Examiner* ran a couple of inches on it. The following day thirty infected women, members of their families, and their friends called Rebecca's apartment desperate for information. Over the next week dozens more called. On some level she assumed that the newsletter would spur meetings, street demonstrations, and eventually a new arm of AIDS activism.

Now it was five years later, and Rebecca was typing out the topography of Desi's life. The newsletter's circulation had grown to nearly ten thousand. AIDS in America had grown blacker and more female, yet no major political movement had been launched to address it. Black leadership had remained largely silent about the epidemic on both the local and the national levels. Few of the AIDS stories in the newspaper focused on the minority epidemic. The ones that did had a tone of inevitability as they glossed percentages of the infected, trends in drug abuse, and sometimes the black church's queasiness regarding issues of sexuality. Few of them captured the lives of the women Rebecca had met. She published one woman's story in every issue of *World*. Many of these women were black.

There was Dawn, whose doctor told her that black women don't last long with this disease; she spent months hiding her illness from her children, washing their dishes with bleach. Another was Vanessa, who had lost her husband and herself to drugs and alcohol; her mother, Della, was dead from AIDS; and her seven-year-old daughter, Nikita, was infected, too. Another was S.T., an infected black entrepreneur who had been single for nineteen years after her divorce because she found it hard to find black men who weren't threatened by her professional and political success. There was a second woman named Dawn, a twenty-five-year-old recovering IV drug user, who prayed over her newborn, Lindsey, who was suffering from pneumonia, "Please, God, if I have to have this thing, fine, if I have to die, fine, I can accept that. I made the mistake. But please,

God, please not my baby. Oh, not my baby. She didn't do anything. She is so innocent. Don't make her pay for my mistakes!" There was Doris, thirty-nine, whose son Jared developed high fevers, ear infections, and colds at ten months. And Monia, who wrote about her life as a runaway: "I'd tell [men] I was from Denver and that I had run away. They'd take me to their house, give me a shower and get me cleaned up. One thing would lead to another and I'd wake up in an empty field. There's a scar on the left side of my mouth where I was forcibly raped by about six guys."

There was Becky Trotter, whose mother's boyfriend and drug supplier had raped and infected her. And LaDonna, who wished sometimes that she and her husband, Paul, could have had a few "normal" years before they found out that she had given it to her son Luke. There was sixteen-year-old Jacki, whose "abuse started in Texas when I was three years old. My grandpa sexually abused me, and I can still remember it like it was yesterday. When I was five he died. But this was only the beginning of my abuse. I've been sexually abused six times by six different men in my family." And Yvonne "Bunny" Knuckles, a mother of two, a grandmother of five, and a thirty-year junkie from West Oakland who wrote, "No, I don't have a lot of money or fine clothes. But I'd love to have the peace of mind."

These women were the invisible heirs of the civil rights movement, its promise and its failure. But they were not activists, and it was not their responsibility to stop this epidemic. They needed support, help, space to breathe, to be embraced in the arms of society. And here was Desi, pregnant with compassion, wanting badly to reach them. But so little was available to help her do it.

———

A FEW MONTHS later Desi sat in a pew at Faith Full Gospel, listening to Pastor Robinson deliver his sermon and waiting for him to mention AIDS. It was December 1996, the week of World AIDS Day, and a year after Monique's death. He read from the Bible and referred to the needs of the congregation. But today those words, which usually moved her, felt empty. Her eyes were swollen, and she was trying not to cry. How could the pastor neglect to mention AIDS? How could he stay silent? He was the one who had pleaded to preside over Monique's funeral. He knew that Desi was infected. If ever there was a moment to bring the disease to the congregation, it was now. And yet he said nothing.

After the service, as people made their way outside, Desi walked against them to the back room where Pastor Robinson kept his office. He was at his desk, his robe unzipped, surrounded by his collection of model cars. Desi stood in the doorway.

"'My people are destroyed,'" she said, reciting Hosea 4:6, "'because thou hath rejected knowledge.'"

"It is not because I have rejected knowledge that I remain silent, Desi," said Pastor Robinson. "It is for lack of knowledge." Then he told her that he had no idea it was World AIDS Day. "Go out and teach us, Desi," he said. "Teach us everything we need to know."

——————

CHAPTER EIGHT

Esther and the King

1990–1997

MINDY FULLILOVE had always dreamed of owning a house with high ceilings and long wooden floors, like the home on South Maple Avenue where she and her brother Josh had grown up listening to their father tell stories of his mythical Harlem character, Homeboy. If East Orange weren't overrun with crack addicts and if Newark didn't resemble the postapocalyptic Los Angeles of Ridley Scott's *Blade Runner,* she and Bob would have searched for that home near their childhood neighborhoods.

Instead they settled for Hoboken, a city of tall, narrow townhouses. Mindy and Bob lived in one of those homes. She named it the Thin House, and she hated it. The Thin House was built like three boxes stacked upon one another. The whole place was only fifteen feet across and was cluttered floor to ceiling with books, clothes, records, and art, so that there was no space to think. When it rained, a chronic leak gathered into a foul-smelling breeding pool for insects beneath the floor. Sometimes Bob would sit in the kitchen and moan, "I hate this house, I hate this house, I can't bear this house."

Mindy did a fair amount of thinking about the Thin House. Something essentially human in her dislike for her home—the way the place constricted her thoughts, her moods, her ability to feel at ease in her own skin—had the capacity to help reveal for her a new way to understand the black experience in America. And something equally important made them unwilling to move to a more comfortable place in Westchester, Stamford, or Englewood. Hoboken was the nearest thing they had to a home. Mindy's mother had settled in the city; her father had organized there; and the owners of Lady Jane's, their favorite restaurant, had christened a drink of champagne and Chambord the "Dr. Full-O-Love."

None of that, though, blunted their hatred of the Thin House. The floorboards had gaps between them, and the biting winter wind whistled up through the cracks to the third-floor bedroom where she and Bob slept next to a window looking out over the branches of an old oak tree. In the winter Mindy could feel the snow before she saw it because it covered the skylight above her bed and darkened the room. On summer mornings she was awakened early by sunlight dappling in through the ceiling. On July 17, 1997—seven years after they left California—she was jolted awake in the middle of the night by a dream.

In the dream she was at a luncheon celebrating the careers of a congressman and congresswoman who had failed to be reelected. At some point photographs were handed around the table. There was one of Mindy's butt. Mindy wasn't heavy, but she had been known to tear pictures of her behind into pieces and throw the tiny shreds into the trash. In this particular photograph her butt dwarfed everything else in the shot. In the dream she was weak with shame. As she looked at this terrible image of herself, this part of her body that she went to great lengths to avoid seeing, she said, "Sustainability is like a big butt: you never want to think about it." She said it again and again and again, until she was lying awake in the darkness in that transparent borderland between dreaming and consciousness. She needed to remember that phrase, that feeling. She pushed back the covers, forced herself out of bed, and wrote down the details.

For a couple of weeks Mindy had been contemplating a speech she was to give in August to the National Catholic AIDS Network, on what could be learned from the epidemic. AIDS had become a black disease. In 1996 41 percent of all new AIDS cases were African American, exceeding the number of whites in the epidemic. Black AIDS patients died faster than whites. Studies showed that blacks didn't take their medications and didn't trust doctors. Meanwhile, the country still hadn't taken notice. One could argue that Mindy had failed as a scientist, a race warrior, and an Esther. She had gone into black America and forecast the suffering of her people; she had stood before the king and asked him to help her prevent it; and he hadn't listened, or she hadn't asked correctly, or her science had been no good, or he had determined that there was only so much he could do. Biologists and virologists had become the white-clad knights of the AIDS wars. *Time* magazine had named Dr. David Ho "Man of the Year" for developing a new drug cocktail that, temporarily at least, could make the virus undetectable in the bloodstream. Certainly that was a triumph, a glimmer of the long-promised magic bullet.

For Mindy, however, AIDS had stopped being about T-cells, or opportunistic infections, or percentages and graphs. She no longer even considered herself an AIDS researcher. For her, AIDS had stopped being about AIDS. The epidemic—its blackness and American society's failure to stop it—was about blacks, whites, God, social hope, poverty, drugs, her father, her children, science, her search for It, everyone's search for It, and her faith in the future. She understood that to stem this epidemic and prevent the next disease, or drug scourge, or housing shortage that attacked blacks in disproportionate numbers, society needed to develop a new language that would transcend the polarizing rhetoric of blame, guilt, and victimhood and would instead enlarge its understanding of how America's racial legacy continued to indelibly shape Americans' experience of those crises. For the last eleven years, Mindy's work had arguably been to develop that language. It had required her to unlearn some of the master narratives she'd come to accept about race, disease, and science and to take a keener look at the obvious in an effort make it out as new again. That process somehow included examining her hatred of the Thin House and her attachment to Hoboken, and it demanded that she pay attention to her dreams.

She didn't sleep the rest of that night. The next morning at the breakfast table she told Bob, "I had the most amazing dream about my butt last night."

"I hope you don't tell anyone about it," he said.

"I'm going to tell the National Catholic AIDS Network," she answered.

———

MINDY FULLILOVE had gone to medical school in Washington Heights—near the peak of the heroin epidemic, and the nadir of New York City's fiscal crisis in the 1970s—and she had practiced clinical psychology in the South Bronx during the early 1980s, when the neighborhood was the poster ghetto for America's inner cities. But somehow that past hadn't prepared her for her return to Harlem. When Mindy and Bob left Berkeley to take up their new positions at Columbia in 1990, the survival rate for men beyond the age of forty in Harlem was lower than in Bangladesh. The vacant lots that dotted the streetscape made the neighborhood look as if it were rotting from its center. Mindy visited the hospital where she had studied medicine and was appalled to find guards posted at the doors demanding identification. The local armory, which she remembered at one time held high school track meets, was now a shelter for homeless men. She watched them walk slowly past her office on West 168th Street, their despair palpable and infectious.

She knew from Ben Bowser's ethnography back in San Francisco, their teen survey, and the exploding rates of STDs in inner cities across the country that crack had exploded on both coasts with the potential to drive the virus through black America. Their model for how crack was accelerating HIV transmission hinged on reports from their teen subjects that young women were prostituting themselves for the drug in alarming numbers. They hadn't, however, been able to get these women to talk openly about exchanging sex for drugs—how pervasive it had become, who was doing it, how women descended into prostitution, or how exactly the practice was changing black teen sexuality. So Mindy decided to hold a series of focus groups. Bob got in touch with Warren Barksdale, an old friend from his days in education who was running a drug rehab program in northern Harlem called Create, and asked him to recruit some of the women he had in treatment for the focus groups.

Mindy arrived at Create on July 30, 1990, for her first foray into the field in New York City. She dressed casually and brought a couple of young research assistants. Create was housed in a spare brownstone, one of hundreds that lined Harlem's residential streets. The meeting room was Spartan, just a circle of chairs, a tape recorder, and a window. The seven women Warren had gathered were in the early stages of recovery, but aside from perhaps some teeth that had gone bad from crack smoke, they looked fairly put together.

Mindy introduced herself and laid out the ground rules: no names, no identifying characteristics. She just wanted their voices. What we're particularly interested in, she said, launching into it, is sexuality and how sexuality has been affected by drugs. The voices came together in rapid fire, "Drugs. Drugs. Drugs, yeah. Drugs, that's true." We think it has been affected by drugs, Mindy agreed. But we want to know your expert opinion, what's really happening. The women were from Bed Stuy, the South Bronx, Harlem, and Washington Heights—the neighborhoods Rod Wallace had identified as epicenters of contagious housing destruction—and they had a certain subjective knowledge base that Mindy wanted to tap.

She asked if their neighborhoods had always been bad. Drugs had been around forever, most of the women agreed. "My father was a dope addict," said one. "I used to peek into the bathroom and see him shooting up. And I'd say, 'Mommy, what is he doing in there?' He comes out sweating. You know what I mean? You could see him with a little Coca-Cola top or something in there cooking something and then he'd have something around his arm and my mother would pull me away from the door and I'd go out on the street. I'd see him nodding up and down, you know, and they nod so good that they don't even fall down. I said, 'That can't be my father.'"

Is your neighborhood the same now as when you were growing up? Mindy asked. No, the women all answered. What are some of the changes? "Oh, God," said one. Is Harlem the same? No. No way. It's worse. Back then, they said, the dope fiends were respectful, clean, and loved. Now there was crack. "The addicts now are not even nowhere like the heroin addicts," started one. "The addicts now, they like monsters." Then all the voices drowned her out in a chorus of agreement. "Right," said the first, breaking through again, "you had the dope fiends and now you got crack monsters. They just walking dead. They don't care about nobody. They don't even care about themselves. It's like they—they—they'd sell their soul."

But it was the younger girls who worried the women most, the ones who were twelve or thirteen years old and already on crack. Not even thirteen, said another, ten, eleven, twelve. What are they doing? Mindy prodded. "I seen them having oral sex. I'm not even lying." There was a wave of agreement: this went on in the park, the elevator, the welfare hotel. "These little girls, you can hear them out in the hallway. I mean you can hear them. And one night this young girl," one woman started, "I heard this young girl, and I swear to God I'm not lying, this young girl said—she walked up and down the hall—and she said, 'I need seventy-five cents. Anybody down?' And this dude said he need one in the bathroom. I'm not going to go into all the explicits, okay? You know?" Could you? Mindy urged her. We would like people to be very explicit here. "She went to the bathroom, and she said, 'I want to give somebody some, anybody I got, I'm gonna give somebody some head. Just seventy-five cents. I need seventy-five cents to get a tray.'" And then another woman said, "They do it for a dollar fifty in my building."

Then the women started describing how people were transformed by crack. Their personalities warped, the color of their skin changed, and they lost respect for themselves. Some in the group wanted to know who was to blame. Was it their fault? Their parents'? Was the moral foundation of the community rotting? The questions hung in the air for a few minutes. Then: "I don't care what kind of upbringing they had. Crack's something that controls your mind." And: "I want to say that I had a good upbringing, okay? And I was a very strong person, and I did a lot of things, you know. That's why I know it can tear a strong woman or a strong man down to their knees. . . . I wore raggedy clothes and shit. And I didn't have fuckin' lights in my house. . . . I used to cry at fucking night because I couldn't stop fucking smoking, you know. I couldn't, you know. I used to beg, 'God, please let me stop. Please.' And I didn't have the fucking will-power to stop, you know. And I didn't have, I just didn't have, if there was help, I wasn't aware. I didn't even care, I just kept smoking the little bit of money I used to get from welfare or whatever. I used to just spend it."

In your opinion, Mindy asked, what's changed about sexual practices in the community? "They have to have sex in order to get drug money. Come on." Is that basically what's happening? There was agreement. Then one woman said, "It's like all the boundaries, there is no boundaries." The women didn't even enjoy sex on crack. They were objects for the men. And they couldn't explain why. "I don't know how it got like this," said one. "Why so many crackheads would stand so low. I don't know why and how it must have been they must have been so desperate for that hit." It wasn't only women, they said—men were selling their bodies, too. And no one worried about AIDS.

I want to get back to your story about living in the welfare hotel, Mindy said, and the young girls being involved with drugs. You said that you had experienced being burned out? "Yeah." Are many of the families burned out? Mindy pressed, referring to people who had lost their homes in fires. "All of them." All of them? What impact is that having on the young girls? "It's traumatic." When you were burned out, how do you think that affected your life? "Living there?" the woman asked, referring to the welfare hotel. Yeah, Mindy said. "It affected my life, oh it affected living in it. First of all, everybody in that hotel—well, most of them— smoked crack, okay. And it was trouble. They like to pick fights with you. It affects my life. I'm—I'm miserable being here. I'm very miserable. Any hotel for burned-out victims, it's no good. I mean, you know the environment. I mean, some people just turn out—some people wasn't probably even like that. And they just, you know, they come in that environment in that hotel, and they just blends, you know. . . . You can't go in the bathroom because they in there turning tricks in the bathtub all day long. . . . Security is never there because security is in the bathroom getting high." So what does this do to the mentality of men? There was some laughter, and then: "I think that they look at women like shit." There was more laughter. "They do, they do. . . . Men put, they put crackheads down. I mean, if you smoke crack, you ain't even worth a damn penny."

After the focus group it was clear that crack was shattering social sexual norms. Even so, the women had described the most troubling behavior from the point of view of observers, not participants. Mindy's qualitative research methods—which were untraditional survey research in that she conducted loosely structured interviews with small but intimate groups of sources—had the potential to close that gap. Practicing qualitative research, in her mind, was similar to practicing magic. When it worked, it opened a window that allowed her to see whatever laws of science, logic, or even popular conception were preventing her from grasping the true contours of a problem. Unfortunately, the outcomes of qualitative research were unpredictable, and Mindy didn't know how to make it work all the time. The best she knew to do was position herself for that serendipitous moment when it did. That had happened with the teen crack dealers at MIRA, and it happened again when Mindy returned to Create for a focus group with a second collection of women.

Mindy had been trained in the South Bronx and wasn't easily shaken in a research setting. But from the start with this second focus group, the explosive energy in the room unsettled her. The women from the first group had apparently spread the word that she could be trusted, that it was okay to tell her their personal stories. "I sucked his dick, right, and he came in my mouth, and I was spitting it out," one woman began, "and he gave me four dollars. I was crying and shit because I knew how bad I [had] gotten. I was like, 'Oh my God, four dollars,' and I was out there beggin' for a fucking dollar. Before, I would never do that shit, and I was doing it for nothing." One by one the women told stories of selling their bodies. When one tried to hold out by saying, "I only did it with someone I knew, never with strangers," the group turned on her, saying she was in denial, that she was refusing to admit that she too had been degraded. "You don't get it," one woman said. Then they were all screaming at her. Mindy had lost control. She wondered if they were going to attack this woman. Stories surfaced of lost children, beatings, and betrayals. "It hurts, it really hurts because you really want to do it," said one woman. "You really want to take care of your children and everything, but the drug is—just constantly—it's like a monkey on your back. 'I want it, I want it, I want it, I want it.'"

This was no longer an equation between prostitution, drug use, and AIDS. These women were describing a wildfire of violence, sex, crack, terror, shame, confusion, addiction, motherhood, divorce, and loss that had everything and nothing to do with AIDS. This was about the social disintegration of inner-city black America.

After the focus groups Mindy was anxious and distracted. She couldn't stop thinking about the second group of women at Create. Young research assistants came into her office, and she made them listen to the tapes, so they would hear the push behind the voices, their searing desperation. Something had gone wrong in these places. These women needed immediate help to understand what had happened to them, or what they had done to themselves. They were clearly traumatized, and their sense of shame was palpable. But what did that reveal?

In the spring of 1991 Mindy embarked on the arduous process of writing her own center grant proposal to NIDA, to investigate women's addiction. At the same time she began putting together a study to measure the rates of trauma among women in recovery for crack at Lincoln Hospital in the Mott Haven section of the South Bronx, one of the city's most severely burned-out neighborhoods. Based on the focus groups at Create, she suspected she might find a few cases of post-traumatic stress disorder (PTSD), which had gained some notice for striking Vietnam veterans. According to the Diagnostic and Statistical Manual's definition of PTSD, the patient had to have witnessed or been threatened by violent death or serious bodily injury in a manner that inspired intense fear, horror, or helplessness. Symptoms included reliving the terror of the trauma in dreams, flashbacks, and hallucinations; emotional paralysis; selective memory loss; detachment; insomnia; irritability; and an inability to concentrate. The disorder was fairly rare among the general public: in one study 43 percent of a sample of Vietnam veterans reported that they had been exposed to a traumatic event, compared with only 5 percent in a civilian control group.

Over the summer Mindy and her team interviewed 105 women at Lincoln. They were on average in their early thirties, 80 percent hadn't completed high school, and almost all had children. Nearly 100 percent had been exposed to a traumatic event. Those kinds of numbers were unheard of in an industrialized country during peacetime. Mindy firmly believed that the epidemics of violence, crack, heroin, AIDS, and trauma were interrelated. Now she needed to figure out how.

In July her center grant proposal was rejected by NIDA. In September she was scheduled to testify before the House Committee on Government Operations. She planned to get the committee's attention with these latest numbers.

CONGRESSMAN John Conyers began the hearing by pointing out that in the early 1970s a presidential commission on drugs had found that the government would have to uncover the causes of drug abuse if it hoped to wage an effective war on drugs. It was now September 25, 1991, and the government, Conyers pointed out, still hadn't developed a body of knowledge on the subject. He had called a series of expert witnesses to Washington that afternoon to determine whether the federal government should fund a commission to investigate the root causes of drug abuse in the United States. His colleague from the Congressional Black Caucus, Charles Rangel, testified first.

Rangel had more questions than answers. Why, he wanted know, were young black men willing to risk death to deal and take drugs? He couldn't believe, as some academics argued, that it was for the money. Did they feel that the world had been so cruel to them that they had no other choice? These young men, Rangel believed, had been left out of the American dream. America's drug policy, he argued, needed to focus on issues like housing, hunger, unemployment, and poverty. He was followed by another black official, New York City police commissioner Lee Brown, who rattled off a list of unsettling statistics: his department had made 87,000 drug-related arrests in 1990; 76 percent of the suspects taken into custody in Manhattan were on drugs at the time of their arrest; and 43 percent of the nation's prison inmates reported that they had used drugs on a regular basis in the month preceding their arrest. Brown didn't mention that HIV was spreading through prisons by rape and consensual sex, that AIDS rates were three to four times higher in the nation's prisons than in the general population, that condoms were not permitted in prison, and that HIV-infected prisoners who were serving short drug sentences were being cycled back into impoverished communities, where they were infecting their girlfriends, wives, and children.

Conyers's voice took on the searching tenor of a man trying to find the reason for a friend's suicide as he prodded each successive expert to explain why, in spite of a multibillion-dollar war on drugs, narcotics continued to plague inner-city America. Eleanor Chelimsky, from the government's General Accounting Office, testified that the United States had spent $10.5 billion on drug control in 1991, but only one-tenth of one percent of that money had been dedicated to researching the reasons that people used drugs. Further, she said, between 1973 and 1990 NIDA, the agency charged with overseeing drug abuse research, had earmarked only 4.6 percent of its research budget to investigate the root causes of the drug crisis.

A law professor from the University of Virginia, who had sat on President Nixon's commission on drugs, testified next that in the 1980s America's federally funded treatment and prevention network was systematically dismantled, leaving the country ill-prepared to confront the duel epidemics of AIDS and crack. He was followed by a legal scholar from UC Berkeley who pointed out that there were increasingly two drug epidemics in America: a middle-class epidemic that was receding, and an epidemic of the poor that was growing in intensity. America's drug problem, he said, dwarfed that of the rest of the industrialized world. By way of example, he pointed out that in 1990 cocaine-related deaths in Los Angeles alone outnumbered all drug deaths in England.

Mindy, wearing a dotted summer dress and large-framed plastic glasses, listened to this last piece of testimony from behind a brown wooden barrister's table. Conyers sat across from her, behind a high bench. To his right was Congressman Frank Horton, a Republican from Rochester, New York, all white hair and careful diction, and Charles Rangel, with his Duke Ellington mustache and cleanly parted steel-gray coif, had taken a seat to Conyers's left. Conyers introduced Mindy by first sending his regards to Bob, who had given a presentation on narcotics and race to the Congressional Black Caucus, then by calling her an expert who he hoped could bring a valuable psychiatric and public health perspective to the proceedings.

"We care about this issue because we work in [this] area," Mindy began. "We work with a very limited amount of money—we bootstrap money to do the kind of research we've been doing, because we think it provides much-needed answers. What I would particularly like to talk about is the work we've done on the disintegration of inner-city America—the collapse of the American city—which we think is intimately linked with substance abuse epidemics that have plagued Harlem, that have plagued Detroit, that have plagued Washington, D.C. Over the past twenty years we've seen a phenomenal process of contagious housing destruction, in which whole neighborhoods have been wiped out in areas of the inner city. Harlem has been completely destroyed; the South Bronx has been completely destroyed; as you know, much of Detroit has vanished from the face of this earth. This process of contagious housing destruction is linked to a loss of adequate municipal services—adequate support—for maintaining populations of urban density. What's very clear from our work is that the process of contagious housing destruction is linked to a whole host of social ills, including an increase in violent crime, an increase in AIDS, and what's most important for this commission, an increase in substance abuse.

"We think that there are two links between the destruction of housing, the destruction of communities, and substance abuse. The first is the loss of social networks. People are embedded in an ecological context—in a community context—and when that context is destroyed, they lose the networks and attachments that they had. And for the poor, it is a fundamental necessity to be attached to your neighbors. For example, when you're poor, you need to be able to borrow a cup of sugar, you need to be able to borrow twenty dollars in order to make it from Monday to Friday. One of our favorite questionnaires is from a study in the South looking at hypertension among black people. One of the things [the researcher found] as a useful question to ask people was 'How often do you have more month than money?' And when you have more month than money, you need to know that there's a neighbor who has twenty dollars that you don't have. And then there's reciprocity, because next month you might have twenty dollars that they don't have. That's how poor people keep going. But as neighborhoods have been destroyed, you don't have that twenty dollars, you don't have that neighbor, and you end up homeless.

"But the second link, which we've begun to study in the last year, is slightly different. And that is not what you lose but what happens to you. And in the process of contagious housing destruction, what happens to you is trauma. People who live in the deteriorating, collapsing inner city are at an extraordinarily high risk to experience traumatic events—trauma including being burned out of your home, being raped, witnessing a murder, seeing a drug deal—phenomenal rates of trauma. As you probably know, Chairman Conyers, there was recently a study done in Detroit which looked at trauma among young people living in that city, and it found that 39 percent of young people surveyed had experienced at least one traumatic event. Of those, 25 percent had PTSD, which as you know is a very debilitating psychiatric illness. Of those with PTSD, fully 43 percent reported a problem with substance abuse, either drugs or alcohol. People take drugs so they can alleviate their pain. We've recently completed some work with women crack users in treatment in New York City. We found that almost 100 percent have had traumatic experiences.

The average number of traumatic experiences is five. And of those who have had traumatic experiences, more than half are suffering from post-traumatic stress disorder. Only two of the women we talked to have had any treatment for PTSD. We—"

"You make it sound so—you make it sound so distressing," Congressman Horton broke in. "As I listen to you, I think, 'My gosh, what can we do?' Have you got any suggestions for what we can do?"

Mindy smiled, almost forlornly. "Excuse me if I make it sound distressing," she said, putting her hand against her chest. "I've spent the summer talking to women about their trauma, and—"

"No, I know it's distressing," Horton broke in.

"It's distressing," Mindy finished.

"I know it is. I'm from New York—not New York City—but I'm the dean of the New York congressional delegation. The mayor has been before me, and others have, and Charlie Rangel, of course, is a member of our congregation." Mindy was leaning forward now, elbows on the table, shoulders slightly hunched, listening. "And I know in these big cities—Detroit is one of them, Chicago—the chairman was just telling me about some of the severe problems they have in Chicago, Los Angeles, every large city's got these problems. Even little Rochester, New York, which is not a big city, has got these problems, too. And we've got these problems in Wayne County, which is a rural county, not as acute, there's no question about that, but what can we do? I mean a commission, that's what we're talking about here today, a commission to look at these [problems] and try to find out what the root causes are, but what can we do? I realize we've got a war on drugs. But in many ways we're really not doing anything. We're not even touching the surface."

"Well, I appreciate your question," Mindy said. "What I think is that a commission throws a spotlight, and that we need a new spotlight on issues of drugs. So I think the commission [would] raise a really great new spotlight: What are the root causes of drug abuse? What I think can be done about it, once we've put the spotlight on the problem, once we've redefined the problem, is that we have to stabilize the social settings in which people live. And I thoroughly agree with you that the collapse of the rural economies has thrown rural America into as much despair as urban America. It seems to me that they are very parallel situations, certainly for those of us who study AIDS, the parallels are very strong."

"Dr. Fullilove," Conyers said, "isn't this whole idea of a commission, looking at root causes and causality, based on the theory that if we did that, we could change our failing strategies, and therefore we would come up with some solutions? . . . We're here on a trail of hope that understanding will lead to the [creation of] a commission, and that the commission will begin to look at root causes and develop a body of knowledge, which hasn't been done, and that that in turn would lead us to doing the right thing, which would lead to a reduction of drug abuse in this country, particularly in that neglected tier that everyone has referred to as the 'inner cities.'"

"What I'm trying to suggest," Mindy said, "is that we've bootstrapped a few thousand dollars here and few thousand dollars there to do the work I'm describing. I think it's work that opens up a whole new way of looking at the problem. If we had more money, we could do more work, we could come up with more answers. That's not to beg the question, but I think—"

"But do you think we need a commission such as what we've been talking about today?" Congressmen Horton broke in. "You've been here for the whole hearing, haven't you?"

"I think that chart is a good reason why we need a new commission," Mindy said, and she pointed to a large white graph that had been set up on an easel by the woman from the General Accounting Office. It broke down NIDA's research budget between 1971 and 1990. The vertical axis was marked in increments of millions of dollars spent and the bottom in years. It looked like a graph of a high-yield security charted over the course of an economic boom: the lines for biological, prevention, and treatment research climbed almost straight up through the late 1980s and into the 1990s. Crawling along the bottom of the chart was the budget for the investigation into root causes of drug abuse in America. It petered out at a slightly lower level than where it had stood in 1975. "NIDA and all these other government agencies are not going to put money into causality research without some major shift in momentum. I think a commission gives us momentum to move in another direction. I think that's what we need." She paused then for a half count, then said, "We're stuck."

"Thank you," said Horton.

"Did you want to add any other comments, Dr. Fullilove," Conyers asked, "or is that an appropriate place—"

"I think you've got me to go to the bottom line."

———————

THAT FALL ANKE EHRHARDT was beginning to draw up a proposal to renew Columbia's NIMH center grant. Mindy and Bob met with her and the center's leadership team to formally propose their research agenda. Mindy told her she wanted to investigate the link between childhood trauma and high-risk AIDS behavior for women in the Bronx. Anke said it was interesting but not fundable. With regard to funding, Anke was probably right. Mindy's proposal was the scientific equivalent of a high-risk bet. There was little established scientific literature to support her hypothesis that a large-scale study would produce significant results. Furthermore, the HIV center was underwritten by soft money from the NIMH, meaning that Anke had to produce results for Ellen Stover if she hoped to have her grant renewed. Ellen Stover, in turn, had to answer to Congress.

Mindy couldn't believe Anke's reaction. Her impasse with Steve Hulley had made sense to her, as his worldview was foreign to hers, but Anke was a politically alive woman, and she'd hired Mindy and Bob specifically because they were rooted firmly in the community. Now Anke was telling her that the research she wanted to conduct—based on data she'd gathered directly from black women in Harlem—wasn't fundable. The meeting grew heated, and by the end Mindy and Bob had resigned their positions with the HIV center. Their jobs with the university were secure, but they were left with only a year's worth of research funding. Mindy was personally devastated. But the conflict with Anke raised a more troubling question: how could the country effectively respond to a rapidly developing public health crisis if the researchers who were marshaled to investigate it were hamstrung by a funding ethos that rewarded scientists for asking incremental questions?

Bob watched Mindy gather her breath and set to work on a second iteration of her NIDA grant proposal with an intensity of focus that was the polar opposite of his frenetic attention span. She studied the language, science, method, and structure of successful proposals. She forced her volunteer staff to work grueling hours, and she spent nights in the office writing and rewriting drafts. On some level he understood: she had faith in science. She believed that it was a correctable institution and that if she simply wrote more crisply and adopted the language of the paradigm more thoroughly, the truth of her arguments would force the veil from the eyes of the review committee at NIDA. But it was hard for him to watch her try, because he knew that she would never get the funding. Baby, he'd say, don't you understand? It isn't about how well you write or say it. We're not fundable; we're not eligible; we're not members of the club. Neither of them had come up through the public health ranks; Mindy was a psychiatrist, and his degree was from Teachers College. They'd published in respected but decidedly second-tier publications like the *Journal of Negro Education* and the *Journal of Traumatic Stress*. They'd been drafted into AIDS work only because Sala Udin couldn't find a black Ivy League doctorate in public health to satisfy Steve Hulley. If we're going to do anything, he told her, it's going to be in spite of—not because of—what these guys give us. Mindy couldn't or wouldn't hear him and insisted that she would eventually get the major government backing essential to an authoritative investigation of the root causes, lived consequences, and relationship between AIDS, drug abuse, and urban decay.

In July 1992 an envelope from NIDA arrived at Mindy's office on West 168th Street. The suite had a chronic atmosphere of focused chaos. Bob's office wasn't much more than a cubicle with a single window and a desk overflowing with articles, CDC reports, letters, and speeches. Mindy's was slightly bigger. The shelves along the near wall were tightly lined with books, focus group transcripts, and videocassettes. Stacks of papers were usually balanced on the bench of seats under the window. Her desk was always a nest of articles, computer wires, and telephone cords.

The package contained twenty or so typed pages of critique. The only word that mattered to her, though, was *no*. She broke into hysterical tears when she saw it. Bob was familiar with the sharp edges of her insecurity, but he rarely saw her lose control, and it frightened him. She picked up the phone and called the chair of the review committee at NIDA. *Why?* she screamed at him. *What did we do wrong?*

The parachute money from Anke was spent, and the only backing they had left was a small grant from the American Foundation for AIDS Research to study the relationship between stress and sex. In the summer of 1993 the foundation refused to renew that, too. Mindy's depression was brightened only by sharp pricks of panic. No funding meant no research; no research meant no public voice; no voice meant failure; failure meant more suffering.

They'd never seriously looked to the black leadership for support. It just hadn't made any sense. While a small community of black AIDS activists had worked tirelessly in virtually every American city hit by the epidemic, the name organizations—the NAACP, the SCLC, the Urban League—had shown only nominal interest in the AIDS epidemic. The Fullloves had, however, developed a relationship with Debra Fraser-Howze, the founder of the Black Leadership Commission on AIDS, a New York–based nonprofit that was trying to bring the black epidemic to the public's attention, largely by capitalizing on the currency of a board studded with black political luminaries like David Dinkins.

Fraser-Howze sent word to the Fullloves that she could scratch up a small grant to fund an investigation into why the black church had been so conspicuously silent on the epidemic. The question seemed relevant. The black church was popularly understood to be the black community's most powerful social advocate and political catalyst, and it seemed to follow that the church should organize and direct the response to the AIDS epidemic, an assumption that fit cleanly with the growing popular belief that the politics, treatment, and prevention of AIDS were the responsibility of the groups hit hardest by the virus. Early on that belief might have been born out of the fact that AIDS was classified as a gay white disease, a distinction that forced the gay community to fight for both resources and civil rights. Thirteen years into the epidemic, though, it had evolved into de facto policy. Gay men, it was understood, were best qualified—could be most trusted—to understand and meet the needs of gay men. Blacks, it followed, knew what it was to be black and understood best what "the black community" needed.

A whole mythology had developed that the black church was some kind of monolithic watchdog prepared to flex political capital on behalf of black Americans. Perhaps that mythology had grown out of the wealth of post–civil rights scholarship that strained to canonize black institutions. Or perhaps church culture was so pervasive on the local level of black neighborhoods that the church's national, political, and cultural reach had become exaggerated. Whatever the reason, the myth had taken on a life of its own and was constantly being reburned into the popular imagination by iconic images of Martin Luther King, the black-and-white schoolgirl smiles of the four children martyred in the 1963 bombing of Birmingham's 16th Street Baptist Church, and Reverend Jesse Jackson gesturing over a storm of cheers at the 1984 Democratic National Convention.

Bob, though, held no illusions that "the black church" was ever going to rise up and exert political pressure on the CDC about AIDS, primarily because he didn't believe any such thing existed. Indeed, even in the 1960s there had been no unanimity within the black faith community about how to conduct an antisegregation, pro-integration, pro–black power movement. When Bob was in Mississippi at the height of the movement, the tension between church leaders, who proselytized for a theology of transcending oppression through prayer, preaching, music, and spiritual catharsis, and those who agitated for political action had divided churches across the South. Bob felt it was a mistake to believe that much had changed. This wasn't to say that the clergy had no role to play in combating the AIDS epidemic. Even the most burned-out, razor-wired neighborhood had a church that provided vital spiritual, social, and even physical support for its members. The more relevant question that needed to be answered was why, if such high numbers of inner-city black men and women were infected with AIDS, so many of them were dying outside the pastoral care of their church ministries.

It was easy to answer that with vague clichés about homosexuality and drug use and the clergy's unwillingness to deal with either sin. While there was some validity to that answer, Bob felt that the clergy's relationship to those behaviors was more fluid. Perhaps by focusing on the often-unspoken compact that black preachers make with God and their congregations regarding what they are and are not authorized to preach about, he felt, he and Mindy would be able to identify a group of clergy who felt comfortable talking about the epidemic.

The scope of the project was modest. Bob and Mindy were friendly with Pernessa Seele, a New York nurse who had founded the fledgling annual Harlem Black Church Week of Prayer for the Healing of AIDS, and she agreed to link them to clergy. Over the fall of 1993 and the spring of 1994 the Fulliloves interviewed fifty-one pastors and ministers. Bob conducted roughly a third of the interviews himself.

The clergy were certainly alive to the reality of the AIDS epidemic. They described it as an "insurmountable problem," a "staggering blow," "devastating," and a "tragedy." One reported that he had buried thirty-four members of his congregation of five hundred. Still, only a handful had established AIDS ministries or developed much of a public voice concerning the epidemic. Some claimed they were overwhelmed by all the other crises that threatened the community. But a more significant number were painfully conflicted over the theological question of whether they should "rescue" sinners from the "consequences" of their sins. "I cannot divorce myself from making people accountable for their actions," said one. ". . . I would rather see a billion bodies dead to have their souls saved." These clergy were caught in an unresolvable antinomy, forced to choose between saving the lives and saving the souls of their congregants. Yet there were clues—both in the history of the black church and in the interviews themselves—suggesting that the clergy had a more pliant understanding of sin than their harder condemnations of homosexuality and drugs intimated.

The modern theological tradition of the black church was still, at its core, informed by its role in the antebellum South, where it had been the only white-sanctioned space in which blacks were afforded a sense of individual dignity. That often-conflicted position fostered a theology that, on the surface, emphasized clear moral readings of the biblical text that were complicit with white social values. But on a more subtle level, it gave birth to a theology that was sensitive to how the contours of social inequality shaped behavior, and more committed to affirming the experience of suffering, than it was bent on condemning sinners. This culture of empathy was still evident in many of the ministers' nuanced interpretations of the drug epidemics that had seized their congregations and to a lesser degree in how they related to gay black men.

Most of the clergy whom Bob interviewed felt unequivocally that drug use was sinful, but at the same time they seemed to understand it as a symptom of a larger social malaise. "Look at NAFTA," said one minister. "You sign an agreement to move capital into Mexico and Canada, you know, and you desert the inner city. Capital's taking flight. Major corporations can hold the city hostage—all they got to do is say we're going to leave. They get all kinds of tax breaks . . . these brothers [who are dealing drugs] are intuitively picking up on that and saying, 'Man, the economic system is rigged; this is what's got to happen; it's every man for himself.' You know? 'I got to get mine.'"

Their views on homosexuality were muddier. The clergy acknowledged that there had always been gay men in the church but felt that while gays' human worth largely transcended the sinfulness of their sexual behavior, it didn't redeem it. Many preached disparagingly about homosexuality while welcoming gay men into the church with the implicit understanding that they were not to self-identify as homosexual. This open-closet policy had been a factor in creating a fluid definition of homosexuality in black culture, where some outwardly "straight" men covertly had "gay" sex. The AIDS epidemic made that contract problematic. Black gay men who were hiding their homosexuality weren't too likely to negotiate condom use, head down to the neighborhood AIDS clinic for an HIV test, seek medical help from a doctor who might call in the family, or turn to the church for help. "What really hurt me," said one minister, speaking of a couple whose son had died of AIDS, "was nobody in the family told me to go to the hospital to see him. They would rather wait until he died and then come to me and say, 'Well, Reverend, you bury him,' not thinking that not only was that bad for him to not have pastoral care and not be able to talk about God and dealing with AIDS, but it's bad for me 'cause I considered him a friend." His sentiment, though well intentioned, was somewhat naïve; open debate about the AIDS epidemic in the church would suggest acceptance of sin or even, as one minister said, "getting on the bandwagon with gays." The code of silence was so strongly enforced that even during Bob's anonymous interviews, some clergy refused to speak about homosexuality unless the tape recorder was turned off.

To Mindy, this culture of empathy and secrecy seemed tragic. And perhaps it was; perhaps the majority of the clergy would never be able to fully reconcile their spiritual convictions with the more pragmatic concerns of public health. And maybe that should have been okay. What role, after all, should the clergy be expected to play as a social welfare, political, or public health institution in a country with a secular government like the United States? Maybe Pernessa Seele could make use of the Fulliloves' data to loosen the culture of silence in the church by reframing AIDS as a story of individual suffering. But Mindy felt it was unreasonable to expect black churches to assume the mantle of AIDS activism. Furthermore, it was unrealistic to expect gay black men to politically organize en masse around the epidemic, intimately engaged as many of them were in a subtle dance of secrecy, acceptance, and exclusion with the clergy, their families, and their lovers.

Bob withdrew further from the research, recognizing that he was never going to be a full-fledged member of the highly funded public health community. In a way, though, coming to terms with that reality was a relief. It had taken him three years of peer reviews, drafts, and rewrites to publish the results of the Oakland teen crack survey—a set of data that he was sure of after three months of research—in *JAMA*. He had neither the constitution nor the patience for that kind of work. He had been raised to be a standard-bearer, and that experience had shaped him into a preacher of sorts in his own right. He needed to be in the street—and figuratively at least, in the pulpit—publicly trying to make sense of and help close the widening rift between the middle-class public, both black and white, and inner-city black America.

He spoke to the CDC, the Congressional Black Caucus, and students at Columbia's School of Public Health. But his message was dark, and it lacked a countervailing optimistic vision. He'd been down to Central Harlem to check out "the mix," as the drug culture was called. The scene itself hadn't shocked him: he'd expected the mall-like atmosphere, the ineffectual policing, and the depravity of the prostitutes. It was the normalcy of it that had disturbed him. He didn't see many outward signs of resistance—people didn't seem angry. The dealing, the gangs, the potential for violence seemed to have become integrated into the ecology of the neighborhood. Crack had become so pervasive that even some of his friends from the movement—functioning people with jobs—were smoking it recreationally. On some level he hoped that the story he told of community disintegration and urban decay would arouse whites and blacks and dispel the notion that this state of affairs was natural in black communities. But privately, his view of the future for impoverished black Americans was bleak.

Perhaps that was because he intuitively understood that it was fundamentally difficult for the American public to make sense of how in the thirty years since the Civil Rights Act—a period that had seen the fall of Jim Crow; the rise of organized busing, affirmative action, African American studies, and Martin Luther King Day; and the election of black officials to federal, state, and local government offices—black America had produced communities that were drug-ridden, violent, diseased, and seemingly asocial. There wasn't any effective American language of race to discuss these things. The shrill rhetoric of racism was stale and ineffectual and increasingly seemed, to many people, not wholly accurate. The politically correct language of cultural relativism—which often strained to pin the most troubling behavior in black communities on cultural difference—could offer insight and certainly had a tempering effect, but it wasn't substantive enough. And explanations that chalked these crises up to poverty were incomplete. In the absence of a fresh language, Bob recognized that the American public would likely insulate itself from these communities, making the conditions that were taking root in them permanent by default.

———

THE AIDS EPIDEMIC in America had reached a critical moment. After the estimated number of annual HIV infections had peaked in the mid-1980s at 150,000, that number had leveled off to 40,000 a year, a rate that would hold steady through the decade and into the next. The problem was that the decrease in new cases was largely due to a dramatic fall-off in infection rates in gay white communities, where preventive strategies had been hugely successful. While it certainly had some effect, prevention was not working nearly so well in black America, where the virus had more entry points and had diffused itself far more thoroughly among both men and women. Consequently the American epidemic was becoming blacker every year.

In scientific circles, AIDS was beginning to be understood as a black disease. The Fullilove's research, and that of doctors, epidemiologists, psychologists, and social scientists at the CDC, the NIMH, universities, and public health departments across the country, had identified and detailed each entry point for AIDS into the black community. Dr. Brian Edlin, the epidemiological intelligence officer in the HIV/AIDS prevention division at the CDC who had been interested in the Fullilove's San Francisco crack data, had submitted a three-year study of crack users in San Francisco, New York, and Miami to the *New England Journal of Medicine*. His results confirmed Mindy and Bob's argument that crack had worked to drive the AIDS epidemic through the inner city.

Edlin's team had interviewed more than two thousand subjects between the ages of eighteen and twenty-eight, over 80 percent of whom were black. The HIV infection rate among crack smokers was a startling 15.7 percent. In New York City 29 percent of the women crack smokers surveyed were infected. In Miami that figure was 23 percent. Edlin's findings were especially shocking when compared with those for the general American population, whose HIV infection rate was estimated to be 0.07 percent. The rates he was seeing in crack users, Edlin believed, were among the highest ever reported in the United States.

John Peterson, Mindy's former colleague at CAPS, had explored how the fluid sexual identities of black men who slept with men often put them at high risk for contracting the virus. Heroin addicts were continuing to spread HIV through dirty needles. And the infection rates in prisons, where disproportionate numbers of black men were serving drug-related terms, continued to be far higher than among the general population. Complicating the matter, none of these people were operating in discrete groups, meaning they were infecting others in their neighborhoods, making the epidemic into a snowball that was slowly gaining size.

At the same time, the decision to classify the epidemic by race had amplified American racial tensions and was crippling efforts to stop the spread of the disease. Magic Johnson's announcement in 1991 that he was HIV-positive had alarmed black America. Surveys showed that blacks believed AIDS was the nation's number-one health threat. Conspiracy theories were running rampant through the black community. AIDS, some thought, was part of a vast federal scheme to wipe out blacks. The government, others believed, was withholding medications or dispensing poisonous ones. Predictably, the Tuskegee syphilis experiment was invoked by academics to explain why blacks had little faith in doctors, and by some blacks as evidence that the government couldn't be trusted. Even Mindy had decided not to publish much of the testimony of the black clergy, because she was afraid it would damn them in the eyes of secular white America.

Did all of this mean that race should be set aside, or ignored, in understanding and combating AIDS? Of course not. Race was the story of America, and that story helped explain why AIDS had merged with a river of other epidemics and was now spreading through black neighborhoods. But if the rhetoric of race was stultifying and divisive, and at the same time race itself remained relevant, then how could the nation engage in a dialogue that would serve to solve the crises gripping African Americans?

Throughout the course of Mindy's investigations into AIDS, crack, and trauma, this question had always seemed to return her to her own conceptual framework for understanding race. On one level, she believed that the twentieth-century black experience was fundamentally shaped by segregation. The popular history of segregation had traditionally focused the black experience in the ghetto through the lens of racism and its destructive consequences. While that wasn't inaccurate, Mindy had always understood the ghetto in richer terms. It wasn't simply false pride and racial animosity that had motivated the leaders of the black nationalist movement to develop a separatist ethos after the institutional barriers to integration had fallen: "The Negro," as her father used to say, "must embrace the ghetto like a mother a child." America was still a country where geography was highly correlated with race. To that end Mindy had spent much of the early 1990s arguing that environment was a much better predictor of disease than race.

Much of her thinking had been influenced by Rod Wallace, the physicist who had shown how the fire epidemic in the South Bronx inflamed the early AIDS epidemic. She'd met with him in 1990, shortly after arriving in New York, and together they had published a series of papers that outlined a theory that linked AIDS to urban decay. For most of the twentieth century, their argument went, the social, cultural, and economic foundations of the African American community had been in a fragile system of grassroots social networks, cheap housing, and unskilled jobs. In the latter half of the century local governments up and down the eastern corridor had failed to invest adequately in the infrastructure of poor black neighborhoods, spurring, among other things, an epidemic of contagious housing destruction that physically decimated ghettos in New York, Philadelphia, Washington, and Newark. The ripple effects of this blight helped to destabilize black urban communities across the nation. Families were scattered, aging housing stock became dangerously overcrowded, and social networks were severed. Simultaneously, the country's evolution from an industrial economy to a technologically driven service economy eliminated unskilled jobs, fueling a wave of black unemployment. The public health consequences could be seen in the soaring rates among blacks of AIDS, syphilis, crack, gonorrhea, tuberculosis, maternal and infant mortality, teen pregnancy, and violent crime.

This sort of macro-structural analysis—unconventional in the field of public health, which traditionally kept its focus narrowed on epidemiological surveillance, health policy, and medicine—was an effective end run around the notion that disease was endemic to poor communities of color. But it didn't seem to move the larger public health community. Perhaps that was because as a stand-alone theory, it was oddly lacking in new insight and pointed toward solutions that, while idealistic, were at once monochromatic, unrealistic, and somehow also predictable: inner cities had to be rebuilt, the poor should be politicized, and the government should subsidize health care and invest in progressive drug rehabilitation programs.

By 1994 this analysis left even Mindy emotionally cold. Part of the problem was that it didn't describe the lived experience of perhaps the most troubling factor in the intersecting epidemics of AIDS, drug abuse, violence, and trauma: the disintegration of black communities. To understand this phenomenon more viscerally, Mindy would have to learn what it felt like to live in these crumbling neighborhoods. From this more humanistic perspective, she began to realize that the story of segregation and the devolution of the American black ghetto had a potentially larger use: it revealed how the human psyche is fundamentally shaped by the physical spaces one inhabits. Developing this "psychology of place" required her to broaden her investigation. Rather than focus strictly on the issue-specific experience of being burned out, as she had done with the women crack users, she began to construct a fuller portrait of these communities that captured their value. Her method was eccentric and decidedly unscientific. She began reading all the psychological literature on "place" that she could get her hands on, and interviewing everyone she met with an interesting "place" story.

In August 1994 she held a focus group with gay men at Housing Works, a New York organization that had been founded in the early 1990s to develop supportive housing for New York City's estimated thirty thousand homeless HIV and AIDS patients. "I've been homeless my whole life," said David, a middle-aged black man with hollow cheeks, bone-thin legs, and a singsongy voice. The phrase caught Mindy's attention, and after the group broke, she asked to interview David later that week one on one. In the interview his fractured description of his life rarely followed a clear line, but it intuitively struck Mindy as important. He was an embodiment of the stories she had been trying to put together. He had grown up in Philadelphia, but his neighborhood didn't exist anymore. He'd been physically and sexually abused as a child and was a crack addict, gay, and infected with HIV. Mindy felt that she and David were lost in the same forest. Come to my apartment, David said, and you'll understand.

David's homelessness was more spiritual than literal. He lived in a single-room-occupancy building in Manhattan's garment district. It had been a monastery at one time, but now David called it Hell Hotel. Derelicts crowded the stairs, drinking beer and passing time. The lobby was dirty, an attendant sat behind a glass window, and if a single lightbulb wasn't dangling from the ceiling, it felt to Mindy that one should have been. She was immediately struck by how his room—furnished with only a bed and a chair—felt impersonal, almost uninhabited. You don't know how long you're going to be here, Mindy said to him. Why don't you make it a home? In the following weeks David found fabrics in the garment district, sewed curtains around his bed, and partitioned the remaining space into a tiny foyer and a living room. Mindy watched and interviewed him, learning about life at Hell Hotel, where cruel and unspeakable things happened after dark: shootings and rapes and drugs, things that she knew repeatedly fractured David's fragile psyche, fueled his drug habit, and probably put the people who lived here at risk for contracting HIV. As she came to know David, she realized that he had spent much of his life in various incarnations of Hell Hotel.

In May 1995 David invited Mindy to travel to Philadelphia to see where he'd grown up. He was born in Elmwood, a once-bucolic community of federal and city government workers on the outskirts of the city where his neighbors had grown peonies and red roses; a close network of churches with ministries like the nurses unit, willing workers, junior and senior ushers, pastoral aid, and choir lent the neighborhood a familial sense of cohesion. Life in Elmwood, David summed up, had been beautiful. When David was eleven, Elmwood was officially tagged as a "slum" and authorized for an urban renewal project. David's family, along with most others in the neighborhood, were pressured to sell their homes to the government, so it could demolish them and build a new development. His family moved deeper into Philadelphia's inner city. David seemed convinced that the loss of their home and neighborhood was the seminal event that destabilized his life.

That spring Mindy was picking through an issue of the *Poverty and Race Research Action Council Newsletter* when she noticed a small advertisement for a newspaper series by Mary Bishop, a journalist for the *Roanoke Times and World News,* titled, "Block by Block: How Urban Renewal Uprooted Black Roanoke." Mindy sent for it and, upon reading it, called Bishop. She explained her project on the psychology of place and told Bishop that she needed to see Roanoke. "Of course you do," Bishop replied. In June 1995 Bob and Mindy flew to Virginia together and stayed at Bishop's home in the city's historic district.

Mary Bishop had accidentally stumbled onto the story of urban renewal in 1993. She was working the weekend shift at the paper and had been assigned to write a small feature on a neighborhood reunion in Northeast Roanoke. She'd heard of the place but not much about it. She put in a couple of calls to the organizers, and they explained the reason for the reunion: their neighborhood didn't exist anymore. She persuaded one of the locals, Charles Meadows, to drive her through the area. Like a lot of the New South, it was now mostly chain stores, fast-food emporiums, and motels. Meadows, though, seemed to be seeing another town.

Where Bishop saw a McDonald's or a Days Inn, he described churches and homes, ones that reminded her of her own neighborhood.

Bishop sensed that she was on to something big. Investigating a bit, she found out that in the 1950s nearly all of Roanoke's black community had lived in the Northeast and Gainsboro sections of town. In the 1960s, under the authority of the federal urban renewal program, both neighborhoods had been almost entirely bulldozed.

Over the following three years, Bishop investigated the fate of nearly every house, church, and business in both neighborhoods. "Government leaders here," she wrote in the opening of one article, "thought urban renewal was a progressive way to clear what looked like slums to them and put in highway, industries and public complexes such as the Roanoke Civic Center. But there was a lack of understanding among those policy-makers—as well as reporters and editors at this newspaper—of what life was really like in black neighborhoods, what those communities meant to people, and exactly what would happen to the families made to leave. Most of all there was little recognition that black families had the same attachment to each other, community and home as everybody else. 'Slum' and 'blight' are words that Roanoke's older white leaders use to describe what they saw in those neighborhoods. Black people who lived there had another word for it: Home."

Bishop took Mindy to meet her sources for "Block by Block." Their memories, while nostalgic and seemingly unblemished by the problems that visit every community, described a 1950s southern black life that seemed warmer, more hopeful, and somehow freer than what they knew now—a life that began to reveal what black Americans had lost in the years during and after civil rights.

IF RACE WAS largely about segregation, and segregation was about place, then the story of urban renewal helps illuminate the social disintegration that underlay the intersecting epidemics of AIDS, drugs, and violence. Eventually, Mindy would come to believe that urban renewal and its parent policies of slum clearance and public housing were among the most destabilizing federal and local programs for black communities in the twentieth century. Ironically, the urban renewal program grew out of an ambitious Great Depression movement to house every American.

In the early 1930s large sectors of the middle class were struggling to pay rent, and a significant number were living in overcrowded tenements in America's central cities. Housing advocates blamed real estate developers for these poor living conditions and argued that the federal government should build affordable housing and rent it to two-thirds of the American public. The leadership of the housing movement, however, was mired in a debate over the best means to accomplish their goals. On one side, conservative reformers and social workers argued that slums were unhealthy and should be cleared, and that new housing should be built in the central city. Opposite them were the self-proclaimed public housers, who felt that tearing down existing neighborhoods would intensify the housing drought; they offered a more expansive vision to decentralize the American city by enticing the poor and middle class out of their tenements and cramped apartments with public housing developed on vacant outlying land. The newly abandoned slums could then be cleared and rebuilt to create a modernist city governed by regional planning that combined the best qualities of urban and country living.

In an effort to unify the movement, the two sides eventually agreed that slum clearance should be a stated goal of the movement but that in the meantime it was more practical to focus on developing inexpensive outlying land for public housing developments. Almost immediately, slum clearance proved to be the more politically potent cause, and in a canny move they made it the centerpiece of their campaign. The strategy helped yield the Housing Act of 1937, which inaugurated the federal government's first public housing program.

The act authorized the Federal Housing Authority to give loans and grants to local housing authorities to develop public housing projects. For every new building constructed, it stipulated that a slum unit had to be torn down. It thereby helped to create what historian Gail Radford would describe as a "two-tiered federal housing policy": the first tier enticed middle- and upper-class Americans to move from the city to the suburbs by encouraging private suburban development through mortgage insurance, while the second tier subsidized limited public housing. Perhaps most significantly, the legislation put an income ceiling on tenant eligibility for public housing. Catherine Bauer, one of the original public housers, feared that confining public housing to low-income Americans would stigmatize the movement and ultimately undermine its political and popular support. Indeed, when the United States entered World War II, Congress directed the entirety of its housing funds to defense workers and barred their use for low-income homes.

By the end of the war there was an intense housing drought. Blacks had migrated en masse from the South to cities in the Northeast and on the West Coast. Many Americans were living in temporary defense housing. Meanwhile, GIs were flooding back into America's cities. In 1945 Harry Truman, a strong advocate of public housing, asked Congress to pass broad housing and urban redevelopment reforms. That year Democratic senators Robert Wagner and Allen J. Ellender, along with Republican senator Robert Taft, drafted the W.E.T. Bill. With a preamble that called for a "decent home and suitable living environment for every American," the housing bill that was introduced sought, among other things, to federally subsidize half a million new units of public housing. The issue of public housing, though, proved too contentious, and the bill was stalled in Congress for three years. In the summer of 1948 Truman trailed Thomas Dewey in the polls, and the prospects for bold housing legislation looked all but dead. Then Truman, in a play to revive his staggering campaign, rebuked the Republican Congress for inaction, called it into a special session, and demanded that it pass the bill. The idea was to box Dewey into the uncomfortable position of either having to come out against public housing in the middle of a housing shortage or to split from his party's platform. It was an effective piece of politicking. The Republicans countered by passing a watered-down version. Truman played it perfectly, putting housing at the center of his fall campaign, and sometime in the early hours of November 5 he screwed his face up into a mischievous smile and waved the *Chicago Daily Tribune*'s mistaken banner headline "Dewey Defeats Truman!" over his head as he celebrated victory.

Truman's election set the stage for the Housing Act of 1949. For six months the new Democratic Congress sparred with Republicans over the substance of the bill. It appeared, though, that Truman had built enough momentum from the election to carry the vote. Then, in a brilliantly cynical piece of political maneuvering, Republican senators John Bricker of Ohio and Harry Cain of Washington added a seemingly progressive amendment to the bill that would ban racial discrimination in all public housing developments. It was a sure way to split the Democratic Party and kill the bill. Liberal northern lawmakers struggled over their position. Southern Democrats simply wouldn't vote for a piece of legislation that essentially collapsed the physical barriers that kept the races apart. Senator Paul Douglas of Illinois, speaking on the House floor, framed the Democrats' final decision to vote against the amendment this way: "I am ready to appeal to history and to time that it is in the best interests of the Negro race that we carry through the housing program as planned, rather than put in the bill an amendment which will inevitably defeat it, and defeat all hopes of re-housing four million persons." The amendment was dead. The Senate passed the legislation, and the House followed suit. But the decision to kill the antidiscrimination provision would have far-reaching implications for black Americans.

The Housing Act of 1949 was a bizarre alloy of New Deal public housing idealism and postwar business acumen. Title I set aside over a billion dollars in loans and grants to help cities buy slums for clearance and redevelopment; Title III was supposed to fund the construction of 810,000 units of low-income housing. In concert, they seemed to aim for a sparkling American city, where the newly housed poor would mix with the middle class both in the newly renovated core and in the suburbs. The new legislation had broad support. There were, however, loopholes that worried a few influential African Americans. Frank Horne, head of the Race Relations Service—a watchdog arm of the Housing and Home Finance Agency (HHFA), which oversaw the country's housing programs—immediately recognized that the Housing Act could be misused to reconfigure the nation's urban racial landscape.

When it became clear that the legislation was going to pass, Horne wrote a memorandum to the HHFA's administrator, Raymond M. Foley, simply titled "The Racial Implications of Title I of the Housing Act of 1949." Race, Horne believed, was bound up with urban blight and the very concept of "slum." The problem with Title I, the slum clearing initiative, was that it didn't do much to protect the people who currently lived in those neighborhoods. City leaders and developers were not mandated to build moderate- or low-income housing in the newly cleared areas. On the contrary, they had quite a bit of latitude to replace slum housing with commercial developments. In fact, they were not required to rehouse the displaced poor at all. As for Title III, the housing initiative, it was potentially even more damaging to blacks. By shooting down the Bricker-Cain antidiscrimination amendment, the Democrats had given local politicians latitude to use public housing as a tool to segregate their cities. In short, nothing in the Housing Act of 1949, Horne wrote, precluded "the possibility of Federal funds and powers being utilized by localities to clear entire neighborhoods, change the location of entire population groups, and crystallize patterns of racial or nationalistic separation by allowing private developers—for whose benefit the legislation is primarily drawn—to prohibit occupancy in new developments merely on the basis of race."

The solution, Horne felt, was for Foley to place race and civil rights at the center of HHFA policy. Otherwise, he warned, the HHFA could be legitimately accused of employing "Federal funds and powers to harden into brick and mortar the racially restrictive practices of private real estate and lending operations.'" Horne's vision was bold; however, the demise of the Bricker-Cain amendment had taken the question of racial segregation out of the federal government's purview and placed it squarely in the hands of local municipalities.

As it turned out, Horne's fears were well founded. Chicago's proposed Project No. 1 was located on a 101-acre section of the city's predominantly black South Side. If approved, it would displace 3,600 black families, of whom only 900 were eligible for public housing. The other 2,700 were to be forced to find new homes in Chicago's scarce private housing market. At the same time, Chicago's Title III public housing effort was running into trouble. The Chicago Housing Authority wanted to build twelve thousand units of public housing primarily on a series of vacant lots on the outskirts of the city. Chicago's city council rejected the proposal and introduced its own plan to build 80 percent of the city's new public housing on already-occupied land, which would force another 9,042 black families out of their homes, nearly 6,000 of whom were also ineligible for public housing. In the fall of 1951 the HHFA approved both Project No. 1 and the council's plan to build public housing on four occupied residential sites.

The situation was worse in the South, where segregationists were able to use the Housing Act as a subterfuge to sift blacks out of integrated neighborhoods. In Baltimore the Johns Hopkins project cleared 956 black family homes and called for the construction of only 178 units for African Americans. Clarence Mitchell, the Washington, D.C., director of the NAACP, said, "What the courts have forbidden state legislatures and city councils to do and what the Ku Klux Klan has not been able to accomplish by intimidation and violence, the present Federal Housing policy is accomplishing through a monumental program of segregation."

By 1952 the 266 "slum sites" chosen for Title III public housing were expected to displace 55,778 families, three-quarters of them black. Title I slum clearance projects called for the removal of 41,630 families, 85 percent of whom were black. And this policy was developed under a Democratic administration that believed in public housing for the poor. Once Dwight Eisenhower was elected, he replaced Foley with Albert Cole, an ex-congressman from Kansas and a long-standing opponent of public housing, who took it upon himself to dismantle the Race Relations Service. He demoted Horne to "special assistant" for minority studies, transferred him out of the HHFA's office, and replaced him with his own man, Joseph Ray, a former member of the black National Association of Real Estate Brokers. It was a shrewd move, as the HHFA's public housing program was potentially threatened by the *Brown v. Board of Education* case.

When the Supreme Court struck down *Plessy v. Ferguson* in 1954, Frank Horne argued that the decision to ban school segregation should be immediately extended to public housing. From his obscure post, though, his voice carried little weight. The HHFA's associate general counsel Joseph Guandolo, invoking the defeated Bricker-Cain amendment, advised Cole that no language in the Housing Act gave the federal government authority to impose racial restrictions on local municipalities that wished to develop public housing proposals. Cole, in turn, resisted using government aid as a "financial club" to pursue nondiscrimination. Instead he felt the country was better served by viewing displacement as a special problem that required targeted minority policies. The Housing Act of 1954 reflected these priorities. The new legislation reframed urban redevelopment as urban renewal and lent cities more flexibility to rehabilitate "slum" areas for commercial development, while requiring that displaced families be relocated in public housing. Since the majority of renewal projects were based in black neighborhoods, the new legislation effectively transformed the country's public housing program into a minority-relocation service. And indeed, by 1957, nearly 90 percent of the displaced families moving into public housing were not white.

Meanwhile, as public housing increasingly morphed into "poor-black-displaced-family housing," the question of where to build it became increasingly explosive. Whites and even working-class blacks didn't want projects put up in their neighborhoods. So most housing authorities built them near older public housing, which cemented urban lines of segregation and concentrated pockets of poverty in the inner city. Most cities didn't think of putting social services on site for the newly displaced or the poor. Many of the projects, particularly in the Midwest and Northeast, were high-rise, institutional examples of brutalist architecture, creating environments that critics charged weren't child friendly.

At the same time the urban renewal projects themselves weren't exactly transforming the American city into the utopia imagined by the public housers of the 1930s. Although some projects had clearly been successful, in 1968 the National Commission on Urban Problems found that two-thirds of America's urban renewal projects took more than six years to complete, with many stretching into a second decade of construction. The much delayed Mill Creek Valley Project in St. Louis destroyed so many city acres that the area became locally known as "Hiroshima Flats." Buffalo's Ellicott project displaced 2,200 black families in 1954; by 1964 only six new houses had been built on the fallow 161-acre site. Eight thousand people, mostly black, were forced to move out of Pittsburgh's Hill District, where Sala Udin had spent his childhood. The city managed to build a civic arena there, but twenty-five years afterward nine acres remained empty. All told, 1,600 of the 2,500 urban renewal projects funded by the federal government targeted black neighborhoods. By the close of the 1960s, blacks had taken to calling urban renewal "Negro removal."

The causes of the AIDS epidemic in black America cannot and should not be reduced to urban renewal, public housing policy, the fires that devastated the Bronx, or contagious housing destruction. The set of forces that fueled the spread of the virus through the African American population clearly also included such complex factors as the nuances of black sexuality, the architecture of the drug wars, gaps in the CDC's prevention and surveillance plan, the crack and heroin scourges, the media's failure to grasp the epidemic's dimensions, the contours of black church culture, and the aftermath of the great southern black migrations, to name just a few. However, the post–World War II history of the black, American, urban landscape did begin to paint a broad portrait of how black communities became such fertile ground for AIDS and the intersecting epidemics of heroin, crack, and violence. And it also started to illuminate why these neighborhoods had become so socially fractured in the years after civil rights that they seemed incapable of coalescing around these crises in a concerted effort to stop them.

Certainly, one could argue that the public health sector's failure to understand how America's urban social history shaped its racial geography—and informed black people's living conditions—undermined its early efforts to prevent the epidemic. When cases of what would later be called AIDS were first reported in 1981, every epidemiologist understood that epidemics spread through geographic spaces. In this respect AIDS was no different from swine flu or polio or the common cold that takes out a fifth-grade class. If GRID and the syndrome killing heroin addicts—nicknamed by some "junkie pneumonia"—were the same virus, the logic went, then infected blacks should have been present wherever there were infected gay men. But while GRID spread to both coasts, junkie pneumonia appeared to be largely confined to the South Bronx and Newark. Few scientists seemed to understand that America's racial geography had bred parallel epidemics of the same disease.

Even as early as 1981 it was probably too late for the CDC to prevent the epidemic from branching into black neighborhoods across the country. But if the public health sector had partnered with urbanists, sociologists, and community leaders, or alternatively if it had understood for itself that contagious housing destruction was simultaneously fanning heroin into a cross-community brushfire and intensifying a housing crisis that forced black families to live literally on top of each other, they would likely have rapidly developed a more focused strategy to prevent AIDS from tightening its grip on black neighborhoods.

There is no single reason why it took so long for the public health implications of urban redevelopment, public housing, and municipal policies to be popularly explored or understood. Maybe it was because much of it was sold to the public as pro-Negro policy rather than a tool for segregation. Perhaps it was because the data suggested the counterintuitive and unpalatable conclusion that black life was in many ways better during segregation. Or possibly it had to do with the fact that the academic worlds of hard science, practical medicine, and social science rarely mixed. While these and other explanations all had truth to them, they—like the struggle to explain why the American public had difficulty framing drug scourges as public health issues—felt incomplete. Something larger, it seemed, about the culture of race in the post–civil rights era made it difficult for many Americans to make the human link between the problems that chronically gripped black America and the enduring legacy of the nation's racial past. The story of Mindy's struggle to get her colleagues to make the intuitive connections between AIDS and crack, then trauma, then social decay, and then the structural history of black neighborhoods offers insight into this apparent disconnect.

AIDS was an epidemic that—like crack, heroin, or even crime—blacks could solve by taking responsibility for their actions. All people had to do to make sure they didn't catch HIV was to use a condom when they had sex, or a clean needle when they shot up. The public health community was never able to come up with a satisfying answer for why it could not get blacks to change these behaviors. The question danced around the epidemic, promising to reveal some awful truth about black sexuality, black civility, or even the very capacity of the black race to survive outside the bounds of institutional control.

Whether Mindy was ready to admit it or not, these issues had run loose through her writing like a threat that she couldn't quite put down. What kind of people celebrate drug use, rape, and murder in their music? What kind of religious leaders silence and reject their sick and dying? What kind of men speak openly about beating their women? What kind of mothers let their daughters give blowjobs in the hallway for a hit of crack? Some had suggested at various moments that poverty was the real culprit. It felt like an equitable explanation, and in the general sense that poverty-is-bad-and-poor-people-suffer-disproportionately-from-everything, it was true. But in the same sense that tired racial language didn't offer much insight into the epidemic, poverty didn't appear to be ultimately predictive of AIDS in the United States, either. After all, there were far more poor whites in America than any other group, and the CDC wasn't publishing surveillance reports that demonstrated AIDS was killing their mothers, children, and husbands in dramatically disproportionate numbers. No, the inevitability of the spread of AIDS into black neighborhoods was quite intimately tied to race. And that was where the conversation seemed inevitably to stall: just before it could circle back in on itself and cast blacks as crackheads, inmates, heroin junkies, sexual animals, and homophobes.

Mindy had tried to enlarge the discussion by exploring the manner in which the crises striking black America were symptoms of a much richer and continuing history of race in America. Yet she didn't seem to be in possession of a safe or publicly sanctioned language to illuminate how they were linked. Consequently, she found herself constantly trapped by the reductive rhetoric of racism, lost in the abstraction of policy and statistics, or self-censored by the danger of exposing the black race to ridicule. Perhaps the problem, though, lay just as much with her colleagues and audience. While conservatives and left-wing activists argued over whether America's race problem was a relevant issue or whether racism was the cause of all the country's problems, most Americans, it seemed, had assumed a far more cautious position, choosing instead to judiciously employ a sensitive rhetoric of cultural relativism that gave weight to the premise that whites should not presume insight into the black experience. This logic, it seemed, was part of what lay behind the impetus in 1986 to create the minority component at CAPS. On one level, the language of cultural relativism gave blacks the space to offer whites insight into how to handle racially sensitive problems. But it was also a sort of nonlanguage that highlighted how, somewhere along the path from institutionalized racism to racial equality, full and honest conversation between blacks and whites had become so fraught with fear and guilt and anger and political sensitivity and morality and pride and shame that the American ability to empathize and employ the full faculty of human logic across racial lines had been compromised.

Mindy was a doctor and a psychiatrist; more broadly, she saw herself as a healer. She had made it her responsibility to close the wound that prevented the white public from understanding black people in the most human terms, so that Americans could construct scientifically sound health and social policy. That task had required her to make sense of and translate the black experience in the post–civil rights landscape. The experience could not be completely reduced to the psychology of place, but the psychology of place seemed to give her the rudiments of a language to engage in a richer conversation that had the potential to cast the black experience in a fresh light and perhaps to open up a more holistic way of understanding and practicing public health.

———

MINDY SAT ALONE in the Mary Garden of St. John's Catholic Church on Cape Cod, in Woods Hole, Massachusetts, and meditated on the AIDS epidemic. It was June 1997, two years after her visit with Mary Bishop in Roanoke, and she had finished the manuscript for *The House of Joshua,* an unusual little book of place stories—her own, her friends', her father's and children's—that were part academic, part memoir, and part journalism. Race, AIDS, crack, Harlem, urban renewal, civil rights, and the South whispered through its pages, but they lived on its margins, background to her more universally human reflection on how we are shaped by the places we inhabit.

She'd come to Woods Hole with Bob, who was in town to attend a meeting of the Institute of Medicine (IOM), perhaps the most respected medical body in the country. She and Bob had never managed to gather significant financial backing, and she had moved far beyond AIDS in her work, yet they had become well-known names in the AIDS world. They had been given a modest three-year CDC grant to examine environmental impacts on public health in Harlem. She had sat on IOM committees and was a member of the CDC's prestigious National Center for Environmental Health's advisory board. *New York* magazine had named her on its list of the city's best doctors, and *Poz* magazine had listed her as one of the leading HIV researchers in the United States. Meanwhile, Bob had also gained entrée into the most elite public health institutions in the country.

When he wasn't teaching at Columbia, he was traveling around the nation guest-lecturing at universities. And her work was always at the center of his message.

At the same time not much had changed. She and Bob were two of only six, maybe seven, nationally recognized black AIDS experts. The CDC had recently written to Mindy asking her to help plan a series of inner-city AIDS interventions. Sure, she said, she'd help in any way she could. There was just one caveat, the CDC said: the structural stuff—housing destruction, poverty, joblessness—was outside their purview. She couldn't talk about the structural stuff? She balked. It was optional, they said. *Optional?* A part of her wanted to scream. But she understood that there was nothing malicious about their request. Rather, she thought, it hinted at something larger about the essential nature of America in particular and human nature in general. In a sense, that was what she was here in Woods Hole to figure out. She had been asked to deliver a talk to the National Catholic AIDS Network in San Francisco about the epidemic and what could help the nation look ahead to the years to come.

On a certain level her message was fairly straightforward. Epidemics threaten the body of a community, and therefore people have a duty to do everything within their power to contain them. Centuries ago Europeans had gone to church and said mass to stop the Black Plague. It ended up killing a third to a half of the people on the continent. But they still prayed, because praying was what they knew how to do. America hadn't done all it knew how to do to prevent AIDS. When the virus materialized in the early 1980s, epidemic response consisted of three well-accepted stages. First, the public health system recognized that there was a rise in cases of a new disease and sent scientists out into the streets to gather data. Second, resources were gathered, in the shape of money, time, will—whatever was necessary to take effective action. Third, people created new alliances to contain the disease. If the United States had followed those steps with AIDS and employed good science along the way, Mindy was sure the epidemic would have been largely contained. The country stumbled, though, over step one, and step two was scattershot. But she believed Americans had particular trouble with the final step. The American public seemed unable to grasp the notion that epidemics arise within a certain status quo, and that containing them requires people to create new ways of being together and helping one another.

The garden was quiet. A stone figurine of the Virgin Mary stood with her head bowed in a thicket of marigold, wild sweet William, Canterbury bells, Madonna lily, and chrysanthemum. Nearby a series of bronze casts depicted the stations of the cross. Mindy read the inscription by Ellen Gates Starr, the founder, with Jane Addams, of Hull House, a turn-of-the-century housing settlement in Chicago. Starr pointed out that on the plaque, which depicted Mary receiving the body of Jesus, the sculptor had managed to show us that Mary's suffering was universal, the suffering of all mothers. And as Mindy sat in this garden, with nothing to remind her of suffering in the midst of flowers and blue sky and gentle breezes, she thought about Christ and how he asked his disciples on the road to Emmaus, "Was it not necessary for the Messiah to suffer these things and then to enter his glory?" Perhaps, she thought, part of the message of the AIDS epidemic was about suffering—and how difficult it is for us to witness and linger with it.

She sat with that thought for some time. A few weeks later she dreamed about her behind. The next morning she knew that she had to tell the National Catholic AIDS Network about it. Because the dream, to her, was a personal metaphor for the human fear of facing the past and confronting the consequences. She thought about how the Western cultural landscape is littered with heroes who looked behind with disastrous consequences: Oedipus tore out his eyes; the wife of Lot looked back and was turned into a pillar of salt. In life, Mindy could tear up the pictures of her behind. But in her dream her unconscious forced her to see the consequences of her behavior. It felt shameful and painful. And it made her realize how her fear of seeing the consequences of the past inhibited her—inhibits the country as a whole—from looking back and confronting the suffering of the present.

The suffering of AIDS in black America was particularly terrible to witness because it forced America to look at how it had purposefully, in her view, left black communities to flounder. Now, as the third decade of AIDS approached, the public was being reassured that it didn't have to look back and see the role that the American story of race continued to play in its suffering, because science had triumphed and the epidemic in the United States had been conquered by new treatments. But while some African Americans would be helped by these treatments, the medications were serving to peel the epidemic apart. Many blacks, Mindy anticipated, were going to continue to die or else suffer from sporadic treatment, because AIDS was happening in black communities that were still falling apart, and the official response, as best she could tell, was that the roots of that crisis could not be looked at. America, Mindy feared, was less a single community of individuals than a collection of communities that stripped and dumped on one another. How, she wanted to know, could the AIDS epidemic help transform that mind-set?

The vehemence of Mindy's position in many ways emphasized her own anger at white America. Sometimes it seemed to keep her from changing that mind-set in herself. At the same time, though, her process of investigating the roots of AIDS, crack, violence, trauma, and urban decay seemed to illuminate, and perhaps even make safe for her students and colleagues and herself, the seemingly dangerous path to undertaking a full and honest examination of the continuing significance of race in America.

Mindy had lingered with the suffering of impoverished black America for most of her professional life. When the suffering seemed interminable, an end unto itself; when it seemed to suggest some unbearable truth about America, blacks, her heroes, her husband, or her mentors; when it made her want to despair and to lash out at NIDA, Tom Coates, Bob for going off and learning French, and what she now considered "the truly sinful scientific organizations" for their failure to act in the face of clear and present danger; when it made her want to stop, turn back, and protect her people from the moral outrage of the American public, she had delved more deeply into the suffering, and sat with it, until eventually it became fresh, raw, new, and then beautiful and suddenly human again. "Was it not necessary for the Messiah to suffer these things?" Jesus had asked the disciples. Perhaps, Mindy thought, she understood now what He meant. Christ had forced the disciples to stay with His suffering. And in staying with His suffering, they had been filled with the fire of the spirit. Maybe, she thought, it is by staying with the suffering, refusing to turn away, witnessing it, that all Americans have the opportunity to feel the full fire of human compassion.

CHAPTER NINE

_____

The Guardians

1997–1998

MARIO COOPER busied himself around his apartment in Manhattan's Union Square. It was April 1997, and he and a group of minority AIDS activists had scheduled a meeting with the Congressional Black Caucus to brief them on the epidemic. After Mario's two futile years of trying to warn his civil rights heroes about the threat of AIDS, his anger had become like a disease, twisting its way through him and slowly grinding into despair. Perhaps it was a family trait. After his parents divorced, his mother had withdrawn behind an impenetrable tapestry of reserve. And sometimes when he visited his father, A.J., the older man would say only five or six sentences over a weekend. A.J. had finally succumbed to his struggle with depression and shot himself in 1969. Some in the family attributed his suicide, at least in part, to the discomfort of being a wealthy black man in segregated Alabama.

Mario's father had had all the trappings of power: the brick mansion, custom built amid the spare family homes of Down the Bay, Mobile's black neighborhood; a uniformed maid who lived on a family property; and the family-owned Christian Benevolent Burial and Insurance Company. People knew A. J. Cooper and recognized the family name. He sent his teenage children away to northern and western boarding schools at the height of Southern racial unrest. Through the 1960s he was part of a small circle of black elite that included a few black business owners, a smattering of lawyers and doctors, and even luminaries like Duke Ellington. It was a tight, clubby world, but also a corner of society whose insularity could remind one that, even with power and old wealth, blacks could never achieve the full flower of southern social status.

Even so, Mario never gave much weight to the notion that Jim Crow had driven his father to suicide. It was too neat an explanation. Depression was a more personal narrative. He thought his father's death had more to do with A.J.'s mother, Sug Johnson, the matriarch of the family. Their relationship seemed to highlight the more internal ways that race could operate in American life. Sug was actually A.J.'s aunt—his mother had died of an intestinal infection when he was seven, and Sug had raised him as her own son and only child. Sug was nearly six feet tall, people said she was more white skinned than light skinned, and Mario wondered if she was illegitimately related to one of Mobile's prominent white families. Sug bought the mortuary in the early 1930s but made her real money selling funeral insurance to black families across Alabama. A.J. helped run the businesses for Sug, but as Mario came to understand it, she summarily rejected his ideas for innovation and growth, as though she feared that if they sought any more wealth and thereby called more white attention to their success, it would be taken away. She never forgave him for marrying Mario's mother, Gladys Mouton—a woman of beauty, drive, and intelligence—who was a Creole Catholic from rural Louisiana. Her resentment was only driven deeper by A.J.'s conversion to Catholicism and his willingness to raise his children in the faith. No, for Mario, his father's depression had had more to do with Sug's paralyzing grip on his ambition, her limited vision of what a black man could and should hope to achieve, her withering disdain for Gladys, and the vagaries of an adopted son's relationship with his mother, than with the legislated indignities of segregation.

In spite—or perhaps because—of Sug's conflicted relationship to race, wealth, and southern society, A.J. and Gladys Cooper understood their responsibility to the civil rights movement and the poor majority of blacks. A.J. raised funds for the construction of Mobile's first black Catholic hospital and frequently gave money to poor blacks on the street. Gladys opened her doors to organizers like Martin Luther King, Julian Bond, and Maynard Jackson. It was a brand of noblesse oblige usually associated with the upper echelons of white society but also often practiced by moneyed black families.

These connections gave Mario and his five brothers and sisters entrée into a black elite that was instrumental in setting the post–civil rights black agenda in politics, academia, and business. His brother Jay helped found the Black American Law Students Association while at New York University and became one of the first black southern mayors, in Prichard, a suburb of Mobile. Mario's oldest brother, Gary, served in Vietnam and became the first black officer in Marine Corps history to lead an infantry company into combat; he became a two-star general, was elected to the Alabama House of Representatives, and then served as assistant secretary of the air force for Reagan. Their sister Peggy, a lawyer, co-founded the Duke Ellington School of the Arts in Washington and, at various points, served on the boards of the D.C. Arts Commission, the American Film Institute, and the PEN/Faulkner Foundation.

Mario, nineteen years Gary's junior, was the baby of the family. He developed his passion for political strategy in his teens, during the early 1970s, staying with Peggy in Washington, D.C., and hanging out at night in her living room while she, Abbey Lincoln, Nina Simone, and other artists and intellectuals debated the civil rights agenda for blacks in the District.

However muddled the civil rights platform became in the 1970s, 1980s, and 1990s, Mario felt that blacks were gaining in America because this close-knit fraternity of legislators, academics, and professionals were wending their way up the staircase of politics. By the time Bill Clinton took office, one could argue that they had evolved into something of a de facto governing body for black Americans, and Mario had faith that they were committed to, and aligned with, the poor majority of blacks. Certainly, their voice helped foster the public illusion of a national black community. The various branches of government made a habit of approaching them on racial matters. They in turn often consulted with one another; took relatively swift and authoritative public positions on issues like welfare reform, drug and housing policy, affirmative action, and public education; and leveraged the power of the black vote to influence national policy.

Now the AIDS epidemic had made Mario doubt this system still served impoverished black Americans effectively. Blacks knew about AIDS, or they should have. David Satcher, the head of the CDC, was black, and so was Helene Gayle, the doctor who ran the agency's National Center for HIV, STD and TB Prevention. How could the black elite ignore the epidemiology? In his weaker moments he wondered if the leaders whom he had grown up admiring had decided that it would be better for blacks in general if America forgot about the distasteful problems of the urban poor and focused instead on their more assimilationist pursuit of middle-class comfort. Or maybe, he speculated, they had simply come to accept the permanence of a black lower class.

Perhaps their failure to recognize the epidemic revealed something about the changing relationship between the black elite and the majority of black America. After all, Mario—himself a gay black man, active in both black and AIDS politics—had been slow to make the connection. It seemed unfathomable that he had been so out of touch. When Mario was growing up, the protocol of segregation had required the Coopers to live amid Mobile's impoverished blacks. While he was always aware that proximity granted him only a window view onto their lives, it helped cement his sense of membership in what he came to understand to be the black community. When he was a kid, that sense of solidarity surfaced in small impulses, as when the limousine would pick him up from school and he'd embarrassedly pull off his uniform in the backseat and tug on a pair jeans as the driver slipped past ramshackle black homes toward his mother's sprawling brick house. As he matured, his sense that he and his family were rooted in black Mobile no doubt informed his enduring sense of responsibility to black America. But like those of many blacks who, after civil rights, ascended to the middle or upper class and blended into white and mixed-race communities, Mario's physical and personal connection to the majority of blacks, who remained in poor black neighborhoods, grew increasingly tangential. Even so, he and other successful blacks were still popularly expected to be alive to the problems that plagued poor black America and to be a voice for insisting upon solutions. The truth, though, was that while his sensitivity to the contours of these crises was amplified by his experience of being black, his knowledge of them, like that of most Americans, was increasingly based not on experience but on what he saw in the media and heard from elected officials. It had taken his own HIV infection for him to feel viscerally bound up in the plight of black HIV victims.

Maybe, he thought, he could use this meeting with the Congressional Black Caucus (CBC) to alert black leadership to the devastating consequences of the epidemic. Louis Stokes, who was hosting the meeting, had helped found the caucus in 1971, with a group of thirteen black representatives that included Ron Dellums from Oakland, Charles Rangel from Harlem, and John Conyers from Detroit. Its ambition was to represent the interests of blacks in every one of the country's 435 congressional districts. Shortly after the CBC was incorporated, Dellums put together an internal report in which he argued that the CBC would maximize its legislative influence if various members convened "brain trusts" of experts in fields like housing, banking, and foreign policy, leveraged their expertise to develop black-friendly positions, and then exercised their influence on the committee level. Stokes had put together the Health Brain Trust in the mid-1970s. He'd used his position on the House Subcommittee on Labor, Health and Human Services and Education to encourage and monitor HHS's 1980s investigation into minority health disparities and most recently had helped negotiate Clinton's apology for the Tuskegee syphilis study.

Maxine Waters, the outspoken chair of the caucus, and a woman Mario had always known to be a political enemy of his mentor Ron Brown, had agreed to show up for the briefing. The caucus's only doctor, Representative Donna Christian-Green, was going to be there, too. The meeting was ostensibly organized to mobilize the CBC to pressure the Clinton administration to lift the ban on funding needle exchanges. In 1989 the Senate voted 99 to 0 to ban the federal government from funding needle-exchange programs, despite CDC surveillance data that clearly showed that blacks were infected more by dirty needles than by any other mode of transmission.

There was, however, a loophole in the law the AIDS community believed that they could take advantage of. Two hurdles had to be cleared to do it: evidence had to be established that needle-exchange programs lowered HIV transmission rates; and proof had to emerge that the programs didn't encourage drug use. Without a uniform set of programs, clearing the first hurdle had been difficult, and the second was elusively subjective. Gradually, though, a body of data had begun to surface. Over the course of the late 1980s and early 1990s AIDS and drug treatment activists had started nearly a hundred locally funded needle-exchange programs. It was a scattershot effort; some programs were overseen by public health and drug treatment experts, while others were guerrilla campaigns run by activists and ex-addicts on street corners or out of vans. The programs' success suggested that they saved lives and didn't draw addicts deeper into addiction.

Even so, the concept of handing out free drug paraphernalia in the inner city remained divisive in black circles. Harlem City Council member Hiton B. Clark had branded it a "genocidal campaign." Congressman Rangel had at one point called it "subsidized addiction and death." The CBC had never taken an official stand on the issue. Dr. Beny Primm had been asked to attend the meeting to lay out the case that a federally funded and monitored needle-exchange program could significantly slow the epidemic. Primm had made his name during the Nixon administration advocating methadone maintenance and was arguably the best-known black drug treatment specialist in the country. For years he'd been publicly opposed to needle exchange. Only in light of evidence that HIV was spinning out from heroin addicts to their families, then through prisons, and back into the general community, had he changed his mind. He had credibility with the caucus, especially with some of the older members who'd been elected in the 1970s, when heroin abuse and its related crime wave threatened the stability of black families and neighborhoods.

At some point after Primm's presentation, Mario figured he'd have a chance to weigh in. The protocol in the community was clear: mainstream black leaders rarely attacked one another, and they certainly didn't accuse their own of callousness toward the poor. If the situation weren't so bad, he'd simply feign admiration for the leaders' long-standing commitment to the issue. But he couldn't afford to let this meeting turn into just another earnest briefing session that generated a press release or some outraged platitudes. If the CBC didn't act now, he feared, AIDS would be subsumed into the morass of crises that chronically festered in poor black America.

On April 29, 1997, Mario met Beny Primm and a group of minority AIDS leaders that included Cornelius Baker of the National Association of

People with AIDS and Miguelina Maldonado of the National Minority AIDS Council at Louis Stokes's office in the Rayburn Building in Washington, D.C. Congresswoman Donna Christian-Green from the Virgin Islands was there. Maxine Waters, the caucus chair, hadn't shown up yet. Stokes led them to a meeting room—and found that another group was using it. Mario was incredulous. Stokes led them to another room. It too was full. Now Mario was angry. How seriously, he thought, could the CBC be taking this meeting if it hadn't even gotten it together to reserve a space? Stokes offered to hold the meeting in his own office. It was furnished with a couple of wingback chairs and a couch, hardly room for all of them. Stokes took a seat behind the desk. Mario mostly listened as Miguelina, Cornelius, and Beny laid out the situation.

According to the CDC, 36 percent of all black AIDS cases could be directly traced to dirty needles. Those numbers suggested that needles were putting everyone in the community—from drug users and prisoners to their girlfriends to unborn children—in jeopardy of contracting AIDS. In September 1996 Congress had asked Secretary of Health and Human Services Donna Shalala to review the scientific literature on needle exchange. In February she'd submitted a report to Congress summarizing two extensive reports by the National Academy of Sciences and UC Berkeley, which found that needle exchange could lower HIV-transmission rates. In March the NIH had published a report indicating that needle-exchange programs could reduce high-risk HIV behavior by 80 percent and transmission rates by 30 percent among intravenous drug users.

Midway through the presentation Maxine Waters arrived late, saying she'd been waylaid at another meeting. Mario grew even angrier. Beny continued putting forward the evidence for needle exchange in his calm, gentle manner. The data, he felt, clearly suggested that the programs prevented HIV infections, and little evidence supported that they affected drug use one way or another. In fact, he believed that properly designed, they could lower drug abuse. The key, he felt, was for the government to actively involve itself in the programs' administration. That would guarantee that they were run by public health and drug treatment experts who could supply the drug addicts with HIV information and at the same time link them to recovery programs.

Everyone in Stokes's office seemed to agree with Beny. Then someone mentioned that the CBC's leadership was especially crucial at this moment in the epidemic. Maxine Waters met that assertion straight on and argued that the CBC had been at the forefront of combating the epidemic. Mario couldn't take it. He believed that AIDS would kill more blacks in the prime of their lives than any other disease. Blacks needed the caliber of leadership that had been provided for years by Kennedy, Pelosi, and Waxman. Waters yelled back that the caucus had been a leading voice on AIDS since the beginning of the epidemic. Blacks, he responded, needed their own "BLACK UP," something, anything, to break the status quo. Waters angrily shot back at him. Mario knew he had alienated everyone in the room, but he was too angry to care anymore.

Miguelina and Beny regarded him warily as they made their way out to the street and hailed a cab. In the car Miguelina turned to him. She didn't want him ever to attend another meeting with them again.

———————

DR. ERIC GOOSBY, the forty-six-year-old black director of the Office of HIV/AIDS Policy, was Donna Shalala's medical expert for needle exchange at HHS. He and Shalala had been over the data ad nauseam. Technically, the decision to lift the ban belonged to her and Surgeon General David Satcher. In reality, however, it was strictly Bill Clinton's call, and the president needed unassailable scientific evidence before venturing into that congressional minefield. The needle-exchange data they had gathered, though convincing, was unorthodox in that it was qualitative, anthropological, and largely based on interviews with drug addicts. Goosby, though, knew that needle exchange would work. He'd seen his first black AIDS patients in 1982 at the South East Health Center in San Francisco's Bayview-Hunters Point and had helped build San Francisco General's Ward 86 into one of the country's most famous and best-equipped AIDS clinics. In the mid-1980s, when doctors at the hospital noticed that IV drug users weren't utilizing the clinic and often didn't make it to the hospital at all until they were rushed to the emergency room near death, he set up an HIV partnership with a series of methadone maintenance clinics, where addicts could get HIV services. Soon emergency room AIDS deaths dropped precipitously. Needle exchange operated on the same premise: methadone clinics could reach junkies—a notoriously submerged population—faster than traditional AIDS programs could, before the virus got into their bloodstream and they posed a public health threat to the rest of the neighborhood. The problem for Eric Goosby was that General Barry McCaffrey, the director of the Office of National Drug Control Policy, was ideologically opposed to the federal government involving itself in needle exchanges.

Goosby was sick of playing politics with the AIDS epidemic. In 1991, shortly after he'd lost his five-hundredth patient in San Francisco, he'd moved to Washington to help implement Ryan White. The epidemic in D.C. was blacker and poorer than that in San Francisco, and the medical care for patients was comparably shoddy. At D.C. General, Goosby heard that when uninsured patients presented prescriptions to the pharmacist, they were routinely told, "We're out of that drug, sorry, see you later." The X-ray department was decrepit and consistently misread potentially fatal symptoms of pneumonia. In his opinion, their radiology was unsophisticated, the microlab was rudimentary, and the staff were unprofessional. His San Francisco patients wouldn't have stood for that kind of treatment. Yet these patients—particularly the black ones—seemed willing to accept it. He didn't believe their passivity was a condition of poverty, having dealt with plenty of poor patients who were perfectly comfortable with their sense of entitlement. The best way he could understand it was through the lens of race.

Many explanations for the uncomfortable relationship between the medical community and blacks focused on the Tuskegee experiment along with a handful of lesser scientific scandals that exploited African Americans. While those events had consequences and threw into relief black distrust of and frustration with the medical community, they seemed to him to oversimplify a far more complex set of circumstances. Other than Bob and Mindy Fullilove's investigations into AIDS, substance abuse, violence, trauma, and the structural breakdown of black communities, few alternative theories shed light on the interface between race, medicine, health, and community. His sense, as a black man, was that African Americans had simply learned how to endure, to retreat from and put up with suffering. He'd seen it often enough in black patients who told him in vacant tones about losing family members to gang warfare, or who chose to spend the night in a chair at home with congestive heart failure rather than check themselves into the hospital. Even that analysis, though, felt incomplete, and Eric didn't have a language to expand on it. As far as he could tell, such a language didn't exist. This, in his opinion, was the big black hole in American medicine.

His office at HHS was charged with overseeing all the federal government's AIDS programs. He wanted the Public Health Service to begin complementing its traditional quantitative epidemiological techniques with a cross-disciplinary approach that employed cultural anthropology, sociology, and urban studies to reexamine questions such as why the AIDS epidemic was continuing to spread through minority neighborhoods; why prevention programs weren't as effective with blacks as with whites or Latinos; why blacks were less likely to take medications and often didn't show up to doctors' appointments; and why they were prone to believe that AIDS was a genocidal government scheme designed to "solve" America's race problem. But he had no oversight authority, and few of the agencies had complied with his recommendations. The NIH, in his opinion, was obsessed with finding the magic bullet in the form of either a cure or a vaccine. Meanwhile the CDC, he felt, had abdicated its public health responsibility to the states in an ill-advised play to advance its reputation as a research institution. Federally funding needle-exchange programs would put the government back in the business of on-the-ground public health. The key was to get the president on board.

In the spring of 1997 Goosby met with Bruce Reed, the president's senior domestic policy gatekeeper. Reed was a boyish, highly energetic former Rhodes scholar who'd drafted the president's crime and welfare reform bills. He told Goosby to draft a memo to the president laying out the argument for needle exchange. Goosby quickly wrote the memo and sent it off. When he got it back from the president, the margins were filled with questions in Clinton's scrawl. He knew then that they had a chance.

AT THE END of July 1997 the Congressional Black Caucus received an eight-page briefing from Mario Cooper. He'd adorned the cover page with quotes that formed a thinly veiled criticism of the CBC. From Alvin Poussaint: "We have to make our response to AIDS have the energy and moral equivalence of the civil rights movement." Then Henry Louis Gates Jr.: "Like the Vietnam War, AIDS is our generation's war." And from Phill Wilson, founder of the National Black Lesbian and Gay Leadership Forum: "Three hundred thousand cases later, I still wonder what has to happen for it to be *our* problem." Then Mario laid out the epidemiology in black men, women, and children. He punctuated his introduction with, "Behind these numbers are your constituents. . . . We need your passion, your energy, and your leadership."

While each point that followed was arguably valid, the tone and the emphasis clearly betrayed Mario's growing distrust of the government and the white AIDS community. Across the board, he wrote, government programs weren't reaching blacks. He traced the problems with Ryan White. The AIDS Drug Assistance Program (ADAP), the federal program that helped the poor pay for medications, gave states too much discretion over who was eligible, which medicines they would reimburse, and how the local programs were designed. In many places—particularly poor southern states, where social welfare budgets were chronically stretched thin—the full phalanx of protease inhibitors simply wasn't available to blacks. Most African Americans, he wrote, "don't know the difference between ADAP and antacid." Compounding the problem, the federal government had little oversight or authority to pressure communities to develop programs that would realistically reach blacks.

The government, he continued, needed to fund research that investigated how to build health care networks that actually met the needs of minorities. The federal government's efforts in biomedical research—a seemingly race-blind field—also needed black attention. Research at the NIH had focused largely on finding treatments and a cure. More measures, he continued, needed to be taken to ensure that blacks were included in clinical trials, a well-known shortcut to receiving cutting-edge treatments. Now the NIH was gearing its research toward developing a vaccine, and black leaders needed to be vigilant that people of color weren't used as "guinea pigs." Prevention, he wrote, was largely guided by the CDC, which doled out the majority of its prevention funds to the states. The recent welfare reform rewarded states with additional prevention dollars if they taught abstinence only, despite the fact that this strategy was evidently often ineffective, particularly among adolescents. Further, many of the existing preventive strategies had been designed and tested with gay white men. The government needed to study and develop new ones that would be effective in black America. Finally, he closed, "African American leaders have virtually ignored HIV/AIDS. We must throw aside the shackles of ignorance, homophobia, and fear, and grasp this window of opportunity."

Maxine Waters couldn't believe it. Cooper was acting as if the CBC hadn't done anything, when it had actually voted favorably on almost every AIDS bill put before the House since the beginning of the epidemic. She had held hearings to investigate if AZT worked differently on blacks and whites. She'd personally called Dionne Warwick to persuade her to become the black community's Liz Taylor. Moreover, Cooper also seemed to be implying that the CBC had lost touch with its constituency and was more concerned with sterile issues like economic empowerment than with the more complicated and often deadly threats that many black Americans grappled with.

Directing that criticism at Maxine Waters was arguably misguided. Born into a family of thirteen in St. Louis, she had begun her career teaching in Head Start and as a congresswoman had fought against welfare reform, the attacks on affirmative action, and three-strikes laws. She'd even personally flown to Nicaragua to investigate evidence that the CIA was responsible for funneling crack into South Central Los Angeles. There were forty-one black men and women in Congress. They were responsible for meeting the needs of more than thirty-four million black Americans who were trying to crawl out from centuries of American slavery, state-governed segregation, racist domestic policy, and poverty. She was willing to fight for measures against AIDS, just as she was prepared to fight for the host of other needs of black Americans. Maybe even more so. After all, her sister was infected with the virus.

———————

ON THE DAY in 1996 when Donna Shalala received news from the White House that the president was going to go against her advice and sign welfare reform into law, she swallowed hard, calmly made the announcement to her staff, and told them simply that they would have to commit themselves to softening its blow to the poor. Two senior members of her office resigned in protest. There were calls in the press for her to do the same. Despite her disappointment, she had resisted the urge to publicly criticize the president. Now, however, in 1997 thousands of American lives were potentially at stake. She felt that the administration needed to set politics aside and lift the funding ban on needle exchange. There would be repercussions from the right, but this decision, in her mind, was worth the political cost.

First she had to figure out a way to get past Barry McCaffrey. The president's czars occupied an unusual space in the White House hierarchy. They weren't as powerful as traditional cabinet members, so their reach was limited, but they did have access to the president and a certain activist independence that was innate to their position as issue-specific problem solvers. McCaffrey was director of the Office of National Drug Control Policy, which had been established by the Anti-Drug Abuse Act of 1988 to implement a national drug strategy and certify the drug-control budget. It had been headed first by William Bennett, who freely invoked war metaphors to describe the government's antidrug efforts. McCaffrey, a decorated veteran of the Vietnam and Persian Gulf Wars, felt it was more appropriate to refer to the drug problem in the public health parlance as a cancer. Shortly after his appointment in 1996, he told the *New York Times* that the country had to start focusing on the root causes of drug abuse, help treat people's pain, and work to preserve the dignity of the afflicted. He stressed that law enforcement had a crucial role to play but argued, "That's not how we're going to solve the problem. We need treatment [and] prevention." McCaffrey's experience with drugs before taking the job had been in controlling the drug trade from Latin America, not in public health. A year after his appointment two-thirds of the government's drug budget was still dedicated to law enforcement and interdiction—roughly the same proportion designated by the Reagan and Bush administrations. Funding needle exchange, in McCaffrey's view, could be confused with a tacit endorsement of drug use.

The best way to maneuver around McCaffrey's ideological posture was to inundate the president with science. So in the fall of 1997 she instructed her staff to flesh out Eric Goosby's memo into a definitive report. Half of all new HIV infections in the United States, the report stated, could be traced to dirty needles, sex with an injection-drug user, or birth to a mother who had been infected through drug use. Over 75 percent of newly infected American children caught the virus through a parent who'd shot heroin with dirty needles. The consequences, it continued, were felt most profoundly in black and Latino communities, where 65 percent of all new AIDS cases were reported between July 1996 and July 1997. Furthermore, the proportion of AIDS cases that could be traced to injection-drug use was only rising. The report then went on to cite a preponderance of studies suggesting that needle-exchange programs not only reduced HIV transmission but guided addicts to recovery programs and mental health services.

Shalala sent the report to each of the government's top scientists. David Satcher, who had recently been nominated to be surgeon general, signed it. So did Dr. Claire Broome, the acting director of the CDC; Dr. Harold Varmus, director of the NIH; Dr. Anthony Fauci, director of the National Institute of Allergy and Infectious Diseases; Dr. Helene Gayle at the CDC; Dr. Margaret Hamburg, the assistant secretary for planning and evaluation at HHS; Nelba Chavez at the Substance Abuse and Mental Health Services Administration; Dr. Eric Goosby; and Alan Leshner, director of NIDA. Shalala figured that some members of Clinton's staff would probably prefer that she give him some political maneuverability and insulate him from the report. But she wanted to pressure the president, so she sent it directly to Clinton and to Vice President Al Gore.

In the early spring of 1998 she met the president and vice president in the Oval Office. For all the public talk about Clinton's highly political relationship with his own convictions, she knew him to respect advisers who stated their positions bluntly and challenged him on issues. So she lit into her argument. Both Clinton and Gore listened intently, interrupting only to ask a few brief, well-informed questions. Clearly, she thought, they'd read the report and understood the science. After about fifteen minutes Clinton raised his hand. Donna, he said, I got it. The meeting was over. She left sure that he did get it, and that Barry McCaffrey wasn't going to prevail on scientific or ideological grounds. The president was too smart for that. Now, she calculated, there was a 50 percent chance he'd lift the ban.

———————

ON MARCH 3, 1998, Beny Primm settled himself into a conference room at the Wyndham Garden Hotel in suburban Atlanta, along with thirty-three black AIDS doctors, advocates, and ministers, for a CDC-sponsored meeting on the epidemic in the African American community. The CDC periodically sponsored briefings like this to update various populations on the latest epidemiology and seek their input. The early ones, back in the late 1980s, were generally rote, careful affairs. CDC staffers typically briefed attendees on the numbers, then receded to the background and let them do most of the talking. The staffers' caution may have been partly due to their sensitivity to the fallout from the Tuskegee syphilis experiment.

After three decades of advising on federal drug policy, Beny understood that most government agencies had been conditioned to cushion their delivery of facts that could be seen as unflattering to blacks. Even considering this delicate context, however, he felt the CDC had been boxed into an overly cautious approach in its handling of AIDS in black America. The agency had advocated for years for states to track and report the names of people diagnosed with HIV. AIDS activists, however, had successfully prevented HIV name reporting in states like California and New York, where the epidemic was concentrated. The AIDS community also continued to stand in the way of any coordinated effort to notify sexual partners of people who had been diagnosed with HIV, a public health method often employed to stanch STD outbreaks. Enforcing confidentiality made sense for gay men, who had careers and private medical plans to protect. That argument, he felt, didn't hold for blacks, many of whom were unemployed, uninsured, or else not covered by Medicaid or Medicare.

AIDS activists had won those confidentiality debates, though, perhaps because their concerns dovetailed neatly with black concerns that any national HIV surveillance and contact-tracing policy would exacerbate black distrust of the CDC and slow efforts to test them. This, in Beny's mind, was backward racial and public health policy. He'd had enough contact with the CDC over the years to know that it wasn't operating from any sort of secret racist agenda. If the public wanted the government to stop the epidemic, it had to grant its leading public health agencies the latitude to engage proactively with blacks, not force them to retreat to a politically correct posture.

Given all of this, it would have been reasonable for the attendees not to expect much from this conference, as they sat back and prepared to listen to the CDC staffers run over the epidemiological numbers. This meeting, however, was different from its predecessors. A few weeks earlier, Helene Gayle had called her staff together and instructed them to take the necessary steps to give this conference a sense of urgency. Beny had been hearing percentages and looking at graphs of the AIDS epidemic for more than ten years. To even the most seasoned public health expert, these statistics could feel empty after a while, fluctuating on and on in a mind-numbing dance with the numbers among whites. This afternoon, though, the CDC's graphs and percentages included one simple new statistic: every hour seven Americans were infected with HIV. Three of them were black. Perhaps it was the ratio that made this fact compelling, or the way it absolutely reduced the epidemic to single human terms. Or perhaps it effectively captured the epidemic's momentum—every hour three more black men, women, and children were infected. In any case, it shocked Beny into the physical reality of AIDS in a new way.

That night a group of the black men and women from the conference met at the hotel bar. They represented a wide spectrum of organizations and regions: Debra Fraser-Howze from the Black Leadership Commission on AIDS; Pernessa Seele from Balm in Gilead; Yvette Flunder from the United Church of Christ in San Francisco; Sandra McDonald from Outreach in Atlanta; and Alexander Robinson from the National Task Force on AIDS Prevention in San Francisco. They started drinking and asking questions. Why were they getting these numbers only now? Why hadn't the CDC done a credible job of warning the information how deeply the epidemic had struck? It must have been holding the information for months or years. We can't trust the CDC anymore. We've got to do something ourselves. "Let's go manifesto," Beny said. Sandra knew of a Kinko's nearby. Pernessa fetched a laptop from her room. The group stayed up until three in the morning drafting a letter to the CDC. The next morning, they agreed, Yvette Flunder would voice their concerns to the agency.

Beny arrived at the conference room at seven-thirty the next morning, and set a copy of the manifesto on each chair. He suspected the CDC staff would actually appreciate it. They'd been waiting for some time for minorities to pressure Congress to invest more in the epidemic. Soon the conference room was nearly full. Yvette still hadn't arrived. Finally Beny was urged to approach the podium. He directed their attention to the manifesto and told them about the meeting in the bar. Then he bluntly stated, "This is a national health emergency." He turned to the CDC doctors and demanded to see Claire Broome, the CDC director, and Helene Gayle immediately. The two doctors came down to the meeting room. They were warm and cooperative, encouraging the attendees to scrap the day's agenda, break into groups, and come up with suggestions for the agency. Unfortunately, they said, they had to catch a flight out of Atlanta to testify before the House Committee on Appropriations to defend the coming year's CDC budget.

On her way out, Gayle pulled Beny aside, and told him that it wasn't particularly productive to publicly undermine the CDC. The policy makers who needed to be pressured were on Capitol Hill. Beny had testified before the committee years ago, when he was director of the Center for Substance Abuse Treatment. Lou Stokes still sat on the committee. So he suggested to Alexander Robinson that they fly to D.C. That night they caught a flight, and the next morning Beny got up early and went to Stokes's office. He'd been a member of Stokes's Health Brain Trust for years. Lou's assistant, Ferdette West, told Beny that the congressman wasn't in. Beny gave her a copy of the manifesto and a series of quick questions that Alexander had prepared for Lou to ask Broome and Gayle. Then he headed to the committee meeting.

The room was nearly full. Beny found one of the last seats near the back. Miguelina came in late and had to stand. Broome and Gayle were called up to a broad wooden witness table. Broome began by outlining the CDC's goals for the budget. Specifically, she highlighted Clinton's stated promise to eliminate minority health disparities by 2010. "It is appalling," she noted, "that the rate of AIDS is more than seven times higher for African Americans than for white Americans."

The committee members questioned the officials about various CDC initiatives. Stokes focused on minority health. He pointed out that in 1985 the Department of Health, Education, and Welfare had issued a report pointing out that blacks suffered disproportionately from heart attacks, strokes, cardiovascular disease, suicide, homicide, and diabetes. Ten years later, in 1995, an update showed that the disparities still existed. Broome had noted in her written testimony that only one percent of the nation's trillion-dollar budget was dedicated to disease prevention. Stokes wanted her to explain to the nation why the president's plan to eliminate disparities was serious and not simply an example of political pandering to minorities.

"I think this goes back to something that we as an agency really believe," Broome answered, "that what gets measured, gets done. And I think the difference is that we now have specific targets, both for the year 2000 and the year 2010, for decreasing and then eliminating the different increased burdens of disease seen in minority populations."

Stokes listened to Broome describe the agency's goals a little while longer, and then he said, "A few moments ago Ms. Pelosi, who sits next to me, showed me your chart."

"We have a big one, sir."

"Could we refer to that for a moment? She was pointing out to me the disparity in terms of the AIDS case rate in persons thirteen years of age, which is shown on this chart. You can see the red block which is marked white, and next to it the yellow block. I understand that in the next hour, seven Americans will become infected with AIDS. Three of the seven will be African American. Is that correct? Let's talk about that chart a moment, so that we can understand what the president is trying to do here."

"Okay. The occurrence of AIDS in African Americans is seven times the rate in white Americans," Broome answered. "And we consider this an indication of an urgent health crisis. The prevention programs—there are two particular areas of activity that we're focusing on. One is prevention of new infections in the first place; and this obviously is a primary goal of CDC AIDS-prevention activities. In the minority community, we have targeted prevention activities . . . in several ways. Most fundamentally, we use the community planning process, which tries to have local areas identify their priority groups and how they should be approached in terms of preventing AIDS. In addition to that, we have directly supported ninety-four community-based organizations to address minority AIDS and HIV issues. In addition to that, as has been noted in previous budget increases, it's very important for us to address the prevention of HIV/ AIDS in populations who use drugs intravenously, and this has affected minority communities disproportionately.

"So we feel that it's very important, because of the increased rates of HIV/AIDS in minority communities, that we be sure our prevention programs are reaching those populations and having an effect. The other major issue for the minority community is being sure that they have access to treatment. As you all know, we've had a very encouraging decline in AIDS deaths nationally. However, that decrease has been much more striking in white groups than . . . in minority populations such as African Americans. We're very interested in working with our colleagues in the health care area to be sure that treatment access is also addressed."

"Would you say from your chart that AIDS has reached what may be described as a disaster area in the United States," Stokes pressed, "as it relates to African Americans?"

"I think that it is a very serious crisis for the African American community. Our surveillance data have identified this, and we are actively working with African American organizations to address it."

———————

DONNA SHALALA met a group that included David Satcher, Tony Fauci, Harold Varmus, Eric Goosby, and her staff at her office on the sixth floor of the Hubert Humphrey Building on Monday morning, April 20. Goosby had received indications from the White House that the federal government would fund a trial series of needle-exchange programs. If they succeeded, then it would fund another group and expand the policy out from there. Melissa Schofield, Shalala's assistant secretary for public affairs, had given the press an informal heads-up that they were going to make an on-air announcement that morning, in the great hall on the building's first floor. Still, Shalala hadn't called a formal press conference. Her deputy secretary of health, Kevin Thurm, had spent Friday at the White House and still hadn't gotten any formal go-ahead from Clinton. The president was in South America, and Barry McCaffrey was with him.

The general hadn't been playing by the informal but well-established protocol that governed internal White House debate in the Clinton administration. Generally in a dispute like this, Shalala and McCaffrey would have met with Reed, who would have mediated their disagreement through a memo to the president that outlined their arguments, summarized the science, and offered a menu of mutually agreed-upon solutions for him to choose from. McCaffrey, though, seemed to believe his congressional charter was to report directly to the president. He hadn't even bothered to meet with the government's top scientists. Then in March two Canadian studies were published that seemed to lend support to McCaffrey's belief that needle-exchange programs promoted drug use; he'd presented the evidence to Congress. The authors of one of the studies had responded in a *New York Times* op-ed that their work had been mischaracterized. But he'd already succeeded in stoking a political firestorm, and Shalala's office had been receiving concerned calls from senators and congressional representatives who had heard through McCaffrey that HHS had decided to lift the ban despite possible scientific evidence of its negative consequences for the drug war. Still, Shalala couldn't believe that the president would be swayed by McCaffrey's studies. Virtually every major medical organization in the country had endorsed her position.

By eight-thirty she was seated with the others at the large conference table in the meeting room in front of her private office. They began going over the fact sheets and press strategy. The best game plan, they agreed, was for her to make the opening statement, then diffuse the inevitable moral subtext by immediately deferring to the scientists. They had been going over it for nearly half an hour when her secretary interrupted them to say that Erskine Bowles, the White House chief of staff, was on the phone.

"Kevin and Melissa," Shalala said, "you want to come with me?"

They followed her past the bookshelves lined with photos of Shalala with Bill and Hillary, framed clip-outs of her favorite political cartoons of her and the president, and her signed Rose Bowl–winning football from her days as president of the University of Wisconsin. Her inner office was simple—a large desk, a computer table, a couple of chairs, and an expansive view of Independence Avenue. She pressed the speaker-phone.

Donna, I've talked to the president, Bowles said. He does not want to make the decision to fund this with federal money. He's concerned that it will send the wrong message about drug abuse to young people.

Shalala felt a wave of disappointment. She was a small woman, with a head of thick clipped brown hair, brown eyes, and a face crisscrossed by smile and age lines. But she had an unrelentingly frank voice that hinted at a subtle, knowing humor. She'd survived the failure of national health care and the establishment of welfare reform, and she'd helped oversee the takedown of Big Tobacco. No part of her believed that Barry McCaffrey had convinced the president that maintaining the ban was good public health policy. This, in her mind, was a strictly political decision. She was sure Bowles wanted her to equivocate on the science, to say that the issue requred further study. But she wasn't going to do it.

Well, Erskine, she said deliberately, I'm disappointed. What I'd like to do is make the scientific determination that needle exchange can lower HIV-transmission rates and doesn't encourage drug use. And I think we have a way to do that.

Okay, he said, but be clear about the federal money.

She looked at Melissa and Kevin. They had been with her for all of her six years in office. This was going to go down on all their private short lists of moments when the administration should have done better. The news was going to be particularly difficult for the scientists. At their level, they were all inured to the political malleability of facts, but the scientists at their core held to the belief that science had the capacity to produce unshakable truths. Shalala was perfectly cast as the nation's top public health official for ethically uncomfortable moments like this one. It wasn't in her nature to explain, apologize, wring hands, or excuse. She was a soldier in the administration. She simply walked back into the conference room and stated the president's decision, and just as she had done after the welfare reform announcement, she reiterated that she was disappointed and said they had to get to work on recrafting the press release.

Everyone present was crestfallen. Goosby in particular felt betrayed. They didn't have much time to dwell on it, though—there were already reporters in the building expecting an announcement that the president had decided to lift the ban. They did have some leeway in what they could tell the press. The ban did not say that funds would automatically flow if the scientific evidence cleared both required hurdles. That meant they could announce the president's decision and still hold that needle exchange was sound public policy—they just had to lift out of the press release every reference to the programs Goosby had proposed. The press, of course, was going to want to know why, if the scientists said needle exchange was good policy, the president still refused to fund it. Kevin suggested that Shalala simply answer that at this time the president felt that local municipalities should be given the discretion to use their own dollars on these programs. It was a lame excuse. But at least it would give cities some moral authority to go forward with their own initiatives and provide an argument to make to states, cities, and nonprofit organizations for funding.

By ten-thirty they had clean fact sheets in front of them. Shalala said she thought they were fine—the best they could do—but she wanted to know what everyone else thought.

People are expecting us to make an announcement, Melissa said, turning to the scientists, concerned that they would publicly balk at the president's decision. Instead of downstairs, on camera in the great hall, she continued, let's do it right across the hall in the conference room with no cameras. I'm thinking that the secretary will have remarks, and no one else will talk. If you don't want to be there, if you have a problem standing there, we understand. But we want you to tell us.

No, we'll be there to support Donna, they all agreed, and support the scientific decision. But we're not going to answer the political question.

"You don't have to," Shalala said. "I'll do that."

A few days later Maxine Waters drafted a letter to President Clinton, signed by eighteen of the thirty-nine members of the CBC, rebuking him for failing to exert leadership on needle exchange. On May 11 she crowded into a meeting room in the basement of the Capitol and mostly listened all afternoon as roughly sixty black AIDS workers from across the country, whom she'd invited at Beny Primm's urging to give her an on-the-ground glimpse of the epidemic, expressed their frustrations. Many of them knew one another and had been working on the front lines of the epidemic for years. And they were angry. They'd been drowned out in public debate, they said, by the gay white organizations. They didn't have the resources to compete at the lobbying table. They'd lost out on Ryan White grants. The caucus, they said, needed to be screaming for attention on Capitol Hill.

Maxine Waters knew how to call public attention to an issue, but these people needed more than press. Four days later she sent a letter to Donna Shalala imploring her to declare a state of emergency in black America. A formal declaration, she wrote, quoting the law, would give the secretary the legal power to "[t]ake such action as [she] deemed appropriate." She then laid out an agenda that included the need to integrate substance abuse and HIV prevention and care, a cohesive strategy to deal with infected prisoners both while incarcerated and after being released, and a campaign to recruit top health care professionals who were willing to specialize in the minority side of the epidemic. But the most telling and substantive item on her agenda was for the government to guarantee a stream of federal dollars into black hands.

Donna Shalala didn't immediately reply to Waters's letter. Over the first weeks of June she consulted with David Satcher about whether the epidemic in black America really constituted a public health emergency. Satcher was not willing to blindly jump into Waters's camp—his feelings on the politics of public health and the epidemic were complex. He had been profoundly disappointed by Bill Clinton's decision not to fund needle exchange, but he wasn't surprised. Satcher had never mistaken him for a man who necessarily governed from principle. Clinton, in Satcher's view, was a pragmatist driven to accomplish the broadest possible agenda. Indeed, he'd always felt the president's unprecedented relationship with the black community had as much to do with his personal manner as his aggressive support of left wing policies.

Satcher's observation echoed that of a number of African Americans who had noted that the president was comfortable around blacks in a way that perhaps only a man who had grown up in the openly racial culture of the South could truly be. It was a form of honesty that seemed to have less to do with being truthful in a technical sense than with what many blacks, including Satcher, noted was his intuitive sense of how to treat people with dignity, by unselfconsciously engaging their opinions, challenging their ideas, and reflecting their experience. One could argue that Clinton had never fully articulated that innate ability into a larger vision for race relations in America. But he had consistently engaged black leaders about policies that impacted their communities. To that end he'd supported Satcher along with Dr. Philip Lee and Donna Shalala in their ambitious plan to abolish health disparities in black communities by 2010. Blacks suffered disproportionately from cancer, heart disease, high blood pressure, hypertension, obesity, and malnutrition.

Satcher, though, believed that AIDS should be treated differently. Unlike those chronic afflictions, it was an infectious disease that could and should be contained by employing strong, uncompromised scientific methods like needle exchange. He'd grown up in rural black Alabama and was alive to the damage this—or another, as-yet-unrealized infectious disease—could do to people living in those conditions. The STD and drug-use data he'd seen suggested that it was just a matter of time before AIDS made its way through the southern black belt.

At the same time he was uncomfortable with the rhetoric of a public health emergency. The scientific definition of such an emergency involved an acute, containable, and short-term set of conditions. He'd sent CDC teams to Africa to contain Ebola, to India to investigate the plague, and to South Carolina to cope with the aftermath of a hurricane, and so he was very familiar with those conditions. AIDS was different. It had been gradually spreading through black America for nearly two decades, had intersected with a series of complicated social problems, and had diffused itself so thoroughly that it had to be viewed through a longer-range lens. Satcher had walked through Harlem with Bob and Mindy Fullilove and agreed with her analysis that AIDS, and the related epidemics of crack cocaine and heroin, had to be understood more broadly in relationship to housing, neighborhood, family, poverty, and community. Miscasting AIDS in black America in the temporary parlance of "emergency," he believed, would give the impression that it could be isolated and quickly repaired. That, he believed, would be a disservice to both black America and the public at large. So he advised Donna Shalala to reject the statement about a public health emergency and urged her to figure out a way to dedicate more resources to the minority epidemic by leveraging HHS's multibillion-dollar AIDS programs.

Over the summer of 1998 political pressure built on the government and on black leaders to do something about the AIDS epidemic. On June 29 the *New York Times* ran a front-page story called "Epidemic of Silence: A Special Report. Eyes Shut, Black America is Being Ravaged by AIDS," which began by citing the latest epidemiology. Public health campaigns, it said, had made dramatic inroads against the epidemic in gay white communities. Those efforts had been less successful among African Americans, accelerating a two-decade-long, proportional shift of the epidemic toward the black population. Fifty-seven percent of new HIV diagnoses were now among blacks. A recent CDC study of thirteen-to-twenty-four-year-olds had found that 63 percent of new AIDS infections in that age group were among blacks. Heterosexual sex had overtaken injection-drug use as the primary mode of transmission in black women. David Satcher was quoted as lamenting the inaction of members of the black clergy. Civil rights organizations had remained relatively quiet on AIDS as well. Neither the NAACP nor the Urban League had put AIDS on the agenda for its annual convention. A spokesman for the Urban League told the *Times* that AIDS was "outside our traditional purview." Louis Stokes told the paper that the silence from the nation's largest civil rights groups was "exasperating."

A week later NAACP president Kweisi Mfume wrote a defensive letter to the *Times* noting, among other points, that in 1992 the organization's board of directors had proclaimed AIDS a public health crisis in the African American community and that it had come out in favor of needle exchange. Then in July 1998 Julian Bond, chair of the NAACP, gave a speech to thirty-five hundred members of the organization wherein he announced, at Mario Cooper's urging, that "AIDS has become a black epidemic."

That same month, in Westchester County outside New York City,

Beny Primm was fixing breakfast at his house when Helene Gayle called. Donna Shalala and David Satcher, she said, felt that public health emergencies were one-act plays, and they weren't comfortable using the term to describe the epidemic in the black community. Possibly, she continued, they'd be willing to call it a crisis, which might in the long run allow them to do more.

Well, Beny said, if that's the best we can do, it would be fine with me, so long as we call some attention to this issue.

He hung up, dialed Maxine Waters, and told her the news.

No, Beny, she said in what sounded to him like powerful-black-mother mode. Don't you dare—you go after this thing, and don't you back down for one minute.

Yes, ma'am, he said.

They're going to ask you to capitulate, she continued, but don't you capitulate, don't bend one iota.

Yes ma'am, yes ma'am, he said, don't you worry. I won't.

The negotiations with the White House heated up over the summer. On September 16 Donna Shalala, in a taped feed, addressed the Congressional Black Caucus's legislative conference, an audience of fifteen hundred African Americans that included civil rights icon Rosa Parks. Shalala sidestepped the breathless language of "public health emergency." "This is a crisis for all Americans," she said, pledging to dedicate an additional $4.9 million for black AIDS programs in the coming year. Louis Stokes quickly noted that negotiations with HHS were still in progress.

The negotiations, though, were actually as much about control as about specific dollar amounts. Stokes and Waters were adamant that HHS guarantee that a significant amount of funds would flow directly into black communities. HHS, however, naturally wanted to integrate whatever new money was made available into its existing programs. There were valid points to be made on both sides. Waters was right that black AIDS organizations, from Harlem to Oakland to the South Side of Chicago, had struggled to compete for government grants with the much wealthier AIDS organizations founded by gay whites, many of which employed full-time staff dedicated to drafting proposals. A wealth of anecdotal evidence suggested that black AIDS patients were less likely to go to AIDS agencies that were popularly identified as gay. Government-sponsored prevention programs had achieved limited success in black America. There were legitimate questions about whether state and local health departments had the cultural know-how to partner with black communities. For all the talk about the black clergy's failure to engage the epidemic socially or politically, the CDC had waited until the late 1990s to seriously partner with the black church, which was perhaps the single most efficient avenue to reach African Americans.

Some at HHS, on the other hand, had reason to feel that opening a parallel funding line was an inefficient way to utilize twenty years' worth of AIDS programs to address the epidemic in black America. Its multibillion-dollar AIDS effort, run now on many levels by African Americans, was designed to utilize state and local health departments to give local communities the resources and flexibility to build sustainable AIDS-prevention and AIDS-care networks. Increasing amounts of money were dedicated to the minority epidemic. And provisions had been worked into Ryan White requiring that the planning councils—through which much of the money was distributed on the local level—reflect the racial makeup of the epidemic.

It seemed, though, that beneath the specifics of this negotiation was a much broader debate about how the federal government—and by extension, the American public—should address crises that were understood to be black. On one level, the Congressional Black Caucus and the administration appeared to agree that blacks were best equipped to and should be granted funding to take on the responsibility of building and implementing AIDS services in their own communities. The tension seemed to center on how far the government's current programs could be trusted to carry out that mandate. Ultimately, Waters and Stokes appeared to win this argument. In October HHS agreed to declare a state of ongoing crisis in communities of color, and to dedicate an additional $156 million to the minority epidemic, much of which would bypass local government and flow directly to organizations that served primarily black and Latino patients. Their victory unquestionably had the symbolic significance of drawing the American public's attention to the fact that AIDS had become a primarily black disease. It also seemed, however, to reinforce a relatively new, politically correct brand of segregation, the consequences of which were not yet entirely clear.

President Clinton's AIDS czar, Sandy Thurman, for one, believed that the design, though not the intent, of the CBC initiative was potentially problematic. Ryan White had been set up to serve all Americans. If it wasn't succeeding, then the administration needed to work with the black community to overhaul it. Instead of doing so, however, the administration had chosen to create a second-tier, parallel funding line, founded on the exclusionary premise that blacks were best equipped to care for blacks and whites to care for whites. The plan, Thurman felt, set a precedent that would inevitably pit these groups against each other. Perhaps worse, it sent a message to white Americans that AIDS in the black community had been addressed and was not their concern. She believed that others in the administration shared her sentiment, but no one would say so publicly.

Taken together, the needle-exchange debate and the Congressional Black Caucus negotiation seemed to highlight parallel challenges in devising solutions to the chronic problems that plagued impoverished black communities. On needle exchange, Sandy Thurman and others in the administration believed that Clinton had been unwilling to lift the ban in part because intravenous drug users were not a powerful or particularly visible constituency who could offer the White House the necessary political cover against the inevitable Republican backlash. With the CBC initiative, quite another set of obstacles had surfaced: the overtly racial nature of the debate had cowed the administration into endorsing a black-devised policy that some prominent members of the administration felt was ill conceived. Whether the policy itself was right or wrong was open to debate, but the fact that members of the administration felt they could not viably oppose Waters without risking being seen as callous, or perhaps even racist, revealed how the culture of race in post–civil rights America severely limited, even between the best-meaning members of both races, the kind of difficult and open conversation necessary to solve the country's most difficult and enduring social ills.

ON OCTOBER 28 Bill Clinton approached the podium in the White House briefing room. He was flanked by a group that included Maxine Waters, Lou Stokes, and Donna Christian-Green on his right, and David Satcher,

Donna Shalala, and Sandy Thurman on his left. Beny Primm looked up at him from the front row of the audience. The president gripped both sides of the podium with his large hands. His hair was almost completely white now, and he appeared to have lost weight. But somehow, here at the height of the Monica Lewinsky feeding frenzy, he seemed to have achieved a certain presence, a binding gravity, that had eluded him early in his presidency.

"Like other epidemics before it, AIDS is now hitting hardest where knowledge about the disease is scarce and poverty is high," he began, gently bowing his head and biting his lower lip, as he was prone to do when trying to convey empathy. "In other words, as so often happens, it is picking on the most vulnerable among us."

The phone rang at Mario Cooper's apartment in New York City later that afternoon. A reporter from the *Washington Post* asked him to comment on Clinton's formal declaration of a state of ongoing crisis in communities of color, and his commitment to dedicate $156 million to minority AIDS programs. Mario's feelings were complex. In a way, this was what he had envisioned when he left the AIDS Action Council in 1995. Yet he felt little joy, partly because the CBC had backed down from the rhetoric of emergency, but partly too because there was something tired about the words, the presentation, and the plan. The CBC, the black elite, had exercised its power—but for what? A couple hundred million dollars? That was a Band-Aid for the much deeper wound that was crippling black America. Moreover, it perpetuated a system of race, supported by both blacks and whites, that could never completely work, either to empower the vast majority of blacks to build feasible separate communities or to guide Americans to achieve the true vision of integration, perhaps best articulated by Martin Luther King when he described an America where whites fully understood that "their freedom is inextricably bound to our freedom." In the absence of any uncompromised, fresh, or substantive conversation on race, perhaps the only hope for the impoverished and increasingly invisible body of American blacks lay with the activists and politicians who were engaged with their plight locally. He paused for a half a beat. He would not be able to completely unpack all those feelings, or get his mind around that thought, for a few years.

"It's a shot in the arm," he said. But then he added, "It's really only chump change for what is going to be needed for this horrible disease."

CHAPTER TEN

The Long Dream

2001–2002

D AVID DESHAZO woke up nervous at six-thirty Tuesday morning, March 6, 2001. Angela Jackson had called the day before to tell him that Rebecca was running a fever. Could she get Rebecca to the doctor? he'd asked. Rebecca's boyfriend, Leon, could drive them when he got off work at five, Angela promised, and if for some reason he couldn't, her uncle would do it. This morning David wanted to believe that they'd made it to Dr. Sherman in Waynesboro or to Dr. Preyear in Mobile, but he couldn't shake a nagging anxiety that Rebecca never got out of the trailer.

He rolled out of bed and braced himself against the cold of the apartment. He'd been trying to save a little money by skimping on heat, and the living room was probably near forty degrees. He choked down a cup of hot coffee, climbed into the Pontiac—its blue paint so faded that it was more of a dust gray now—and headed down historic Dauphin Street toward Mobile AIDS Support Services. He pulled into the parking lot of the MASS building, a single-story cinder-block box crammed with case files, drug-assistance-program applications, and bills. When he got inside, he put on a pot of coffee and glanced at his watch. Seven-thirty. The Jacksons usually didn't stir until at least ten. He picked up the phone and dialed their number. Sara answered and passed the receiver to Angela before he could ask any questions. They had never made it to the hospital.

"How high is the fever?" David asked.

"One-oh-four point two."

"Okay, Angela. I'm gonna leave in just a few minutes."

David grabbed a couple of toys for Rebecca's son, William, and headed for the car. He couldn't fucking believe they hadn't made it out of the trailer. Well, yes, he could: how the hell were they going to explain to the uncle that Rebecca had to go to the emergency room without having him ask what's wrong? Of course that didn't clarify why Leon, who knew she was infected, hadn't shown up after work to take her. David pulled onto Highway 45, heading north toward Choctaw County. It was nearing eight o'clock. If everything went smoothly, he'd have her in the hospital by twelve-thirty. Of course, if he'd been able to get her the home health services she so obviously needed, she might already be there now. This whole case had been a nightmare, from that first November afternoon five months ago, when he'd found her huddled over the stove with pneumonia and Sara seven months pregnant, in that rusting tin box they called a home.

He'd gone back up there probably ten times in November alone. The girls had been getting their primary care in Waynesboro from two general practitioners, Dr. Sherman and Dr. Powell, and their HIV care from Wayne General Hospital's infectious disease doctor. David had spoken with all three. Sherman and Powell seemed okay. But David could tell that the infectious disease doctor was fed up with Rebecca from the start. And in a way he didn't blame him. She didn't take her medicine, had stood him up for God-knew-how-many appointments, and checked herself out from the hospital against his orders. David suggested that they put her on some antidepressants. "She won't take them," the infectious disease doc said angrily. Eventually David was able to convince him to sign home health orders, which guaranteed that a nurse would check in on Rebecca once a week. Then he went to Sherman for the mood pills.

On November 19 he'd got the call that Sara had gone into labor seven weeks prematurely. She'd been rushed to Waynesboro. From what David was able to gather, they'd refused to take her because they didn't have facilities for a premature birth. He suspected they didn't want to deliver an HIV-positive baby. Was that paranoia? Probably. Waynesboro sent her in an ambulance to USA Women's and Children's Hospital in Mobile, where she gave birth to a baby girl, Felicia, who weighed in at four and a half pounds. When David got to the hospital, a nurse, citing the policy for publicly insured patients, told him the hospital was going to discharge her within forty-eight hours, with a bus ticket back to Choctaw. He managed to get her one more night.

After Thanksgiving he had driven to the trailer to meet Rebecca's home health nurse for her first intake. The nurse didn't show up. David called the Choctaw County Health Department. Nurse Ratched, as he liked to call the woman in charge there, told him that they had received an anonymous call warning them that Rebecca planned to bite and infect anyone who came on the property. It took him another couple of weeks to schedule a second appointment. The nurse showed up that time, but when David pulled up to meet her at the trailer, Angela told him she had left. Apparently, Angela said, the nurse had called the infectious disease doctor at Wayne General to confirm some information and had been told that he had dropped Rebecca as a patient for missing appointments. Without a supervising doctor the nurse couldn't take the case.

Things just got more complicated from there. Over the first couple months of 2001 he couldn't persuade Rebecca's boyfriend, Leon, to test at the clinic. Sara had been turned down for disability, which meant no Medicaid and no additional income to pay her electricity bill or buy propane for the trailer. No electricity meant that she couldn't plug in the electric blanket he'd brought for the baby, Felicia. And it was pretty hard to advocate for her when he couldn't even tell people that he worked for an AIDS organization. Eventually he was able to cut a deal with the guy who sold propane in Gilbertown, by posing as a United Way worker. At least he had gotten Rebecca enrolled with Dr. Preyear at USA Hospital in Mobile. Preyear, a black doctor, seemed to connect with her. But he was in Mobile, which meant that on mornings like this one, David had to drive two hours each way to get her to that office.

With one hand on the wheel, David dialed Dr. Preyear's office on his cell phone. He wanted to make sure that there was a room and a friendly staff waiting at the hospital. Diane, Preyear's assistant, told him that Preyear was at another clinic. David quickly briefed her on the situation, and she promised to page the doctor. David pulled into a Hardee's and picked up four sausage biscuits. He forced one down, threw the rest onto the front seat for the Jacksons, and tried to calm himself. At ten-thirty he pulled up to the trailer. William was standing on the weathered porch in a pair of blue rubber boots. *He looks like he's about to stomp through a mud puddle,* David thought, remembering his own kids, Kate and Daniel, as toddlers. He knocked on the door, and Angela yelled to come on in.

The trailer was in its usual state of clutter with pillboxes, clothes, and toys scattered across the floor. Rebecca was lying on the couch, eyes closed.

"I'm almost ready, Mr. David!" Angela called from the back of the trailer.

"No problem—just be sure to get her Medicaid card. We're gonna need that!" he yelled back. Then he turned to Rebecca. "Good morning, Rebecca." No response. He pressed his hand against her forehead. It was pulsing hot and sweaty. He hunted around and found the digital thermometer he'd bought them. "Rebecca, open your mouth, I need to check your fever." She didn't move. "Rebecca, it's David," he said, his accent twisting his own name into *Die-vid.* "I need you to open your mouth up." Still no response.

"Open your mouth up for Mr. David!" Angela yelled.

Rebecca looked up at David. Her eyes were glazed and dull.

"This is David," he said again, so as not to scare her. "Put this under your tongue." It instantly registered 102.7, then started climbing: 103, 103.5, 104, 104.3, 104.7, 105. David started to panic. At 105.2 and rising, he pulled it out. There was no reason to see any more. He glanced around for the bottle of liquid Tylenol he'd picked up from the pharmacy a few visits ago and found it on the floor, empty. William started opening and closing the front door: *slam, click; slam, click.*

Angela walked in. She had on a black-and-white dress that made her look almost as if she were ready for church. "Quit slamming that door!" she screamed, then knelt down next to Rebecca. She pulled a gray hooded sweatshirt over her daughter's head and laced her tennis shoes, forcing a smile for David.

He headed out to the car and got the backseat ready for Rebecca. *God,* he thought, *I hope she doesn't die before I get her to Mobile.* He went back inside and asked Angela for the car seat for William. Sara had taken it to Butler that morning. *Why the hell was Sara going to Butler when her sister was probably dying on the couch?* He didn't have time to get pissed about that. "Look, Angela," he said, "this ain't safe. But we don't got any choice. If we pass a cop, you'll just have to pull William down below the dash so I don't get a ticket." Then together he and Angela carried Rebecca out to the car. The cold air felt crisp against his face, and he could feel her burning up through her sweatshirt. They gently laid her on the backseat, and he wrapped an old beige electric blanket around her, then draped his leather coat over her chest.

Angela balanced William on her lap in the front. David pulled the Pontiac onto the dirt road. After a while he told Angela that he was going to stop off and get some more liquid Tylenol. Then Angela told him that Rebecca hadn't been able to hold any food down in nearly twenty-four hours.

That was why Rebecca rarely took the medicine she was prescribed— it all made her sick to her stomach. She couldn't to go outside to throw up, because she didn't like people to see her ill—neighbors, friends, and cousins would all start talking. She could sense that they avoided the trailer. She hated how the sickness had stolen her curves. She wanted to have more babies, like Sara, and be a schoolteacher, or a nurse, or maybe work on girls' hair. Her mother thought she was good with hair.

David pulled into the Exxon station at Gilbertown and picked up some soda for William and Angela; nothing for Rebecca. Angela and David started talking about a recent day when he'd taken Rebecca to the clinic. On the way back to the trailer, he'd said that if she were his daughter, they'd be knocking on the doctor's front door pleading for help. Then he had started insisting that Rebecca take her medications. "Rebecca," he'd said, "I don't want you to ever forget that HIV wants you dead." He had kept on repeating it. Finally, Rebecca hadn't been able to stand it anymore and had blown up: "You talk too much! This conversation is over!"

"Later," Angela said, chuckling at the memory, "Rebecca told me, 'Mr. David's okay, but he gets on my fucking nerves telling me that HIV wants me dead.'"

David turned the music down on the stereo and half-leaned back. "Look, Rebecca," he said softly, "I'll try not to get on your last nerve this morning." Then he was talking to Angela again. "The reason we butt heads is because we're so much alike. I'm hardheaded, stubborn, and I want my way."

"You're right," Angela said.

David plugged a mixed blues tape into the stereo with Derek and the Dominos, Albert King, ZZ Top, Stevie Ray Vaughan, and Joe Cocker. They drove on for a while.

Rebecca's throat was completely dry and hurting. She gathered her energy and stirred for the first time. "I want something cold to drink."

"Okay, Rebecca, we're coming into Chatom," David said. He pulled into a gas station, climbed out of the car, and came back a few minutes later with a ten-ounce bottle of orange juice and a bag of ice. "If it comes up, just aim for the floor," he said, layering it with paper towels. Then he encouraged her to try to get a little juice down. She took a few sips, but there was no ice in it to soothe her throat. David didn't have a cup, so he put some ice in a paper towel and suggested that she use it to cool her head. She refused.

"Well, as you drink the juice, you can put some in your mouth. It might make you feel better."

Rebecca felt the door close, and they drove on. Then her stomach seized up. She gagged and vomited a stream of clear fluid onto the floorboards. Then everything went dark.

David turned into the ER of USA Hospital in Mobile at about twelve-thirty. He parked illegally, bolted out of the car, ran up through the sliding electric doors, spotted a technician, and asked her to follow him outside with a wheelchair. They walked around to the backseat, where they found Rebecca passed out. She had a fever of one-oh-five point two, two hours ago, he told the woman. She's got an infectious disease, and she's here to go through PRO at Dr. Preyear's request. PRO stood for physicians referral office. He didn't know exactly what it meant, except that Dr. Preyear's office had phoned ahead to warn the hospital that they were coming, so Rebecca didn't die in the waiting room. The technician paused. She was an older white woman, probably pushing sixty.

"What kind of infectious disease?" she asked carefully.

David started to panic. Angela was in the front seat holding William. The windows were still rolled up. He stammered. And then he said, "She's got AIDS."

The woman did an about-face and walked back through the electric doors. David waited helplessly in the cold for a short eternity. What was the technician going to do? How would they treat Rebecca? This was the horror of AIDS: the not knowing, the paranoia. The woman returned wearing a pair of plastic gloves, and gently the two of them shook Rebecca awake and awkwardly lifted her into the wheelchair. Inside, David told the woman at the admit desk that Rebecca had managed to put down a bit of OJ, which he thought might have lowered her temperature a bit. She put a thermometer in Rebecca's mouth—it came out at 104.9. Next came blood pressure: seventy-seven over thirty-seven. One-twenty over eighty was normal. David asked again about PRO.

"I know what you need, sir," the nurse told him. "There's a different form for that, and I'm working on it."

A second nurse walked up. "Give us a minute, please?" she said curtly. David shut up and took a seat. People were milling about the ER, but it wasn't as hectic as he'd seen it on other visits. A nurse walked up and asked him if Dr. Ramsey was Rebecca's doctor. Ramsey ran the AIDS clinic at USA. David told her that Ramsey had seen her but had put Preyear on the case.

"Well, she's too sick to go to PRO," the nurse said. "We need to get her into a room as soon as possible."

David relaxed for the first time that morning. He turned to Angela and told her that he had to check in at the office, and asked if she was going to be okay.

"Yeah, we'll be all right," she said.

From the car David dialed Preyear's office. Diane put him through to the doctor's cell phone. Preyear picked up, and David started quoting vital signs. The connection clicked in and then out again. Finally Preyear said, "David, I'm right nearby. I'm coming over now." *Praise be,* David thought to himself.

He swung by his own apartment, ate a microwaved Lean Pocket, then headed over to the MASS office.

At MASS one of the administrators and a local black minister were putting together posters for the Black Church Week of Prayer for the Healing of AIDS, which Pernessa Seele had developed into a nationwide event. "Y'all want to head to USA and knock some nurses around with me?" David asked, half-smiling. They laughed. He checked messages, then briefed a couple of the administrators on Rebecca's condition. The mood in the office was grim. They had had news yesterday that the governor hadn't included some sort of minimum state match for the federal ADAP in next year's state budget. David didn't have all the details yet, but from what he could gather Alabama stood to lose a block of its federal AIDS funding. He couldn't think about that now. He had to get back to the hospital.

Back at the ER, he found Dr. Preyear writing Rebecca's case notes at a desk in the hallway outside her room. Technicians, medical students, internists, and patients were milling about.

Preyear was a tall, soft-spoken man with a gentle demeanor. Rebecca was complaining of chest and head pains, Preyear said, which worried him. They wouldn't know much until they'd seen pictures of her brain and chest. He'd ordered a CT scan, chest X-rays, and blood tests. She needed to be stabilized for twenty-four hours before she could be moved to a regular room.

"Dr. Preyear, is there any chance she won't be admitted?" David asked. He could feel the paranoia rising him up in him, an awful alloy of fear and anger. *Preyear was a doctor of osteology. What if some asshole M.D. overrode him?*

"No, David. She's very sick."

"What do you think of the prognosis?" David asked.

"David," Preyear said, almost sighing, "I think it's real poor."

"Why do you say that?"

"Because of these recurrent pneumonias," he said.

David excused himself and walked down the hall to Rebecca's room. She was lying in the bed. A thin oxygen line had been run up her nose. An IV drip was pulled up next to the bed, still unhooked. "How you doin'?" David asked gently.

"I'm hurtin'," Rebecca said. "Where's the man with the medicine?"

"I don't know," he said, and turned back into the hallway to get Preyear. "She's complaining of head and chest pain. Are you gonna give her something?"

"We got it coming, David."

An internist in his early forties and a younger woman, whom David took for a medical student, walked up. Preyear wheeled around in his chair, introduced David as Rebecca's case manager, and began running over her case history. Preyear was so soft-spoken that David literally had to lean his head in between them to try and figure out what was going on. Rebecca's CD4 count was only fourteen; a healthy person's might reach the thousands. David followed the three doctors into Rebecca's room. Her eyes were closed, and tears were streaming down her cheeks. The medical student and the internist gently started taking a family medical history: cancer, diabetes, heart disease—standard questions, but all ailments for which Africans Americans are disproportionately at risk. Last menstruation? A year ago. Do you smoke? I haven't had a cigarette in over a month. Drugs? No. Drink? I quit drinking. When? January.

Meanwhile, Angela was in the waiting room trying to control William. She was a woman who, at first glance, looked, in David's words, like someone who had been "rode hard and put up with." She'd waited years for her husband to get out of prison in Texas; she'd lived on food stamps; she had back pain and leg pain; and she'd drunk her way through whole stretches of her life. Her eyes squinted a little, so that sometimes they looked half-closed. She was heavy around the cheeks and chin, and her hair was dry and often half teased out so that it looked as if she'd put a little straightening grease into it, then had a few beers and gone to bed for the night and not fixed it in the morning. Sometimes it was hard for people to see past those things. But then, if one looked again, she had smile lines that betrayed the wisdom of a woman who didn't cry easily and who knew her daughters, understood how stubborn they were, and was willing to lie, sometimes maybe even to herself, to protect them. She would take William, if Rebecca died. But then, Angela never believed that Rebecca would die anytime soon.

Not much had happened for the first couple of years after Rebecca and Sara were diagnosed. Then one day in 1998 Sara announced, "You gonna be a grandmother." Angela told her she'd better not be lying, because that was how rumors got started. Then Sara took her into the next room, where Rebecca was fevering. Rebecca had hidden her pregnancy for six months. Angela loaded her into the car and drove her to Dr. Sherman in Waynesboro. He immediately transferred her to Mobile, where she stayed in the hospital for six weeks. Rebecca was too sick to have the baby naturally, so they delivered William by c-section. After the operation the doctors called Angela into a private room and asked her delicately about the future: What were her plans? Would she be able to look after William? She could tell they were trying to be sensitive; she understood what they were getting at, and she started to cry in front of them. She hated that, because she didn't want them to think she felt sorry for herself. Rebecca probably wouldn't make it to nineteen, they told her. Maybe, she thought, they just weren't used to seeing strong families, and that was why they were so quick to give up on her daughter. Then the doctors separated William from the other babies, which bothered her. She didn't suspect racism; she knew it was because Rebecca had AIDS. But it did make her hate taking Rebecca to the hospital.

Now Angela looked around the waiting room. David appeared from a door behind the admit counter.

"How you doin', Angela?" he asked.

"I'm okay."

"Did you meet Dr. Preyear?"

"Yeah, I met him. He seemed real nice."

"Angela, she's right where she needs to be."

"Yeah, I know that," she said, her tone distant.

"Look, I don't know that they're gonna let you stay in the room."

Angela said she'd made arrangements with her mother and asked David to drive her and William there.

Angela's mother lived in a mostly black working-class neighborhood just a few blocks from the hospital. William sat on Angela's lap. They drove quietly for a while. Finally, Angela told David that today was her birthday, then added that on her last birthday, her trailer had burned down.

"Gee, Angela, I'm sorry, I didn't know that," he said, gently. "Happy birthday." They were quiet again for a few more blocks. Up ahead, Angela's mother's house came into view. "Angela," David said, "I'm going to be with you until this crisis is over."

Once Angela and William were safely inside, David turned around and headed back to USA. He found Rebecca looking more comfortable, with the IV hooked up and running into her arm. Look, Rebecca, he told her,

going to put you on a floor where the nurses are going to be watch-
real close for about twenty-four hours. And they're going to be
running some tests. Once you're stabilized, they'll move you to a regular
floor. Do you have any questions about where you are, what's going on, or
what the plan is?"

She smiled, and it melted him. "Will you pull the blanket up on me a
little?" she asked.

"I'm gonna say good-bye," he said, and felt suddenly connected to her,
as though for all their distance, she was suddenly his daughter. "But I'll be
back tomorrow to check on you."

It was nearly four in the afternoon, and David felt like his head was too
full. *Screw going back to the office,* he thought, and headed home instead.
He put on yet another pot of coffee, stuck the Allman Brothers album *Eat
a Peach* on the stereo, and listened to Dickie Betts sing to him about a
woman who made him feel high when she showed him her love. He planned
to have that song played at his funeral. After that he played Diana Ross's
Lady Sings the Blues. He called his eighteen-year-old daughter, Kate, and
made her promise to have lunch with him the next day. He made more
phone calls that night—Bobbi, his swing-dancing partner; Janie, a nurse
friend; his twin brother, John—just searching for some kind of reassurance.
Finally, a little after eleven, he made himself go to sleep. At two A.M. he
jerked awake, looked at the clock, and forced himself to go back to sleep.

At three A.M. he was up again. *Fuck.* He pulled back the covers and
staggered into the living room, which looked half like a teenager's dorm
and half like a southern gentleman's study. He leaned back in a turn-of-
the-century rocking chair and lit a cigarette. In the dark the white on a
skull-and-crossbones flag he'd tacked up over a cherry antique dresser
was barely visible. He felt anxious. For the past two years he had driven
through forests and countryside that were hardwired into his speech,
thoughts, and manner in ways that even he had trouble understanding.
Yet he had done it very much as an outsider, trying to penetrate a black
world that at once overlapped every inch of his own and at the same time
was peopled by men and women whose thoughts, language, and families
were untouchable, perhaps even invisible, to him.

For much of that time he had been lost in a kind of racial borderland.
He knew now that he had crossed some sort of boundary, although he

wasn't exactly sure how he had done it. It certainly wasn't by being politically correct or culturally sensitive. He was a man, after all, who had recently offended the white director of MASS by unselfconsciously referring to some of the old men who hung out at the stores in his territory as "porch monkeys." Maybe it was actually his innate lack of caution, his lack of pretense, that gave him the freedom to try to understand Rebecca in the same complex, and perhaps even flawed, ways that he viewed his own daughter, Kate.

He took another pull on his cigarette, squashed it out, and made his way back to the bedroom, where he drifted into a dream. He was sitting on a beach in Mississippi, staring out at the emerald-green Gulf of Mexico. The waves were peeling off, glassy and clean. He pulled off his shirt and dove headfirst through the breakers. Then in an instant the waves doubled in size, and he was being sucked into their teeth by a twisting riptide. He began swimming parallel to the shore, as he had been taught, to escape the undercurrent. Between breaths he screamed at the people on the beach for help. No one paid any attention to him. He couldn't tell if they didn't care or didn't hear him. The waves were smashing over him now. He kept paddling and paddling. Then he was on the shore, gasping for breath. He looked around and realized that he didn't recognize the beach, which was deserted. He started to panic, paused, and then said to himself, *This is a dream, David. It's time to get up.*

He opened his eyes and lay for a moment in the predawn darkness. It was a little past six. There was no use trying to sleep anymore. He prayed for tolerance and for God to help him make it through the day. He was at his desk by seven, looking up at a photo of his two children, Kate and Daniel. *Jesus,* he thought to himself, *I'm lucky.* Precisely nine years ago he'd burned out on social work, quit his job at the psychiatric hospital, and moved to Orange Beach, right across from the Gulf, to work as a prep cook in his brother's restaurant.

The phone rang. It was Angela. She wanted to meet him at the hospital. He grabbed his keys and headed out the door.

David's boss, Kathy Hiers, was arriving at work when he pulled out for the hospital. She had recently received the news from Randy Russell at AIDS

Alabama, the state's mother AIDS organization in Birmingham, that Governor Don Siegelman had put only $500,000 of state money toward the federal AIDS Drug Assistance Program in his new budget. The state's waiting list for ADAP had grown into the hundreds. According to the Governor's Commission on AIDS, the Alabama state legislature would have to kick in $6 million to get everyone who qualified on the program. Complicating the matter, according to CDC surveillance data, the state had officially become home to one percent of the nation's AIDS patients. That threshold triggered a clause in the Ryan White Care Act that required the state government to pay 25 percent of the $8 million in Ryan White money it received, or else lose significant chunks of the federal funding. This year the state could probably cover the match through a stipulation in the law that allowed it to count the money the state health department was already spending on its HIV/AIDS programs. That would work only for a year or two, though, because the amount of money the state was required to match automatically increased with each successive year it stayed above the one percent threshold.

Kathy knew their main ally in the legislature was State Representative Laura Hall, who had written a $6 million amendment into the budget that would provide enough additional funding to wipe out the waiting list for ADAP. The state Ways and Means Committee, on which Laura sat, was going to vote on it on Wednesday in Montgomery. Randy had organized a rally for that morning at the statehouse, to support Laura. Kathy distributed a memo urging everyone in the office to make the drive to the rally.

Laura Hall was at first shocked and then angry when she got the news that the governor hadn't put enough money into ADAP to guarantee life-saving medications for infected people. She had just finished four months of chairing his AIDS commission. The latest information on the epidemic was dire. AIDS in America had unequivocally become a black epidemic. The disease was spreading most rapidly through the South, large parts of which were impoverished, had thin social entitlement programs, and possessed few resources to fight AIDS.

There were a number of reasons for the epidemic's move into the South. In a massive reverse migration, 630,000 blacks, according to the

U.S. Census, had moved to the region between 1990 and 2000. Slow-burning epidemics of crack cocaine and speed were festering across the region, and services for those infected were uneven. In places like rural Alabama, high alcoholism, STD, and teen pregnancy rates were threatening to intersect with and foment the epidemic. Perhaps most significantly, though, AIDS had diffused itself through black America, and the South was disproportionately black. Alabama faced a particularly difficult road. The state had no Title I cities, which meant it was completely dependent on Title II money, and the bad economy, which was beginning to drag down the nation, had hit the state hard.

Laura had run for and been elected to the state legislature in 1993, partly as a way to help herself get over Ato's death. She hadn't done much about AIDS, though, until Randy Russell approached her to sponsor a Medicaid waiver for AIDS patients. That initiative failed, but their partnership flourished. Together they had lobbied the governor to put the state's first $500,000 into ADAP. Now, if he didn't sign on to at least $2 million, she was willing to threaten Siegelman politically.

On Friday morning, March 9, three days after David had picked up Rebecca, he called the hospital and asked for her. She'd been discharged. He didn't know if she'd been sent home because she was legitimately better or because she was a publicly insured patient, or if she'd checked herself out. He couldn't bring himself to believe Preyear would let her be discharged prematurely. It wasn't above Rebecca, though, to run from that place as soon as she could take a step under her own power. He called the Jacksons' trailer. No answer. That didn't mean much; their phone was out half the time. So on Monday, March 12, he decided to drive up there and take a look for himself. From the car he called Preyear's office. Diane told him the doctor wasn't in. David asked what medications Rebecca was supposed to have brought back with her. She didn't know, but she'd ask the doctor. Rain beat steadily against the windshield; on the radio the DJ announced tornado warnings for Mobile and the surrounding counties.

David arrived at Tornado Road and found that the rain had turned it into a river. He gunned the Pontiac's engine down the half-mile of muck.

There was no sign of anyone in front of the trailer. He was about to get out of the car when he caught himself: he was wearing an AIDS Walk shirt. He zipped up his jacket and, squinting against the rain, ran up the porch and tried the door. Sara was drinking a Budweiser in the living room, and Angela was sorting laundry in the kitchen. William, Benny Jr., and Felicia were screaming and playing.

David fixed his eyes on Rebecca, who was sitting on the living-room couch with Leon. She had on a pair of jeans and a T-shirt that looked as if it had been dragged through the yard. She was thin but looked more alive than he'd seen her in weeks. "How you doin', Rebecca?" he asked carefully.

"I'm doin' just fine," she said, dissolving into a smile.

"They picked out rings, David!" Sara burst out from the kitchen.

The rain was still pinging against the metal trailer. David knelt down in front of Rebecca, took her hand, and noticed that she was wearing a tiny diamond ring. He felt like crying, laughing, and collapsing all at once. Leon was standing next to him by the television. He was Rebecca's age but didn't look much older than fifteen, with his slender frame and thin mustache. David had been so pissed at this guy for not showing up when Rebecca was fevering, but now it occurred to him that maybe he really did love her. "That's real pretty. Congratulations, Rebecca," he said. "Can I come to the wedding?"

"You can if you want to," Rebecca said. He'd probably be the only white person there.

"Have y'all got a date?"

"It's going to be sometime in June," Angela said.

"I think it's probably going to be June tenth," Leon said.

June 10 was the anniversary of David's first marriage. "I been married and divorced twice, so I ain't no expert," he said, "but I wish y'all the best." He took a breath and asked Angela what medicines she'd brought back from the hospital. She set down her laundry and brought him over a little white paper bag. Inside he found what he thought was a steroid to build up Rebecca's lungs and more antibiotics for the pneumonia.

"Rebecca," David said, "you got a follow-up with Dr. Preyear next Tuesday."

"I ain't going to Mobile to see any more doctors," Rebecca said evenly.

"I think it's probably in your best interest to have that follow-up," he said, falling into his stubborn, preachy tone.

"I'm not going to Mobile to see any more HIV doctors," Rebecca said angrily.

"Rebecca, you need to go to your doctor," Angela said.

Rebecca repeated again that she wasn't going to go.

"I got two boots on, and if I need to put on a third one, I will," Leon said, threatening to kick her in the ass if he had to.

Soon everyone was screaming. William hit Benny. Sara smacked William across the butt. David threw his hands in the air as if he were being robbed, and when he could get a word in, he turned to Leon and said, "I really think this is between you and your fiancée." After about ten minutes they all retreated to their respective corners. David didn't push it any further. He at least felt confident that the family would force Rebecca down to Mobile, even if she was too scared to go on her own.

Carefully, David redirected the conversation to Leon and Rebecca's sex life. They insisted they were using condoms. But when David asked Leon again if he'd been tested, his answer was still no. Rebecca and Leon seemed as if they'd had enough of him and excused themselves, saying they had to head down to Gilbertown to pick up some groceries.

"There's gonna be a meeting on Wednesday in Montgomery about families living with HIV," David said, before they could leave. "Rebecca, Sara, I'd like y'all to come up there with me and bring the children." The trailer was suddenly quiet. David turned to Sara. "Remember those two times that I filled the propane tank?" He was referring to the occasions when MASS had paid for the fuel to heat her trailer. "That's what this is about."

"You can tell them that I'm doin' just fine," Sara blurted out, and abruptly stood up from the couch. Rebecca was quiet.

Oh hell, David thought, *I done stepped in it again.*

"What about you, Angela?" he asked. She was folding clothes on top of the freezer at the back of the kitchen.

"I can't go, David."

"Angela, what do you want me to tell those politicians?"

"You tell them not to forget about us, David," Angela said.

Leon and Rebecca headed for the door.

"Leon will get her to her appointment, David," Angela said reassuringly.

David hung out for another forty-five minutes or so and talked to Sara. He had back-burnered her case to focus on Rebecca. From what he could gather, she had managed to get Medicaid for Benny Jr. but none for herself. He wanted to get her on the waiting list for ADAP, and he needed to get her to Mobile to see the HIV doc to have her blood work done. He'd managed only to get her to the children's clinic to have Felicia checked out. So far Felicia's blood work was clear, but it would be a year before they were sure. Finally, he said good-bye and headed home.

Butler, Gilbertown, and Silas faded into sheets of rain. It looked to David like a tornado had touched down in McIntosh and ripped open an elementary school. Its roof sat in the playground a hundred yards off the road. *God,* he thought, *I hope there were no children inside.* A thicket of twisted pine trees and huge oaks had been broken in half like matchsticks. He drove on. Somewhere between Silas and Grove Hill his cell phone rang. It was Dr. Preyear. Rebecca's T-cell count had been only ten when she left the hospital, he told David. They needed to get her on antiretrovirals. David asked which ones. Preyear mentioned a few, but it was so complicated and there were so many names that they were gone from David's mind moments after Preyear uttered them. All he knew was that if she didn't take the medications she was going to die.

Randy Russell glanced down the hallway of the statehouse. It was Tuesday afternoon. Lobbyists, state representatives, and the departmental staff were frantically negotiating the fine points of the state's budget. Randy himself was frenzied. Tomorrow the House Ways and Means Committee would vote on Laura's resolution to add $6 million to the ADAP budget. Most of the community-based AIDS organizations in Alabama were sending clients to rally for it. He'd scheduled a press conference for the late afternoon, at which the Governor's Commission on AIDS would publicly release its report.

His top two priorities were to eliminate the waiting list and to get the state to start paying for the federal match. His political game plan was simple: press hard for the $6 million, and tell the legislators and the governor that the state stood to lose its Ryan White Title II funding if it didn't make the minimum match. That, of course, meant omitting to mention the provision that allowed the state to count the already allocated dollars toward the match. But that was a risk he was willing to take. Life-saving medications, in his opinion, should not be considered an optional cost for the state government. Furthermore, paying for the federal match now would establish a precedent and make it harder for the legislature to balk at paying it in the coming years, when the size of the bill would be even harder to swallow.

Randy had tried to exert some pressure on the governor through the press. On Thursday the *Mobile Register* had run a front-page story that Alabama stood to lose $8 million in AIDS funding if it didn't come up with the match. On Friday one of the governor's spokesmen had said that he would try to find "most" of the $2 million match. That was hardly a guarantee, but earlier in the day Randy had given the commission's report to a couple of the governor's aides, and he thought he'd seen a glimmer of passion in their eyes as they looked it over. They'd promised to put it directly in Siegelman's hands. But when he'd pressed them to get the governor to meet with him, they'd alternately told him that Siegelman was out of town, still had to weigh his options, and had another engagement. Randy had left them his cell phone number but hadn't yet received a message.

Maybe, Randy hoped, Laura Hall would be able to persuade the governor to meet with them before the press conference. Randy turned his attention to the infected black woman who was standing next to him and talking; to State Senator Roger Bedford. Yeah, you've got AIDS; I've had cancer; I've survived a car wreck, Bedford was telling her. I appreciate what you're going through. Cancer is awful.

Was this what AIDS had come to at the dawn of the new century? Infected mothers standing in statehouse hallways trying to convince legislators that medication was a necessity? Randy tactfully extricated the woman from the conversation. He figured they had Bedford's vote anyway. After all, he was a family-values Democrat.

That same afternoon David drove out of Mobile, planning to spend the night at his twin brother John's in Prattville, near Montgomery, a short drive from the statehouse, and meet everyone in the morning for the rally. He hoped he could trust Leon to get Rebecca to Preyear's on his own. He crossed the Tombigbee River into Clarke County, where he had grown up. On a whim, he decided to head over to the local radio station in Jackson and see if he could get the DJ to put him on the air. Jackson was a quiet town; the Baptists had always kept and probably always would keep it dry. The radio station was a three-room affair. The two women at the front desk eyed David's MASS T-shirt warily as he pushed through the front door. He introduced himself and said he wanted to get on the radio and warn folks about the AIDS epidemic. They stared at him silently for a ten count, with what felt like bald hatred. He hadn't gotten one of those looks in a few months. He smiled slowly. "You know," he said, "nice people get HIV, too."

Randy Russell woke up early Wednesday in his hotel in Montgomery. He took a last look at the speech he'd written for Laura. They had grown so close that he felt he could almost crawl inside her mind and channel her thoughts. He scrawled a note to her across the top of the script that they'd have to do some quick rewriting if they landed the meeting with the governor. It was still early. He had enough time before meeting everyone at the church to see if any word had come from Siegelman's people. He picked up Kathy Hiers, and they drove over to the statehouse. The sky was broken, and rain beat softly against the windshield.

Randy had burnt-red hair, a square jaw, and a mustache. He was in his early forties, beginning to fill out in the jowls and around his middle, but he carried the extra weight well on his tall frame. He'd been an employee with the Birmingham Symphony Orchestra when he'd started volunteering at AIDS Task Force Alabama in the early 1990s. The work felt meaningful, so he'd gone back to graduate school to get his master's in social work and then built the agency into AIDS Alabama. Eventually, he'd grown frustrated with much of Birmingham's AIDS community, many of whom seemed to equate AIDS advocacy with gay advocacy.

He'd quickly learned that the trend in AIDS policy—in most health policy, for that matter—was to let states, cities, and even neighborhoods raise, ask for, and spend money for health care as they saw fit. At one point in the AIDS epidemic that idea had held merit. Indeed, he could make a fairly strong argument that there would have been a lot less suffering in San Francisco if the local gay leadership had been making the decisions at the NIH or the CDC in the early 1980s. But that system wasn't workable now. AIDS was moving into resource-poor communities, there was no effective network for information dissemination, and the epidemic was fading from the national consciousness. In 2000 the Institute of Medicine had come out with a report that said the CDC needed to develop a new national plan to combat the epidemic as it took deeper root in communities of color.

Alabama presented some serious challenges. The average AIDS patient in the state was black, made less than $560 a month, and probably wasn't too public about his or her HIV status. Randy's people estimated that there were two thousand infected in Alabama who hadn't even tried to get medical care. The state's public health officer, Dr. Don Williamson, hadn't named HIV in the state's top-ten list of health concerns. And the head of the state's HIV/AIDS department had made it clear to him that she didn't feel it was appropriate for her to lobby the governor for ADAP funding. In fact, Randy had found out that the state was going to have to start making the match only at an ADAP meeting he'd voluntarily attended in the spring of 2000.

Randy felt that America needed some kind of national umbrella organization, akin to the American Cancer Society or the American Lung Association, with lieutenant agencies in every state and satellite offices in cities like Mobile, Selma, and Winter Park, Florida. Those institutions did not double as "black" or "gay" or "Latino" advocacy organizations. Rather, they were successful because they functioned in the interest of the public health. Randy had tried to build AIDS Alabama on that model. He'd linked up the state's nine community-based organizations and positioned AIDS Alabama to assume the role of flagship organization if a national foundation was put together. At the very least, he hoped he'd built a network that could survive after he burned out. So far, though, he and Laura had been the only real political advocates in the state. A part of him wondered what would happen to the state's infected population if he quit or if Laura lost her reelection bid.

Randy parked the car, and he and Kathy made their way into the state-house. It was hot, and he was sweating through his suit. They hunted around for the governor's assistant, hoping for some word on their status with Siegelman. There was no sign of her. Maybe she was at a staff meeting, or maybe she hadn't even made it into work yet. Any hope for a meeting was pretty much in Laura's hands now. Randy had to get back to the church, brief the advocates, get them to the statehouse for the one o'clock Ways and Means Committee vote, meet the Governor's Commission on AIDS at two-thirty, and then make the press conference by four.

David arrived at the church in Montgomery at a quarter to ten. The bus that MASS had rented was already there. He said hello to everyone. Kathy and Randy drove up soon afterward, and he followed them inside. David counted a hundred people, the majority from MASS. Randy laid out the game plan. They were to divide up into two groups. Those who weren't comfortable talking should pin red ribbons to their clothes, crowd the Ways and Means Committee meeting, and silently wait out the vote. The rest were to head up to the seventh floor and knock on the senators' office doors. Everyone who talked to the senators, Randy said, should stress that they needed $6 million to wipe out the ADAP waiting list. David paired off with Nick, a young Jesuit volunteer who helped MASS process medication applications, and one of Nick's friends who'd come up for the rally. Kathy assigned them ten senators and gave them hand-outs that Randy had prepared with the epidemiological surveillance data from each of their districts.

David followed the MASS van to the rally. He had to leave early so he could make it to Butler that night, to do a radio interview in the morning. The higher-ups at MASS had instructed everyone to wear their churchgoing clothes. His gray hair was starting to crawl down the back of his neck, and he was wearing dirty jeans, a MASS T-shirt, a windbreaker, and his rose-colored glasses. *Screw it,* he thought, *I'm a fieldworker.* He parked and walked three blocks, past Jefferson Davis's Confederate White House, to the towering cement statehouse. He ran up the steps, past Randy and Kathy, who were doing a television interview in the rain, and rode the elevator up to the seventh floor, where he met Nick and his buddy. They worked their way down the list alphabetically. *God,* he thought, *we got balls to ask for $2 million for AIDS out of a general fund that's so tapped that they're cutting all the sports, music, and theater programs in the public schools.* His own son Daniel's life centered on playing in the high school music program. He himself might have been against putting all this money toward the disease, if he hadn't seen it up close.

"When I heard that the governor left the two million dollars out of the budget," State Senator George Callahan told Nick, "I called him myself and told him it wasn't right."

The senator's office was small and had a blue Bush campaign poster still tacked to the wall. "What we need is six million dollars to wipe out the waiting list," David said.

"Well, you got to understand," Callahan cautioned, "we got limited resources, and the general fund is in proration."

"Medication is a necessity," Nick said.

David glared at Nick. Maybe that was how they talked to politicians in Washington state, but Nick was in Alabama now, where high school science books were stickered with warnings that evolution was only a theory, and the state supreme court chief justice had got himself elected by barnstorming the countryside in an old blue Cadillac, promising to bring more religion to public life. You didn't push a southern politician into a corner on AIDS. You were polite to your adversaries, even if you found their positions distasteful. "Thank you, Senator, for your support," David said, hustling Nick out of the office.

"You were kissing his ass, David," Nick said.

"Look, you guys are going to be leaving the state of Alabama," he said, trying to control his frustration. "I got to live here."

Laura Hall looked toward the door. The committee room was packed, nearly overflowing with AIDS patients. Most of them were black. She thought of Ato. She had gotten the votes for the $2 million, but there was no chance for the $6 million. Still, that was the first step to wiping out the waiting list. Now it would go to the House floor. If it passed there, it was headed to the Senate, where it would go through the same process. But ultimately she needed to get the governor on board. When Laura still hadn't been promised a meeting with him that morning, she'd called his assistant and threatened to filibuster his economic stimulus initiative. She knew that could prove politically problematic for her in the 2002 election, but it seemed like a small sacrifice. An hour later she had gotten the word that Siegelman would talk with her and her allies after the committee meeting.

She spotted Randy at the door. He signaled for her, and she discreetly excused herself and made her way over to him. Randy pressed the speech into her hands.

"We got the meeting with the governor," she said.

"You're kidding."

"No, it's at three-thirty."

"Laura, our press conference is at four."

"I know, but what are we going to do? We've got to go to the governor."

"I guess they'll wait."

"I guess they will," she said, beaming.

They walked into the governor's conference room early. The ceiling was sculpted, and an antique table that could seat twenty dominated the floor. The governor's desk was at the far end, bookended by the American and Alabama flags. The governor came in behind them. He was tall, with steel-gray hair. Laura said hello and introduced him to Randy. The meeting was a mere formality—Laura knew that the governor would not risk his economic stimulus bill. They posed for pictures. Randy stressed the $6 million need. Siegelman promised $2 million, then asked how their press conference had gone.

"We're actually keeping them waiting," Randy said.

"You mean you haven't been yet?"

"We'd actually love for you to come down and join us."

"Actually," Siegelman hedged, "I've got some appointments."

"Well, we've really got to scurry," said Randy, trying to contain himself, "because we've got about four hundred people waiting to hear what you've said."

The governor paused.

"Don't worry," Randy said. "We'll tell them it was good."

Randy's assistant, Sharon, had a car waiting for them downstairs. Randy and Laura shielded themselves from the rain and pushed into the backseat. They drove the two blocks to the press conference, at the Alabama Activity Center down the street from the Supreme Court building, and ran from the car to the lobby. Laura patted herself dry, then heard the murmur of the crowd from the conference room. It gave her a chill. She took Randy's arm, and together they peeked into the packed hall. There were hundreds of people. Many were black. She looked at Randy, and they basked for a moment. "This is your show," he said. "Don't you dare call on me." Then he pushed through the doors. Laura barely heard his introduction.

"We've just come from a meeting with the governor," Laura declared, "and he's pledged to find the two million." The crowd stood and cheered. Then she told them about her son, Ato, feeling as if he were there with her.

After her speech she found herself alone, waiting in line for the buffet table. A black woman in her mid-fifties approached her with her son, whom Laura recognized as one of the AIDS patients who had lobbied the legislature. Laura took a deep breath. The woman was, like Laura, five and a half feet tall, with hair coloring to cover up the gray. The young man was Ato's age, if Ato had lived.

"I want to thank you for your courage," the woman started.

Laura's insides were quivering. She wanted to cry out that she had hidden her son's disease, that this woman was the one who was brave for bringing her family into the open. But she stopped and looked at the woman's son. She felt grateful that he was alive and here. And then, for a moment, her own grief gently receded.

David was somewhere on State Highway 85 heading toward Selma. He was still buzzing from his afternoon in Montgomery. The road stretched out in front of him like a gray river, edged by open pastures and farmland. Every so often he passed a sign commemorating Martin Luther King's march from Selma to Montgomery. He felt as if he were with them now. At the same time he wanted to know how it came to be that he was fighting for medications to save the lives of the same people whose freedom the civil rights workers had marched for three decades ago. He didn't really know if Americans cared much about the South anymore.

Indeed, the South seemed to exist now mainly in lowercase. When other Americans did think about it, they were often peering at iconic, rough-grained images of tenant farmers, shotgun shacks, fire hoses, and burning crosses. Surely that was because they wanted to honor those who had suffered and the heroes who delivered them from oppression. Americans also seemed drawn to those images, however, because they reminded and reassured them that they were a people who stared down hatred and injustice. In that sense, reflecting on them was a redemptive process that worked only so long as Americans believed that the Old South was somehow a place physically, culturally, and socially separate from the rest of the country. The veneer of the "New South" had made it possible for even the South itself to participate in that process.

Perhaps, though, this process of redemptive reflection obscured Americans from fully seeing themselves and how, in their effort to move past racism, they'd failed to address the more enduring and substantive consequences of the country's racial past. The South, with its fine-tuned civility, its self-determination, its moral certainty, and its bald willingness to say what the region was and what it stood for, had always powerfully mirrored the core of the American national character. For a long time David had thought that AIDS had led him into a foreign and unknown world, but the Alabama he had seen remained what it always had been: a startling, beautiful, complex, and in many ways honest reflection of America and what it had become.

ON THE MORNING of April 24, 2002, Sara Jackson opened her eyes, grasping at the strands of a nightmare. In the dream Leon and Rebecca were asleep up the road in the front room of her parents' trailer. Rebecca looked thin on the bed, and her chest was heaving. Leon stirred awake, and Rebecca stopped breathing. Then he was on top of her, his mouth against hers, breathing, breathing, breathing, and screaming for Angela and Robert. Then Sara's father was knocking at her door. Half asleep, she met him in the darkness.

"Rebecca's gone."

"Tell me you're playin'," she said, her voice rising in anger, "'cause this ain't no playin' situation." Then her feet were running up the road, brushing dirt and grass, her face framed against the night sky. Tears ran down Sara's cheeks. She felt sick all at once, as if she needed to throw up.

Then she was holding Rebecca in her arms, her body so frail now that she had taken to dressing in children's clothes. Sara shook and shook her sister. Maybe, she thought, she was in a deep sleep. But her baby, her big baby, didn't stir. Sara was crying harder now, and through the tears she sang, "'Hush little baby, do not cry, Mama's gonna sing you a lullaby.'" Then the paramedics were there in the trailer. And they were listening to Rebecca's heart. No sound.

Sara rolled over in bed. The sun was peering in through the trailer window. Benny Sr. was next to her, his arms and shoulders, a mass of granite muscle, spread across the bedclothes. "I dreamed that my sister was gone," she said. "I dreamed that she passed away."

"Baby," he said, "that wasn't no dream."

The morning of Rebecca's funeral was bright and thick with humidity. Rebecca's son, William, stood on the deck before his grandma's trailer, the hood of a blue-and-yellow jacket draped over his head like a Superman cape. His eyes were like almonds, and his full cheeks, pulled down over his chin, made him look like a small man. The porch had finally fallen down, replaced by a makeshift wooden deck with two rickety steps, held up by a couple of cinder-block bricks. A brown Datsun was parked in front of the trailer, its side mirror melted from the fire that had burned down the old trailer. A black wig lay in the dirt next to its rear right tire. A deflated child's swimming pool with a puddle of dirty water lay in the front yard. William didn't look sad, just open, like a child watching.

Sara walked up the road wearing a black dress, barefoot. She yelled hello to some of the guests who were arriving for the funeral procession. She looked strong, and her hair was highlighted red in the front and gelled so it stood on point. Fred from the trailer next door walked up, holding Felicia over his shoulder. After a time Angela came outside, smiling and friendly, her hair pulled back tight, a brush of bangs swept across her forehead. She hugged a couple of guests and said it was lovely for them to have come. David walked over, and they hugged. His gray hair was long in the back, and his shoulders looked hunched under his powder-blue blazer, but his eyes were clear behind his rose-colored glasses.

William climbed down off the deck, traced his hand along the edge of the Datsun, and made his way toward his great-grandmother's cottage. He'd shed the Superman hood; his hair was cut tight to his head so that it was just a shadow across his scalp. Dust kicked up off the road onto his silk vest, which was decorated in a paisley pattern of tiny racing cars. His great-grandmother's boyfriend, Paul, a tall man from Detroit with a square jaw, wearing a pinstriped suit hanging loosely from his lean arms and hollow legs, greeted him on the front steps. Paul bent over, tied William's shoes and dusted him off, then went back inside to finish dressing himself. William plopped down onto a worn porch chair and stared off over the rail, across the road, through the barbed wire, past the cows wandering in the luminous ocean of grass, and off into the forest. He'd told his grandma that he wasn't a baby anymore. He was a boy. He was three and a half years old, and he knew his mama was dead.

Soon Angela had him bundled into the seat of a car, and the funeral procession pulled out from the trailer. The cars crawled in a slow parade up a gentle hill. The forest gave way to a thin veil of trees along the road; behind it the woods had been clear-cut. The trees left behind were white and dead against the lush undergrowth. The cars made their way toward the church. By the roadside vultures, their long necks and small heads arched out from heavy black bodies, watched the procession pass.

The cemetery lay on one side of a country road. Some of the gravestones were nothing more than deteriorating metal posts sticking up from the ground, like the remnants of a rusting shovel or soda can that one might find on an old farm. Others were newer white stones, carefully nestled in the grass. On the other side of the road stood a hearse, its black paint and chrome fenders swirling in the sunlight, backed up to the front doors of the church. It was a new building, whose redbrick facade gave it a hollow look, almost like a movie set.

Angela and Robert entered the church through the double doors and made their way up the center aisle toward a long silver coffin. Rows of polished pews stretched out on either side of them, and the floor beneath their feet felt thin under its green carpet. White metal pull blinds kept the country heat from overwhelming the sanctuary. Angela and Robert took a seat one row back from the front on the left.

Sara followed behind them, her eyes fierce as she laughed and talked in a strong confident bellow. William entered with Leon; his eyes were wide, and he was calm and still. They sat together in the front row on the far right side of the church, next to David. Sara's son, Benny Jr., was one of the last inside. Benny Sr. got him to the door, and then the child started screaming. "Come on!" Benny Sr. said, and jerked him by the arm. Benny Jr. caught hold of the doorjamb. His daddy grabbed him by the waist and pulled him until he was parallel to the floor and shrieking. Benny Sr. yanked until Benny Jr. finally couldn't hold on anymore, and he carried him to the front, where they sat down next to Leon and William.

Angela grasped Robert's arm. A large man approached her and asked if she'd like one last chance to see her daughter's body. She turned to Robert to see if he'd come up there with her. He shook his head no. She hunched forward, and her hips and thighs sent ripples across her dress as she neared the casket. Her expression didn't change much as she looked down at her daughter. Rebecca's eyes were closed; she looked almost asleep, delicate and open. Angela turned around and curled back down next to Robert. A woman from the church asked if anyone else wanted a final viewing. A few mourners rushed up to the front and snapped pictures of Rebecca. Then they gently lowered the coffin lid as one of Rebecca's cousins sang. The woman from the church asked if anyone wanted to speak. There was an awkward silence. A baby cried.

David stood up. "I—I'd like to just say that there's a lot of love in this family," he started.

An old thin man mumbling something about a goddamn white guy drowned his voice out. Angela looked over her shoulder, caught her cousin Bill's eye, and stared him down coldly. David was family—his skin color had nothing to do with it. He'd suffered with that girl as if he were her father. Bill kept mumbling. He was drunk. David's voice trailed off. He ducked his head and returned to his seat next to Leon. Reverend Williams approached the pulpit.

Funerals aren't the time to preach, he began. Still, he wanted to talk about finding Jesus. He couldn't determine if Rebecca was headed to heaven or hell. Only God could make that decision. But he did know that Rebecca had had her chance. And it wasn't too late for everyone there. Angela's grief turned to a hot, almost violent anger. She bored her eyes into the reverend's. He was talking about Job. *How dare he!* she seethed. *Rebecca prayed, she prayed for God to take her, to end her suffering. She loved God. She was just too sickly to come to church.*

Leon was weeping and clutching William. David's eyes were red and swollen. They were the only two crying openly. William's eyes were wide, and he sat straight up in Leon's lap. Leon was his daddy now. Angela continued to lock eyes with the reverend. Folks had died young in this country for as long as people had been here, but this was a different kind of death. Why was Rebecca gone? Angela wanted to know. Why did she have to suffer? If anyone let Rebecca down, she believed, it had been her.

After the eulogy a woman from the church in a cotton dress, tall and skinny, woodenly asked the mourners who were seated in the aisle to leave first with their chairs. Then the men from the family carried Rebecca's silver casket to the hearse. Sara followed behind. She made it to the front door. The heat was all around her, rich and stifling. Sweat beaded up on her brow. And then suddenly her strength gave out. "I can't, I can't, I can't!" she cried, her voice clear and raw, piercing the summer air. A girlfriend collapsed her arms around her like a tourniquet. Rebecca, her sister, her baby, was gone, gone, gone! And she couldn't watch them put her into the ground. "No!" she screamed.

Monday afternoon Sara sat alone in her mother's trailer. Tornado Road was quiet. The mourners had left. She had curled up in Rebecca's bed every day since her death to be close to her. Rebecca had been so angry. She and Leon had postponed their wedding half a dozen times because she was too ill to take her vows. A fungus had eaten at her brain, and she finally refused to take her medicine altogether. At the end she was like a bomb waiting to explode. She couldn't understand why her doctor had given up on her. What'd she done wrong? she'd ask her mother. Angela had tried to explain that some people just don't like other people; they aren't patient and don't have any business being in the medical profession. Maybe, Rebecca sometimes thought, it would be better just to give up and die. That way the pain would be gone. But then she'd think of William and that she had to live long enough to see him get on that yellow bus to school.

Sara felt the same way. She knew she should go to the doctor now— for her children, for her mother, and for herself—and that she had to take her medicines. But sometimes her infection made her feel too angry, too alone, to face that ordeal. She didn't deserve to have this thing, she thought. A part of her believed that Satan had made her sick and that only the Lord could help her. The heat was almost unbearable. She looked out the window. The skies had opened, and it was raining. She watched the water beat against the dirt road, transforming the clay into a soft river of red mud. She knew it was God, and that He was washing Rebecca's footprints from the face of the earth, freeing her from its pain, so she could be delivered into heaven.

EPILOGUE

On a cloudy November afternoon in 2000 I boarded a plane in San Francisco and flew to Mobile to find out why so many black people were dying of AIDS. I didn't know what I was going to find. And quite frankly, I was worried that I would fail to uncover many new answers. For more than a year I had been trying to understand why blacks were dying from AIDS. I had heard many explanations, but most of them felt abstract, tired, and far away. I had found the epidemic, like black America itself, to be searingly vital and at the same time elusive, ephemeral, and hidden. I hoped to find some clarity in the murky landscape of the American South.

I changed planes in Atlanta and rode the indoor airport subway to my connecting flight to Mobile. My gate was almost deserted. As I walked down the ramp to my plane, I listened absently to the singsongy accents of two middle-aged white men—good old boys—headed home from a weekend of beer and golf. The confident tenor of their voices was at once attractive and unsettling. On the plane a large coal-black middle-aged man sat down next to me. With a tinge of embarrassment, I stuffed the copy of *Black Like Me* I'd been reading into my carry-on bag and shifted awkwardly in my cramped seat so I could take full measure of him. His small head seemed perfectly balanced on a spiraling mass of chins, belly, and thighs. I thought he looked tired and wondered how he would feel if he knew I was studying him. As we taxied down the runway, I asked him if he was from Atlanta. He looked at me through cloudy red eyes and told me he had been in Georgia on business and was headed home to Mississippi. I said something nondescript about my work in Mobile. Much to my relief, he didn't ask me to elaborate, though if he had, I don't suppose

I would have said anything about my interest in AIDS and blacks. I suspect it would have made us both feel vaguely ashamed, and he probably would have felt obligated to inquire what I was after, a question that at the time had no clear answer.

Early on in my research I often avoided telling people that I was writing about AIDS and black America. I felt a little uncomfortable about it, and more than a few of the people to whom I described the project seemed worried that I might actually be writing more about race than disease. I think most of us are anxious that race still somehow defines us. Yet at the same time, it seems, few have a strong sense of what the word means anymore. Race is confusing and exciting, a concept that, like right and wrong, is vital, dangerous, all encompassing, and perpetually just out of reach. Perhaps that's why so many people I met in the course of writing this book seemed to prefer the idea that I was writing about sex, drugs, gay culture, public health, politics, or religion. Those are issues that I could at least take safe positions on without inadvertently condemning myself or my audience.

Quite frankly, I was more comfortable speaking about those issues, too. After all, on the day I met my agent she told me—with the refreshing honesty that is her trademark—that whites aren't usually offered book contracts to write about blacks. Indeed, when I met fellow authors and academics writing about subjects with seemingly racial themes like inner-city education, drug abuse, and prisons, the actual issue of race was rarely central to their investigations. AIDS, though, was unique among the chronic ills commonly understood to afflict black neighborhoods, because by the time I got on the story in 1999, it had been designated as a largely black disease by the government, the public health community, and even the Congressional Black Caucus. I was going to have to explore what about this epidemic made it black.

During my first interviews with the people who would inhabit this book, my questions often focused on the narrow issue of oppression and victimhood, which has always been a central theme of the American racial debate.

Do you trust the doctors? I asked Desi Rushing. Do you experience them as callous about your needs or those of your family?

What about Tuskegee? I asked Bob Fullilove.

Are the black elite refusing to own up to AIDS because they want to protect the larger reputation of the race? I asked Mario Cooper.

While they all had opinions on these subjects, their responses were mostly flat, and their answers nearly monosyllabic, as though these issues—each of which peppered seemingly every newspaper account of the black epidemic—were peripheral to their experience.

Only when I steered my questions more personally toward what had brought them to AIDS, or alternatively to what had brought AIDS to them, did their tone became urgent and their answers unpredictable. Their memories were nonlinear and often tied to the epidemic only by their intuition: Bob Fullilove's parents teaching him to pronounce his words so that they sounded white; Desi smoking crack to blunt her pain, and her sense that something essential was wrong with her world; Mario struggling out of his school uniform and into a pair of jeans in the backseat of the limousine as he was being driven to his parents' mansion in Mobile's black ghetto. Their memories were raw and occasionally so painful that some of my sources would put off our interviews for weeks, even months, at a time.

So when I arrived in Mobile, a year after starting this book, all I thought I had was a pastiche of powerful fragments that by themselves seemed to have little to do with AIDS and everything to do with race, and yet were so universal in their humanity that they felt almost completely race blind.

I planned to use my two weeks in Alabama to drive through the poorest rural counties north of Mobile with David deShazo. I had been talking with him by phone on and off for a couple of months and knew him only by his smoky southern Alabamian drawl. He had told me about rural ghettos, crack-infested towns in the woods, filth and poverty that made his skin crawl. His Alabama sounded like Africa. But it wasn't Africa that had attracted me to David. It was the words he chose to describe the rural South: forgotten towns settled after the Civil War; AIDS tests under the pecan tree on the hill; "niggers" and "faggots"; general stores; holy rollers and preachers; azaleas and sweet gum trees. Perhaps, I thought, I would find the source of the AIDS epidemic in this heartland of the American civil rights movement.

On my third day with David we drove out to the Jacksons'. Rebecca was desperately ill, but I was immediately struck by Sara's openness. We had been there less than two hours when she showed me the scars from where she'd been shot. Like all the people I met in the course of my research, she seemed to have something urgent to share, even though she wasn't quite sure what it was or how it was tied to her disease or to her dying sister who lay on the couch next to us.

When I returned home to California, I realized that the story I wanted to tell—that I believed needed to be told—was in fact this confusing collection of fragmented memories and impressions. In that sense, this book is not an exhaustive investigation of the black AIDS epidemic. Rather it is an exploration of the interior experience of the black AIDS epidemic, lifted from the minds of the people on the front lines of public health, politics, urban America, the black elite, and the American South.

Three years later AIDS, it seems to me, has forced each of the people in this book to unsparingly confront the legacy of America's racial past. The process for each of them—Mindy delving into the roots of the epidemic, David returning to the heartland of the civil rights movement and engaging with the Jacksons, Desi raised in the chaos of the urban landscape, and Mario confronting the boundaries of the black elite—has been psychologically, intellectually, and spiritually dangerous. Yet while they all have struggled at times with anger and frustration, rarely have I heard them fall back into the old paradigm of blame and righteousness. Rather, they have struggled—with varying degrees of success—to develop a richer language to make sense of and share their experience.

Mindy has continued to use the psychology of place as her central metaphor to describe the black experience. Shortly after she delivered her speech to the National Catholic AIDS Network in 1997, she was invited to speak to some residents of two Pittsburgh housing projects that were slated to be torn down. After her speeches the women of the community took her to a cocktail hour with their city councilman—Sala Udin. Mindy hadn't seen him in nearly ten years. In 1998 Mindy and Bob accepted invitations to become visiting professors at the University of Pittsburgh. Her experience there launched her into a five-year investigation of how urban renewal changed black American life, a project that has culminated in a contract for a book she has tentatively titled *Root Shock: Upheaval, Resettlement and Recovery in Urban America.* While the epi-

demic in this new work is central to the story she tells of David, she treats
AIDS as a symptom of a much larger process of community destruction
and disintegration. And she uses urban renewal as a window through
which to explore what happens to people, and by extension the country,
when their neighborhoods are destroyed. Even now, though, Mindy continues to wrestle with her language when talking about her own experience of race, often falling back on metaphors and anecdotes to express
her points.

Mario Cooper has struggled to articulate a vision for the future of
black political leadership. He stayed active in the AIDS community for a
year or two following the Congressional Black Caucus initiative. Gradually, though, he has become disillusioned with national black politics and
leaders and remains deeply conflicted over the role they now play in advocating for the larger black community. Sometimes he will cast them as
deeply committed, passionate leaders who made great strides during the
Clinton presidency but remain overwhelmed by the breadth of issues
they are expected to lead on. Then in another conversation he will sum
them up as a group who on the whole have come to accept the permanence of a black underclass and have chosen instead to represent the
interests of middle-class black Americans. Often he returns to the notion
that local black politicians are the ones who will ultimately lead against
the crises, like AIDS, that continue to strike the poor.

Laura Hall is still in office and has found her voice by publicly telling
and retelling the story of Ato's death. She is one of a small cadre of state
and local southern black politicians who are outspoken on AIDS. In 2003
she helped win $2.9 million from the Alabama state legislature for AIDS
services and medications, and in 2004 she is working for nearly $5 million.
She sits on the board of the Black AIDS Institute and remains chair of the
Governor's Commission on AIDS. She recently wrote an editorial in *USA
Today* encouraging a more open dialogue among black women about sex.

David deShazo is still plainspoken and eccentric. He spends much of
his week driving through the same rural counties above Mobile talking
about sex to just about anyone who will listen. Most of the locals know
him now and often chuckle when he pulls up in the Pontiac. He's taught
himself to play his acoustic guitar, which he often keeps in the backseat
of the car. Most of his songs are blues and country, with titles like "Dirt

Road Fever," "Ride the Anger," and "A Time to Heal." He plans to keep his AIDS job for another year or two, then wants to move to Nashville to try to make it as a country singer.

Desi remains healthy and still orders much of her life through her faith and relationship to God. Shortly after she told her story to Rebecca Denison, she joined the staff of WORLD, becoming a peer advocate for infected women. Pastor Robinson has supported her AIDS work and helped her develop a flourishing AIDS ministry at Faith Full Gospel Church. Her story has been featured on Black Entertainment Television and local Bay Area newscasts, and she often recounts it in public schools, Christian churches, and AIDS forums. She has repaired her relationship with her father, Harold, and has come to understand his behavior through the lens of alcoholism. In the spring of 2001 she introduced Harold's childhood best friend, retired congressman Ron Dellums, for a lecture he delivered on the global AIDS pandemic. Her son, Ken, has also been saved and is training to become a minister. Desi eventually resigned her position at WORLD—a secular nonprofit organization—so she could have more freedom to integrate her Christian message with her AIDS work.

In the spring of 2003 she spoke about HIV to a class at McClymonds High School in Oakland. Like many public schools in Oakland, it was largely minority and underfunded. The day she spoke there a fire drill interrupted her presentation. All the classrooms on her floor emptied out of the school. Once outside Desi gathered as many students as she could and started telling her story. It poured out of her—her drug use, her rape, Monique's death. The kids began firing questions at her about sex, and family, and child abuse, and drugs. To Desi it felt as though they were talking not just about AIDS but about everything. Afterward it struck her that they were the children of her generation—the children of crack-heads and broken families.

Perhaps, though, it would be more accurate to describe them as the children of the heirs of the civil rights movement. Judging from her description, many of them were struggling, as she had, to come up with a language to describe and make sense of an America that didn't feel right to them. It seems to me that Sara and Rebecca Jackson were members of that new generation.

Shortly after Rebecca died, Deborah, a black infected woman who worked as a peer advocate at Mobile AIDS Support Services, drove Sara to Mobile to have her blood worked up at the University of Southern Alabama Hospital. The results were encouraging: her T-cell count—the number of disease-fighting white blood cells in her bloodstream—was near the level one might expect to find in a healthy person, meaning that her immune system was still strong enough to fight off infection. She had recently been approved for disability insurance, and with proper monitoring and medication it was reasonable for her to expect to live relatively symptom free for years. Soon after she received the results, though, Sara cut herself off from Deborah, David, and the rest of the social workers at MASS. Perhaps she will one day decide to reconsider that decision. Or perhaps, as David believes, she won't resurface until her HIV infection progresses to full-blown AIDS, and she shows up in the emergency room near death.

I first came to Alabama to discover why Sara, her sister, and thousands of blacks like them seemed fated to die from AIDS. Nothing about Sara suggests to me that she experiences herself as a victim. She is self-possessed, defiant, at times angry, sure of her decisions, and seemingly unselfconscious about her blackness. Yet she, like Rebecca, is also in many ways invisible: she lives in a place that has faded from the popular American imagination, and she has slipped through the cracks of nearly every American public institution. Even when David—a man whose unusual innocence seems to know few racial boundaries—first met the Jacksons, he seemed to be talking to them as if he were shouting across an unbridgeable racial chasm.

After nearly four years of trying to piece together the impressions, emotions, and memories of my sources, I have come to believe that the nature of that chasm—more than the architecture of any specific social policy—lies at the bottom of the black and white failure to stop the spread of this epidemic. It seems to me that AIDS—its blackness, and the way it has intersected with civil rights, drug abuse, policing, religion, politics, public health, housing, religion, sexuality, sin, and virtue—has offered the country an opportunity to forge a new American language to engage in a fresh conversation on race that has the potential to close the chasm. For much of the past twenty years, however, the epidemic has had the opposite effect: regenerating a narrow debate conducted either in a rhetoric of racism that makes whites into oppressors and blacks into victims of oppression, or in a language of cultural relativism that too often reduces whites to passive actors and blacks to unknowable others. In the absence of a new language, the much richer, more vital, and continuing story of race in the post–civil rights era has been obscured. That perhaps, more than any callous disregard for human life, has kept the contours of this very public disease secret. I am confident that opportunities to forge this new conversation have and will continue to be presented, whether by the enduring social problems of AIDS, crime, and drug abuse, or by some new epidemic that has yet to materialize, or by the daily ways blacks and whites encounter each other. The questions I am left with now center more on what risks the members of both races are willing to take to engage in it, and what potential it holds to change the nature of life in the rural and urban landscape, not just for people like Sara, but for all Americans.

Notes

Each chapter in this book is based on extensive interviews both with the people who are featured in the narrative and with a host of public health experts, doctors, policy makers, academics, social workers, AIDS advocates, and, most important, people infected with HIV, their friends, and family members. Wherever possible I corroborated, contextualized, and filled in gaps in their memories with scholarly articles, journalistic coverage, government reports, and personal papers.

PROLOGUE: TORNADO ROAD

3. *Sara Jackson:* The names and identifying characteristics of the Jackson family and their friends have been changed.

CHAPTER ONE: SMOKE

10. *more people were infected in the region:* All proceeding HIV and AIDS statistics that appear in the book come either from CDC surveillance reports or from other publications put out by the CDC media office, unless otherwise noted. CDC surveillance reports are available online at *www.cdc.gov.*

10. *population of Choctaw County, Alabama:* All proceeding demographic information that appears in the book is taken from reports by the Bureau of the Census, U.S. Department of Commerce, unless otherwise noted. Census Bureau publications are available online at *www.census.gov.*

19. *a high incidence of teen pregnancy:* Population Resource Center, *Executive Summary: Teen Pregnancy Rates in Alabama,* online at *www.prcdc.org.*

19. *Crack associated with HIV:* Brian R. Edlin et al., "Intersecting Epidemics—Crack Cocaine Use and HIV Infection Among Inner-City Young Adults," *New England Journal of Medicine* 331, no. 21 (1994): 1442.

22. *He carried a list of statistics:* In October 2000 the Kaiser Family Foundation published a Capitol Hill Briefing Series that reported that the CDC estimated that 800,000 to 900,000 Americans were infected with HIV. Sixty percent of them, it esti-

mated, citing the *New England Journal of Medicine,* were not receiving regular medical care. An estimated 46 percent of Americans with HIV, it continued, had annual incomes below $10,000. See Kaiser Family Foundation, "Capitol Hill Briefing Series on HIV/AIDS," 2000, online at *www.kff.org.*

23. *a case in a Mississippi town:* Centers for Disease Control, "Cluster of HIV-Infected Adolescents and Young Adults—Mississippi, 1999," *Morbidity and Mortality Weekly Report* 49, no. 38 (1998): 861–63.

25. *Between 1990 and 2000 the number of infected people living in Alabama:* Richard Holmes, M.P.H., director of HIV/AIDS Branch, Alabama Department of Public Health, communication to author, 20 August 2000.

25. *The average AIDS patient in the state:* AIDS Alabama, *Statewide Needs Assessment Results* (Birmingham: Censeo Research Services, 1999), 5.

25. *Only a scant few:* Ibid., 77.

26. *Ten states had capped enrollment:* National Alliance of State and Territorial AIDS Directors and AIDS Treatment Data Network, *Fact Sheet: AIDS Drug Assistant Program,* online at *www.kff.org.*

26. *Just to wipe Alabama's ADAP waiting list clean:* The $6 million figure was calculated by AIDS Alabama and later endorsed by the Governor's Commission on AIDS.

CHAPTER TWO: ALLIED

30. *Dr. Mindy Thompson Fullilove:* My interviews with Mindy were greatly informed by her semiautobiographical series of meditations on the psychology of place. Mindy Thompson Fullilove, *The House of Joshua: Meditations on Family and Place,* ed. Sander L. Gilman (Lincoln: University of Nebraska Press, 1999), 31–32.

31. *a leader of the burgeoning black labor movement:* Ibid., 13.

31. *forced her to desegregate the Orange school system:* Ibid., 45–53.

32. *At Columbia University College of Physicians and Surgeons:* Ibid., 80.

32. *She had published articles in two of the country's:* Steven Shea and Mindy Thompson Fullilove, "Entry of Black and Other Minority Students into U.S. Medical Schools: Historical Perspective and Recent Trends," *New England Journal of Medicine* 313 (1985), and Mindy Thompson Fullilove and Tyrone Reynolds, "Skin Color in the Development of Identity: A Biopsychosocial Model," *Journal of the American Medical Association* 76, no. 6 (1984).

37. *In August 1969 Dr. Robert DuPont:* "Drug Wars," produced by Brooke Runnette and Martin Smith, reported by Lowell Bergman, *Frontline,* Public Broadcasting System, October 9, 2000. Available online at *www.pbs.org.*

37. *Nixon had campaigned hard on crime:* Eva Bertram et al., *Drug War Politics: The Price of Denial* (Berkeley: University of California Press, 1996), 105.

37. *murder and burglary rates in the District:* "Drug Wars."

37. *Nixon took the gamble:* Ibid.

37. *Then in 1971 Congressman Robert Steele:* Ibid.

37. *"Drug traffic is public enemy number one"*: Bertram, *Drug War Politics*, 106.

38. *The number of cities with federally funded treatment services*: Ibid., 89.

38. *Nationally, treatment and prevention worked*: Joan F. Epstein and Joseph C. Gfroerer, *Heroin Abuse in the United States: OAS Working Paper* (1997), online at *www.health.org/govpubs*.

38. *Nixon was in a delicate position*: "Drug Wars."

39. *There were 1.8 million lifetime heroin users*: Office of National Drug Control Policy, *National Drug Control Strategy Update: Estimated Number of Users of Selected Illegal Drugs* (2003), online at *www.whitehousedrugpolicy.gov*.

42. *Margaret Heckler, head of the Department*: Jon Cohen, *Shots in the Dark: The Wayward Search for an AIDS Vaccine* (New York: W.W. Norton & Co., 2000), 6.

42. *When four cases of swine flu were identified*: Elizabeth W. Etheridge, *Sentinel for Health: A History of the Centers for Disease Control* (Berkeley: University of California Press, 1992), 247–67.

43. *They found that the men knew about AIDS*: Randy Shilts, *And the Band Played On: Politics, People, and the AIDS Epidemic* (New York: Penguin, 1988), 260.

43. *Ordinarily the doctors and epidemiologists at the CDC*: Etheridge, *Sentinel for Health*, 43.

44. *the scientists at the National Cancer Institute*: Cohen, *Shots in the Dark*, 7.

45. *the scientific community felt that infectious diseases*: Gregory L. Armstrong, Laura A. Conn, and Robert W. Pinner, "Trends in Infectious Disease Mortality in the United States During the 20th Century," *Journal of the American Medical Association* 281, no. 101 (1999): 61.

45. *the blood banks were worried that the agency would jeopardize*: Shilts, *And the Band*, 220.

51. *As far as Mindy knew, no AIDS researchers had gathered*: When MIRA was launched, Mindy hired her husband to review the extant literature on AIDS in minority communities. See Robert E. Fullilove, "Minority Communities and AIDS: A Review of Recent Literature," *Multicultural Inquiry and Research on AIDS* 1, no. 2 (1987).

51. *The first cases of what would come to be known as AIDS*: The first years of the CDC's AIDS investigation were discussed in my interviews with several sources. But the definitive journalistic account of this period is Shilts, *And the Band*.

54. *Little action had as yet been taken against AIDS in Alameda County*: M. Garcia-Soto et al., "The Peculiar Epidemic, Part I: Social Response to AIDS in Alameda County," *Environment and Planning* A30 (1998): 731–46.

54. *In fact, barely anything substantive had been written about black sexuality*: Eugene Crayton Jr. and Richard B. Goodjoin, "Black Sexuality: A Preliminary Review of the Literature," *Multicultural Inquiry and Research on AIDS* 1, no. 4 (1987): 2–3.

55. *"Medical studies" at the turn of the century*: W. Michael Byrd and Linda A. Clayton, *An American Health Dilemma: A Medical History of African Americans and the Problem of Race: Beginnings to 1900* (New York: Routledge, 2000): 410–11.

55. *In the weeks leading up to the first day of school*: Fullilove, *House of Joshua*, 49.

55. *the story of Esther*: Ibid., 52.

CHAPTER THREE: THE HEIR

63. *Between 1950 and 1960 the city's black population had grown:* William L. Nicholls II and Earl R. Babbie, *Oakland in Transition: A Summary of the 701 House-hold Survey* (Berkeley: Survey Research Center, University of California at Berkeley, 1969), 6.

63. *During that same period nearly one-sixth of the city's whites:* Ibid., 5.

63. *unemployment had swollen to 7.7 percent:* Ibid., 110.

65. *At the end of the 1930s the city emerged as the Bay Area's:* Ibid., 3.

65. *In 1940 Oakland's shipbuilding and manufacturing companies:* Ibid.

65. *Between 1940 and 1946 600,000 people moved to the Bay Area:* Ibid., 3–4.

66. *The rush of migrants transformed Oakland:* I owe much of my description of Oakland during World War II to Marilynn S. Johnson, *The Second Gold Rush: Oakland and the East Bay in World War II* (Berkeley: University of California Press, 1993), 144–50.

66. *Then, almost as suddenly as the war had reinvented:* At the close of the war more than 50 percent of Oakland's black community was living in temporary housing projects, 90 percent of which were either structurally substandard, unsanitary, or overcrowded. Nicholls and Babbie, *Oakland in Transition,* 4–5.

71. *According to a* Newsweek *article on black youth:* Peter Goldman et al., "Black Youth: A Lost Generation?" *Newsweek,* August 1978, 22.

73. *Desi tried to fight through her feverish haze:* This is a classic symptom of sero-conversion, the process by which a person becomes HIV-positive.

75. *"I killed you":* After Eddie McKnight raped Desi, she found out that his real name was Larry Hunt and that he had been using the alias to provide cover for an ear-lier offense. Years later she heard that he had died of AIDS. Alameda County Court records document that Larry Hunt was convicted of purse-snatching in 1980, and was sentenced to one year of county jail and an additional two years of parole. He was arrested again in 1987 for skipping out on that parole sentence. This arrest was fol-lowed by a series of parole violations for testing positive for cocaine. These violations led to a jail sentence in 1990. By 1991, according to court records, he was in the final throes of AIDS: Kaposi's sarcoma lesions covered his body and were threatening to move into his left eye; he was showing signs of AIDS-induced dementia; his white blood cell count was falling precipitously; he was losing his memory; and he was chronically fatigued. "All medical indications," a nurse from the Alameda County Health Care Services wrote in a letter to the court, requesting clemency, "indicate that he is unlikely to live more than a year."

CHAPTER FOUR: FIRE

80. *"Man, where you from?":* Quoted in Benjamin P. Bowser, "Crack and AIDS: An Ethnographic Impression," *Multicultural Inquiry and Research on AIDS* 2, no. 2 (1988): 1.

81. *The older residents, who had settled there in the 1940s*: Benjamin P. Bowser, "Bayview–Hunter's Point: San Francisco's Black Ghetto Revisited," *Urban Anthropology* 17, no. 4 (1988): 384.

84. *In New York City syphilis rates had shot up*: Robert Pear, "Sharp Rise Found in Syphilis in U.S.," *New York Times,* 4 October 1987, A1.

84. *Penicillin-resistant cases of gonorrhea*: Sandra K. Schwarcz et al., "Crack Cocaine and the Exchange of Sex for Money or Drugs: Risk Factors for Gonorrhea Among Black Adolescents in San Francisco," *Sexually Transmitted Diseases* 19, no. 7–13 (1992): 7.

84. *there had been a sharp rise in chancroid*: Michael Specter, "Factor in AIDS' Spread on Rise in U.S.; Chancroid Linked to Heterosexual Transmission of Virus in Africa," *Washington Post,* 11 December 1987, A12.

85. *Under his leadership it had won a $7.1 million supplemental grant*: Mindy Fullilove, "AIDS Prevention Research Funded," *Multicultural Inquiry and Research on AIDS* 1, no. 4 (1987): 1–2.

85. *HIV incidence had been reduced*: Thomas J. Coates et al., "Behavioral Factors in the Spread of HIV Infection," *AIDS* 2S (1988), online at *www.caps.ucsf.edu.*

90. *Mindy and Gail decided to pool their resources and put together a joint study*: Robert E. Fullilove et al., "Risk of Sexually Transmitted Disease Among Black Adolescent Crack Users in Oakland and San Francisco, California," *Journal of the American Medical Association* 263 (1990): 852.

90. *The results from a preliminary sample were ominous*: Mindy Fullilove and Robert Fullilove, "MIRA Crack Project: Preliminary Report," *Multicultural Inquiry and Research on AIDS* 2, no. 4 (1988): 1.

91. *Bob and Mindy estimated conservatively*: Benjamin P. Bowser, Mindy Thompson Fullilove, and Robert E. Fullilove, "African American Youth and AIDS High-Risk Behavior: The Social Context and Barriers to Prevention," *Youth and Society* 22, no. 1 (1990): 58.

91. *Newly proposed federal laws stated that possession*: Tom Kenworthy, "Mandatory Terms for Possession of Crack Added to House Bill: Five Grams Would Yield Five Year Sentence," *Washington Post,* 17 September 1988, A4.

92. *Yale psychiatrist and pharmacologist Robert Byck appeared*: Beverly Xaviera Watkins, Robert E. Fullilove, and Mindy Thompson Fullilove, "Arms Against Illness: Crack Cocaine and Drug Policy in the United States," *Health and Human Rights* 2, no. 4 (1998): 45.

92. *Byck listened to a line of witnesses*: I owe my description of Byck's testimony and Paly's trip to Peru to Gary Webb, *Dark Alliance: The CIA, the Contras, and the Crack Cocaine Explosion* (New York: Seven Stories Press, 1998): 23–37.

93. *Coca paste, Jeri wrote, "is the main drug"*: Quoted in ibid., 28.

93. *Chemically, basuco, freebase, and powdered cocaine*: Jesse Katz et al., "Tracking the Genesis of the Crack Trade," *Los Angeles Times,* 20 October 1996, A1.

93. *a person could only sniff so much cocaine powder*: Ibid., 28. See also National Institute on Drug Abuse, Research Monograph 50, *Cocaine: Pharmacology, Effects,*

and Treatment of Abuse, ed. John Grabowski (Washington, D.C.: Government Printing Office, 1984).

94. *"Number one, find out about it":* Quoted in Webb, *Dark Alliance,* 35.

98. *"The Crack House of today":* Quoted in Marsha F. Goldsmith, "Sex Tied to Drugs = STD Spread," *Journal of the American Medical Association* 260, no. 14 (1988): 2009.

98. *From a public health perspective, they were making:* Despite the fact that no large-scale public health campaign had been launched to prevent crack users from becoming infected with HIV, officials at the CDC were beginning to go to the newspapers to warn the public about the possible link between crack and AIDS. See Peter Kerr, "Syphilis Surge with Crack Use Raises Fears on Spread of AIDS," *New York Times,* 29 June 1988, B1.

99. *The behavioral prevention strategy promoted by Tom Coates:* Ron D. Stall, Thomas J. Coates, and Colleen Hoff, "Behavioral Risk Reduction for HIV Infection Among Gay and Bisexual Men: A Review of Results from the United States," *American Psychologist* 43, no. 11 (1988): 884.

99. *Senator Daniel Patrick Moynihan was accused by the left:* Jacob Weisberg, "For the Sake of Argument," *New York Times,* 5 November 2000, 48.

99. *In 1960 78 percent of black families were headed:* Helen Gasch et al., "Shaping AIDS Education and Prevention Programs for African Americans Amidst Community Decline," *Journal of Negro Education* 60, no. 1 (1991): 91–92.

101. *In 1986 Mindy and Bob had flown to Newark:* Mindy T. Fullilove, *The House of Joshua: Meditations on Family and Place,* ed. Sander L. Gilman (Lincoln: University of Nebraska Press, 1999), 1.

102. *The first clue came to her when she read an article:* Rodrick Wallace, "A Synergism of Plagues: 'Planned Shrinkage,' Contagious Housing Destruction, and AIDS in the Bronx," *Environmental Research* 47, (1988): 1–33. See also Rodrick Wallace, "Minority AIDS and 'Planned Shrinkage' in New York City," *Multicultural Inquiry and Research on AIDS* 3, no. 1 (1989): 1ff.

102. *There were credible estimates that as many as one in five black men:* Bruce Lambert, "New York City Maps Deadly Pattern of AIDS," *New York Times,* 13 December 1987, A1.

CHAPTER FIVE: INVISIBLE

123. *grandson Darren's stroller:* Darren was Janeka's infant son.

124. *"My son died of AIDS":* Quoted in Catherine S. Manegold, "The Surrounding Scene—Demonstration, 10,000 Protesters Demand Help for People with AIDS," *New York Times,* 15 July 1992, A9.

125. *"walk the streets of this city":* Quoted in "In Their Own Words: Excerpts from Dinkins Remarks to Convention," *New York Times,* 14 July 1992, A12.

CHAPTER SIX: FRACTURED

129. *"Frankly," Fowler wrote, "the Democratic Party continues to be seen"*: Don Fowler, letter to Ron Brown and Mario Cooper, quoted in Cooper memorandum to Brown and Alexis Herman: 13 November 1990.

129. *"the Democratic leisure class"*: Quoted in Robin Toner, "Democrats in New York—Party Leadership: 1992 Ticket Puts Council of Moderates to Stiff Test," *New York Times,* 15 July 1992, A6.

129. *Sure, Jackson had held back his endorsement*: Maureen Dowd and Frank Rich, "Garden Diary," *New York Times,* 13 July 1992, B1.

131. *In March 1993 Mario helped organize a meeting between Clinton*: Karen De Witt, "Washington at Work: Gay Official Has the Look of Apple Pie and the Outlook of a Revolutionary," *New York Times,* 24 April 1993, A10.

132. *The CARE Act, named for the teenage hemophiliac*: My understanding of the reauthorization of the Ryan White CARE Act was greatly informed by Elinor Burkett's reporting in *The Gravest Show on Earth,* which both filled in blanks and corroborated the events recounted to me by sources including Mario Cooper and Doug Nelson. See Elinor Burkett, *The Gravest Show on Earth: America in the Age of AIDS* (New York: Houghton Mifflin, 1995), 141–68.

132. *the hundreds of thousands of Americans living with AIDS*: Boyce Rensberger, "HIV Estimates Reinforced by Random Tests," *Washington Post,* 14 December 1993, A13.

133. *Naturally, many had rewarded their own agencies*: Burkett, *Gravest Show on Earth,* 147.

133. *accusations of favoritism, homophobia, and racism*: Ibid., 146–151.

135. *The CARE Act was divided into a series of titles*: For more information on the various titles of Ryan White, see *www.dhhs.gov.*

137. *in June 1994 he hand-delivered a letter*: Russell D. Feingold, Herb Kohl, Ernest F. Hollings, Patrick J. Leahy, Dave Durenberger, Jim Sasser, Jeff Bingaman, and Daniel Akaka to "Colleague" (Dear Colleague Letter), 13 July 1994.

137. *Ted Kennedy's office warned the CAEAR coalition's lobbyist*: Burkett, *The Gravest Show on Earth,* 160.

137. *AIDS wasn't as complicated in the Midwest*: Ibid., 161.

137. *Title I cities like Detroit*: Ibid., 161–62.

140. *While it was true that the majority of black AIDS infections*: José Zuniga, "Has a Rift Opened Among the AIDS Lobbying Groups?" *The Washington Blade: The Gay Weekly of the Nation's Capital* 26, no. 28 (1995): 1, 25.

141. *In June 1995 Pat Christen wrote to Mario*: Pat Christen to Mario Cooper, 13 June 1995.

141. *Mario's reply was short and blistering*: Mario Cooper to Pat Christen, 21 June 1995.

142. *In his letter of resignation he implored the board*: Mario Cooper to AIDS Action Council, 3 November 1995.

142. *The new bill, however, did not repair many of the inequities:* House Committee on Commerce, Subcommittee on Health and Environment, "Prepared Testimony of Janet Heinrich, Associate Director Health Financing and Public Health Issues Health, Education, and Environment," 11 July 2000 (Washington D.C.: Federal News Services, 2000).

144. *The NAACP had five hundred youth councils:* Mark Schoofs, "Blackt Up! African Americans Confront Their Worst Health Crisis: AIDS," *Village Voice,* 5 November 1996, 45.

144. *"There ain't nothing we can do":* Quoted in Derrik Z. Jackson, "Black Indifference on AIDS," *Boston Globe,* 9 October 1996, A27.

145. *That AIDS had eclipsed homicide as the number-one killer of:* Sara Rimer, "Blacks Urged to Act to Increase Awareness of the AIDS Epidemic," *New York Times,* 23 October 1996, A16.

145. *"In part because of the traditional homophobic tendency":* Quoted in ibid.

CHAPTER SEVEN: SURFACING

165. *Dawn:* Dawn, "I Learned to Show Love to My Kids," *Women Organized to Respond to Life Threatening Diseases* no. 5 (September 1991): 1–3.

165. *Vanessa:* Vanessa, "AIDS: It's a Family Affair," Ibid., no. 58 (February 1996): 1–2.

165. *S.T.:* S.T., "One Day at a Time," Ibid., no. 8 (December 1991): 1–2.

165. *A second Dawn:* Dawn "Lindsey," Ibid., no. 7 (November 1991): 1–2.

166. *Doris:* Doris Butler, "Jared: A Mother's Story," Ibid., no. 17 (September 1992): 1–3.

166. *Monia:* Monia Perry, "To Survive Is a Victory," Ibid., no. 23 (March 1993): 1–2.

166. *Becky:* Becky Trotter, "So Let's Talk!" Ibid., no. 32 (December 1993): 1.

166. *LaDonna:* LaDonna Love-Kretchmer, "A Very Special Child," Ibid., no. 35 (March 1994): 1–2.

166. *Jacki:* Jacki, "Speaking Out About Sexual Assault," Ibid., no. 38 (June 1994): 1–2.

166. *Yvonne:* Yvonne Knuckles, "People Said I Couldn't Change," Ibid., no. 39 (July 1994): 1–3.

CHAPTER EIGHT: ESTHER AND THE KING

168. *Mindy Fullilove had always dreamed of owning a house:* Mindy T. Fullilove, *The House of Joshua: Meditations on Family and Place,* ed. Sander L. Gilman (Lincoln: University of Nebraska Press, 1999), 131–42.

169. *In 1996 41 percent of all new AIDS cases:* Centers for Disease Control, *Fact Sheet: HIV/AIDS Among African Americans* (2003), online at *www.cdc.gov/hiv/pubs/facts/afam.pdf.*

170. Time *magazine had named Dr. David Ho:* Christine Gorman, "The Disease Detective: As the AIDS Epidemic Unfolds, Dr. David Ho Had a Knack for Asking Just the Right Questions," *Time,* December 1996, 56.

171. *the survival rate for men beyond the age of forty*: Helen Gasch et al., "Shaping AIDS Education and Prevention Programs for African Americans Amidst Community Decline," *Journal of Negro Education* 60, no. 1 (1991): 85.

171. *Mindy visited the hospital where she had studied*: Fullilove, *House of Joshua*, 1–3.

176. *post-traumatic stress disorder (PTSD)*: See American Psychiatric Association, *Diagnostic and Statistical Manual of Mental Disorders*, rev. 3rd ed. (Washington, D.C.: American Psychiatric Association, 1987), 247–51.

176. *The disorder was fairly rare among the general public*: Mindy Thompson Fullilove, Anne Lown, and Robert E. Fullilove, "Crack 'Hos and Skeezers: Traumatic Experiences of Women Crack Users," *Journal of Sex Research* 29, no. 2 (1992): 284.

176. *Over the summer Mindy and her team interviewed*: Mindy Thompson Fullilove et al., "Violence, Trauma, and Post-Traumatic Stress Disorder Among Women Drug Users," *Journal of Traumatic Stress* 6, no. 4 (1993): 533.

176. *Congressman John Conyers began the hearing*: This account of the hearing is based directly on a videotape (titled *Root Causes of the Demand for Drugs in the U.S.*) of the testimony presented before the House Committee on Government Operations, Subcommittee on Legislation and National Security, September 1991.

177. *Brown didn't mention that HIV was spreading through prisons*: AIDS rates in prisons would continue to grow relative to the general population. By 1994, they were seven times higher than among the public. See Peter M. Brien and Allen J. Beck, "HIV in Prisons, 1994," *Bureau of Justice Statistics Bulletin* (1996), online at *www.ojp.usdoj.gov/bjs/pub/pdf/hivip94.pdf*.

186. *"I cannot divorce myself"*: Quoted in Mindy Thompson Fullilove and Robert E. Fullilove, "The Peculiar Epidemic, Part II: African American Clergy Struggle with AIDS," unpublished manuscript.

186. *Yet there were clues—both in the history*: Mindy Fullilove and Robert Fullilove, "Health Good versus Moral Good: Solving the Antinomy," *Current Issues in Public Health* 1 (1995): 119–21.

186. *The modern theological tradition of the black church*: This material was culled from interviews and from Mindy Thompson Fullilove and Robert E. Fullilove, "Homosexuality and the African American Church: The Paradox of the 'Open Closet,'" in *Though I Stand at the Door and Knock: Discussions on the Black Church Struggle with AIDS*, ed. Julia Walker (New York: Balm in Gilead, 1997); published in *American Behavioral Scientist* 42 (1999): 1–9.

187. *"look at NAFTA"*: Quoted in Fullilove and Fullilove, "The Peculiar Epidemic, Part II," 16, 17.

187. *Their views on homosexuality were muddier*: Fullilove and Fullilove, "Homosexuality and the African American," 1–9.

187. *"What really hurt me"*: Quoted in Fullilove and Fullilove, "The Peculiar Epidemic, Part II," 21.

187. *perhaps the majority of the clergy would never*: Fullilove and Fullilove, "Homosexuality and the African American," 9.

189. *The politically correct language of cultural relativism:* The Fulliloves note that the wealth of post–civil rights academic literature, which has focused heavily on the attributes of black institutions and cultural contributions, has "failed to assess accurately the processes that signaled decay and destruction." See Mindy Thompson Fullilove and Robert E. Fullilove III, "Understanding Sexual Behaviors and Drug Use Among African Americans: A Case Study of Issues for Survey Research," in *Methodological Issues in AIDS Behavioral Research,* ed. David G. Ostrow and Ronald C. Kessler (New York: Plenum Press, 1993), 119.

190. *doctors, epidemiologists, psychologists, and social scientists:* This book does not attempt to document the important work of every black AIDS activist and researcher; there are too many names to list here. However, I would like to acknowledge a few: Phill Wilson of the African American AIDS Policy and Training Institute; Pastor Preston Washington and Canon Frederick Williams of Harlem Congregations for Community Improvement; Cornelius Baker of the Whitman-Walker Clinic and the National Association of People with AIDS; Ernest Hopkins of the San Francisco AIDS Foundation; Bishop Carl Beam, a longtime Los Angeles–based AIDS activist; his brother Joseph Beam, who died of AIDS after publishing a number of works by gay black writers; Norm Nickens, a founder of the National Minority AIDS Council; Surgeon General Jocelyn Elders; and Keith Cylar of Housing Works.

190. *Dr. Brian Edlin, the epidemiological intelligence officer:* It should be noted that participants in Edlin's study had never injected drugs. Brian R. Edlin et al., "Intersecting Epidemics—Crack Cocaine Use and HIV Infection Among Inner-City Young Adults," *New England Journal of Medicine* 331, no. 21 (1994): 1422.

190. *the general American population, whose HIV infection rate:* Brien and Beck, "HIV in Prisons, 1994."

190. *John Peterson, Mindy's former colleague at CAPS:* For Peterson's work on black male homosexuality, see John L. Peterson and Gerardo Marín, "Issues in the Prevention of AIDS Among Black and Hispanic Men," *American Psychologist* 43, no. 11 (1988); John L. Peterson et al., "High Risk Sexual Behavior and Condom Use Among Gay and Bisexual African American Men," *American Journal of Public Health* 82, no. 11 (1992); and John L. Peterson, "AIDS-Related Risks and Same-Sex Behaviors Among African American Men," *AIDS, Identity, and Community: The HIV Epidemic and Lesbians and Gay Men,* vol. 2 of *Psychological Perspectives on Lesbian and Gay Issues,* ed. Gregory M. Herek and Beverly Greene (Thousand Oaks, Calif.: Sage Publications, 1995).

190. *Conspiracy theories were running rampant:* "The AIDS 'Plot' Against Blacks," *New York Times,* 12 May 1992, A22. See also Elinor Burkett, *The Gravest Show on Earth: America in the Age of AIDS* (New York: Houghton Mifflin, 1995), 182–83.

191. *Race was the story of America:* Mindy explores these issues in Mindy Thompson Fullilove, "Perceptions and Misperceptions," *Journal of the American Medical Association* 269, no. 8 (1993); and "Deconstructing Race in Medical Research," *Archives of Pediatric Adolescent Medicine* 148 (1994).

191. *"The Negro . . . must embrace"*: Quoted in Fullilove, *House of Joshua*, 29.

191. *a theory that linked AIDS to urban decay*: See Mindy Thompson Fullilove, "Death and Life in the Great American City," *International Journal of Mental Health* 28, no. 4 (1999–2000); Robert E. Fullilove and Mindy Thompson Fullilove, "HIV Prevention and Intervention in the African-American Community: A Public Health Perspective," in *The AIDS Knowledge Base*, ed. P. T. Cohen, M. A. Sande, and P. A. Volberding, 3rd ed. (Philadelphia: Lippincott Williams and Wilkins, 1999); Rodrick Wallace, Mindy Thompson Fullilove, and Deborah Wallace, "Family Systems and De-Urbanization: Implications for Substance Abuse," *Comprehensive Textbook of Substance Abuse*, ed. J. Lowinson et al., 2nd ed. (Baltimore: Williams and Wilkins, 1992); and Mindy Thompson Fullilove and Robert E. Fullilove, "What's Housing Got to Do with It?" *Focus, A Guide to AIDS Research and Counseling* 5, no. 12 (1990).

193. *New York City's estimated thirty thousand homeless*: See *www.housingworks.org*.

194. *a newspaper series by Mary Bishop*: Mary Bishop, "Urban Renewal's Untold Stories," *Roanoke Times and World News*, 29 January 1995, A1; "Veteran Son Shocked Couple Left Before 'Renewal,'" *Roanoke Times and World News*, 2 April 1995, G1; "Residents Get on Record About Wells Avenue Project," *Roanoke Times and World News*, 30 July 1993, B3; "Roanoke's Hidden History Interviews Reveal Glimpse of Early Black Life," *Roanoke Times and World News*, 16 January 1994, 1; "A Walk Along Wells Avenue," *Roanoke Times and World News*, 27 February 1994, 1; and "The Loss Still Stings," *Roanoke Times and World News*, 29 January 1995, 10.

195. *"Government leaders here"*: Bishop, "Urban Renewal's Untold Stories," A1.

195. *the story of urban renewal*: For an excellent in-depth discussion of this history, from which I gathered the historical information in this section, see Jon C. Teaford, "Urban Renewal and Its Aftermath," *Housing Policy Debate* 11, no. 2 (2000): 443–465; Alexander von Hoffman, "A Study in Contradictions: The Origins and Legacy of the Housing Act of 1949," ibid.: 299–326; and Arnold R. Hirsch, "Searching for a 'Sound Negro Policy': A Racial Agenda for the Housing Acts of 1949 and 1954," ibid.: 339–341.

201. *two-thirds of America's urban renewal projects took more than six years*: See Mindy Thompson Fullilove's forthcoming *Root Shock: Upheaval, Resettlement and Recovery in Urban America*.

CHAPTER NINE: THE GUARDIANS

213. *Gradually, though, a body of data had begun to surface*: Department of Health and Human Services, "Fact Sheet: Needle Exchange Programs: Part of a Comprehensive HIV Prevention Strategy" (1998), online at *www.hhs.gov/news/press/*.

214. *"genocidal campaign"*: Quoted in Cathy J. Cohen, *The Boundaries of Blackness: AIDS and the Breakdown of Black Politics* (Chicago: University of Chicago Press, 1999): 333.

215. *In February she'd submitted a report to Congress*: Donna E. Shalala, "Needle Exchange Programs in America: Review of Published Studies and Ongoing

Research," report presented to the Committee on Appropriations for the Departments of Labor, Health and Human Services, Education, and related agencies, 18 February 1997, 5–11.

215. *could reduce high-risk HIV behavior:* Department of Health and Human Services, "Fact Sheet: Needle Exchange Programs," 3.

217. *At D.C. General, Goosby heard:* Ronald Bayer and Gerald M. Oppenheimer, *AIDS Doctors: Voices from the Epidemic, An Oral History* (Oxford: Oxford University Press, 2000), 241.

218. *Congressional Black Caucus received an eight-page briefing from Mario Cooper:* Mario M. Cooper, "The AIDS Crisis Within the African American Community," paper presented at the Congressional Black Caucus Briefing on AIDS, Washington, D.C., 29 July 1997, 1.

221. *There were calls in the press for her to do the same:* David Corn, "The Coward," *Salon* April 1998, 1–2.

221. *"That's not how we're going to solve the problem":* Quoted in Christopher S. Wren, "New Drug Czar Is Seeking Ways to Bolster His Hand," *New York Times,* 17 March 1996, A18.

221. *two-thirds of the government's drug budget:* Michael Massing, "Winning the Drug War Isn't So Hard After All," *New York Times,* 6 September 1998, A48.

222. *flesh out Eric Goosby's memo into a definitive report:* "Needle Exchange Programs in America: Review and Evaluation of Scientific Research," report prepared by the Department of Health and Human Services, unpublished.

222. *Shalala sent the report to each of the government's scientists:* David Satcher, Harold Varmus, Claire Broome, Anthony Fauci, Helene Gayle, Margaret Hamburg, Nelba Chavez, Eric P. Goosby, and Alan I. Leshner to Donna E. Shalala, 20 April 1998 (date of public release).

225. *Then he headed to the committee meeting:* See House Committee on Appropriations, *Budget for Centers for Disease Control: Hearing Before the Subcommittee on Labor, Health, and Human Services and Education,* 105th Cong., 2nd sess., 5 March 1998.

227. *Goosby had received indications from the White House:* John F. Harris and Amy Goldstein, "Puncturing an AIDS Initiative: At Last Minute, White House Political Fears Killed Needle Funding," *Washington Post,* 23 April 1998, A1.

230. *A few days later Maxine Waters drafted a letter:* Congressional Black Caucus to President William Jefferson Clinton, 24 April 1998.

231. *Four days later she sent a letter to Donna Shalala:* Maxine Waters to Donna Shalala, 15 May 1998.

233. *On June 29 the* New York Times *ran a front-page story:* Sheryl Gay Stolberg, "Epidemic of Silence: A Special Report. Eyes Shut, Black America Is Being Ravaged by AIDS," *New York Times,* 29 June 1998, A1.

233. *A week later NAACP president Kweisi Mfume wrote:* Kweisi Mfume, "Letter to the Editor: Poverty Is Scourge Behind Global AIDS Epidemic," *New York Times,* 11 July 1998, A10.

234. *The negotiations with the White House heated up:* Leroy Whitfield, Esther Kaplan, and Shana Naomi Krochmal, "The Fire This Time: After Years of Indifference, the Nation's African American Leaders are Finally Tackling the Epidemic in Their Midst," *POZ,* January 1999, 64.

237. *"Like other epidemics before it":* Quoted in *HIV/AIDS and African Americans,* a videotape produced by the National Minority AIDS Council in Collaboration with the National Institutes of Health, Office of AIDS Research, November 1999.

237. *"It's a shot in the arm":* Quoted in Amy Goldstein, "U.S. to Begin Minority AIDS Initiative: $150 Million Campaign Targets Blacks, Latinos," *Washington Post,* 29 October 1998, A3.

CHAPTER TEN: THE LONG DREAM

250. *In a massive reverse migration, 630,000 blacks:* Although in 2002 the AIDS epidemic in the South was still heavily concentrated in cities, the proportion of infected southerners living in rural areas had slowly grown through the 1990s. Public health researchers have theorized about a "two-wave" spread of AIDS into the rural South. The first wave was introduced by gay men and intravenous drug users who had been infected in cities and then moved to rural areas, perhaps to be with family. This wave precipitated a second wave of infections that are largely being spread sexually. See Amy Lansky et al., "Human Immunodeficiency Virus Infection in Rural Areas and Small Cities of the Southeast: Contributions of Migration and Behavior," *Journal of Rural Health* 16, no. 1 (2000): 20–30.

251. *Slow-burning epidemics of crack cocaine and speed:* Centers for Disease Control, "Risks for HIV Infection Among Persons Residing in Rural Areas and Small Cities—Selected Sites, Southern United States, 1995–1996," *Morbidity and Mortality Weekly Report* 47, no. 45 (1998): 976.

257. *the Institute of Medicine had come out with a report:* Institute of Medicine, "No Time to Lose: Getting More from HIV Prevention" (2000), online at *www.iom.edu.* For further coverage see Lawrence K. Altman, "A Report Harshly Criticizes the Federal Policy on AIDS," *Washington Post,* 28 September 2000, A18.

Acknowledgments

My deepest gratitude goes to each person who appears in the pages of this book. Not only did they give generously of their time, but they displayed courage in openly sharing the intimate details of their lives and work in service of a fuller conversation about some of the most difficult and enduring issues facing this country. The list of people who helped shape my thinking on the epidemic but whose stories I did not explore in the manuscript is too extensive to write here. There are a few, however, whom I wish to acknowledge at this point. Kenneth Raphael, the first infected person I asked to participate in this project, died of AIDS in the early stages of my research. However, his story, which I told in the proposal for this book, was instrumental in moving first my agent, and then my editor, to take on this project. Thanks also to David Schulman, an AIDS attorney in Los Angeles, who patiently tutored me over many phone calls on the history of the epidemic; Robert Sember, a South African, whose elegantly articulated ideas on AIDS in the American South helped me see freshly the richness and texture of the material I gathered in Alabama; Pastor Preston Washington of Harlem, who gave me a raw glimpse of what the epidemic looked like from behind the pulpit; Jane Silver, who gathered a trove of documents that both informed and corroborated my reporting on needle exchange; and Sean Strub, who advocated for this book in the foundation world.

Every idea requires time for its fullest development. I am deeply grateful to the Open Society Institute for providing the critical funding that allowed me to devote my undivided attention to this subject.

While all books are truly collaborations between a writer and their wider community of colleagues and peers, this axiom is never more true than for a first book. The professional expertise and wisdom of every one of the following are present in these pages. Andrew Miller, a true editor in the classic sense, who took a risk by going to bat for this book at Grove Atlantic, took another by taking it with him to Pantheon, and then dedicated an unimaginable number of hours to insightfully poring over every sentence in the manuscript; Kris Dahl, my extraordinary agent, who took a flier on me when I had no track record and gave me four years of sage advice, as well as

Acknowledgments

representation above and beyond any rational expectation, all the while exhibiting humor and patience—without her this book would not have been published; Samuel G. Freedman, my teacher and first editor, who imagined this book when I approached him with the glimmer of an idea, then lit the tunnel with his vision, and unmercifully closed the door behind me; Brad Foss, my confidant, fellow writer, editor, critic, and true friend, who helped burnish every chapter; Mary Kay Martin, who gave generously and gently of her time and editorial pen to help my sentences read with the rhythm in which I heard them in my head; Jonathan Schorr, who showed me that it could be done, and then encouraged me to join him at the finish line; G. R. Anderson Jr., my brother in mind, who reminded me what I do well, and then showed me his writing, unknowingly challenging me to do better; Sonji Jacobs, who gave of her time and insight in helping me craft the proposal; Gayane Keshishyan and Kerry Donahue, first-rate journalists and friends, who offered unfailing insight and humor at my lowest moments; Michael Shapiro, who gave me the first sentence of my epilogue when I feared that I didn't even have a book; Roger Cohn, for believing in this topic and giving me my first magazine assignment to write about it; the entire staff at Pantheon and Random House, every one of whom treated this book with extraordinary care and attention to detail; the editors at *The Oxford American*, who helped make the Alabama material come alive on the page; and Richard Scheinin, who ushered me into journalism, and then into book writing.

Ultimately, however, this book belongs to my friends and family, a few of whom went far and above the call of duty to support, encourage, and whip me through these four years: Abra Levenson, who, at the end, flew across the country on three days' notice and worked twelve hours a day to help me finish the project; Rhys Levenson, who never wavered and who taught me to take the heat; Judy and Steve Ross, who housed and fed me too many times to count; Scott Brenner, who gave generously of his invaluable expertise and time; Lucille Levenson, who supported first my father and then myself in taking on challenging projects; Peter Lundgren, for his generosity, love, and inspiration; Vic Lundgren, who set the standard; Paul Bracke, who patiently and honestly guided me around some of the most difficult obstacles; Jean-Paul Leonard, who helped make it possible for me to live in New York and also granted me a computer to complete the book; the generous crew at Angry Monkey for use of their office space and equipment; Wes Lovy, who first told me to take on this topic and then advised me to make it into a book; Ellie Carmody, who many years ago helped me believe in my convictions; Bonnie Settlage, who drew me through the wilderness; and Lawrence Cohen, a medical anthropologist, who shaped my approach to journalism.

Index

abstinence, 144, 220

ACT UP, 132, 164

ADAP, *see* AIDS Drug Assistance Program

AIDS:
  African origins of virus in, 143
  believed to be genocidal government scheme, 190–1, 218
  education about, 19, 99
  first known cases of, 51–2, 202
  groups hit hardest by, made responsible for politics, treatment, and prevention, 184
  isolation of virus in, 44, 46
  local control over programs for, 256–7
  statistics on, 22, 50, 134, 139, 144, 145, 169, 189, 224, 233, 277*n*–278*n*
  stories of families affected by, *see* Hall family; Jackson family; Rushing, Desiree
  suffering of, 207–8
  see also HIV

AIDS Action Council, 128, 134, 237
  Ryan White reauthorization and, 132, 133, 137, 138, 140, 141–2

AIDS Alabama, 25, 249–50, 256, 257

AIDS Clinical Trial Group, 164

AIDS Drug Assistance Program (ADAP):
  in Alabama, 25–6, 245, 250, 251, 254–5, 256–61
  state caps on, 26
  state discretion in, 219

AIDS Project Los Angeles (APLA), 138

AIDS-related opportunistic infections (AIDS-OI), 139

AIDS Resource Center of Wisconsin, 135

AIDS Task Force of Alabama, 256

Alabama, 3–29, 140, 238–68
  challenges faced by AIDS workers in, 19–20, 257
  culture of secrecy in, 14–15, 17, 22
  funding for AIDS programs in, 25–6, 245, 249–51, 254–61, 273
  Governor's Commission on AIDS in, 25, 26, 250, 254, 258, 273
  heterosexual transmission of HIV in, 23
  inadequacy of AIDS programs in, 25–6
  invisible rural communities of, 20–2
  profile of average AIDS patient in, 25, 257
  racial divide in, 22–3

Index

Alabama (*continued*)
   Ryan White grants and, 250, 251, 255
   statehouse rally in, 250, 256, 258–61
   statistics on HIV/AIDS in, 25
   story of family affected by AIDS in,
     see Jackson family
Alcohol, Drug Abuse, and Mental
   Health Agency, 50
American Foundation for AIDS
   Research, 184
American Psychiatric Association,
   91–2
anal intercourse, 42, 43
Anti-Drug Abuse Act, 221
Army, U.S., 37, 50
AZT, 16, 23, 111, 112, 220

Baker, Cornelius, 140, 214–15
Balm in Gilead, 224
Baltimore, urban renewal projects in,
   200
Barksdale, Warren, 171
Barnes, Mark, 140
Barry, Marion, 127, 128
basuco, 92–3
Bauer, Catherine, 197
Bayview-Hunters Point (San Francisco),
   research on crack in, 79–84, 85, 90
Bayview-Hunters Point Foundation, 40,
   50–1, 80, 82, 94
Bedford, Roger, 255
behavioral prevention strategy, 98,
   99–101
   gay community and, 43, 98, 99, 220,
     233
   ineffective in ghetto context, 99–101,
     104
behavioral research:
   NIMH funding for, 43–6, 47

   see also Center for AIDS Prevention
     Studies; Multicultural Inquiry and
     Research on AIDS
Bennett, William, 221
biomedical research, 218, 219
Bishop, Mary, 194–5, 205
Black AIDS Institute, 273
Black Church Week of Prayer for the
   Healing of AIDS, 145, 244
black clergy, 110–11, 145
   culture of silence and, 187–8
   Fullilove's research on, 184–8
   homosexuality and drugs condemned
     by, 185, 186–7
   inadequate response to AIDS
     epidemic ascribed to, 158–60,
     166–7, 184–8, 203, 233, 235
   lack of unanimity among, 185
   mythology surrounding, 184–5
black elite, 128
   Cooper's attempts at mobilization of,
     141, 143–5, 211–16, 218–20
   Cooper's upbringing amidst,
     209–11
   Fulliloves' research and, 184
   inadequate response to AIDS
     epidemic ascribed to, 144–5,
     165, 211–12, 233
black family, deterioration of, 99
Black Leadership Commission on AIDS,
   184, 224
black nationalism, 36, 67, 191
Black Plague, 206
black power, 67
blacks:
   AIDS statistics for, 22, 50, 134, 139,
     144, 145, 169, 224, 233
   disproportionate health risks for, 226,
     246
   medical community distrusted by,
     169, 191, 217–18, 219